BSW
Tha

**LIBRARY**

CHRISTIE HOSPITAL NHS TRUST

*DO NOT REMOVE THIS CARD*

DEMCO

# Fractionation
in Radiotherapy

# Fractionation in Radiotherapy

**Howard D. Thames**

Department of Biomathematics,
M.D. Anderson Hospital and Tumor Institute,
Houston, TX, USA

and

**Jolyon H. Hendry**

Department of Radiobiology,
Paterson Institute for Cancer Research,
Christie Hospital and Holt Radium Institute,
Manchester, UK

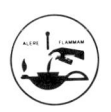

*Taylor & Francis*
*London—New York—Philadelphia*
*1987*

| | |
|---|---|
| UK | Taylor & Francis Ltd. 4 John St., London WC1N 2ET |
| USA | Taylor & Francis Inc., 242 Cherry St., Philadelphia, PA 19106-1906 |

Copyright © H. D. Thames and J. H. Hendry 1987

*All rights reserved. No part of this publication may be reproduced, stored in a retrieval system, or transmitted, in any form or by any means, electronic, electrostatic, magnetic tape, mechanical, photocopying, recording or otherwise, without the prior permission of the copyright owner.*

**British Library Cataloguing in Publication Data**

Thames, Howard D.
  Fractionation in radiotherapy
  1. Cancer — Radiotherapy
  I. Title  II. Hendry, Jolyon H.
  616.99'40642    RC271.R3

ISBN 0-85066-374-1

**Library of Congress Cataloging in Publication Data**

Thames, Howard D.
  Fractionation in radiotherapy.

  Includes bibliographies and index.
  1. Radiotherapy. 2. Radiation—Dosage. 3. Radiation injuries. I. Hendry, J. H. II. Title. [DNLM:
  1. Radiation Injuries—etiology. 2. Radiotherapy—adverse effects. 3. Radiotherapy Dosage. WN 250 T366f]
  RM849.T47 1987   615.8'42   87-10059
  ISBN 0-85066-374-1

Typeset by Mathematical Composition Setters Ltd, Salisbury, Wiltshire
Printed in Great Britain by Taylor & Francis (Printers) Ltd, Basingstoke, Hants.

# Contents

| | | |
|---|---|---|
| *Foreword* | | vii |
| *Chapter 1.* | **Radiation-induced injury to tissues** | 1 |
| 1.1. | Patterns of cell renewal in tissues | 1 |
| 1.2. | Effects of radiation on cell production | 6 |
| 1.3. | Pathogenesis | 10 |
| *Chapter 2.* | **Evidence for target-cell depletion as determinant of tissue response** | 22 |
| 2.1. | $D_0$ values: functional or *in situ* colony assays | 23 |
| 2.2. | Altered fractionation and dose rate | 38 |
| 2.3. | Slopes of isoeffect graphs | 46 |
| *Chapter 3.* | **Response of tissues to fractionated irradiation: effect of repair** | 53 |
| 3.1. | Damage and repair after low-LET radiation | 54 |
| 3.2. | Damage and repair after high-LET radiation | 62 |
| 3.3. | Tissue response to fractionated irradiation | 64 |
| 3.4. | Repair kinetics | 82 |
| 3.5. | Response of normal tissues to low doses | 89 |
| 3.6. | Hyperfractionation | 95 |
| *Chapter 4.* | **Proliferative response to radiation injury** | 100 |
| 4.1. | Proliferative response following single and fractionated doses | 101 |
| 4.2. | Proliferation during fractionated or low-dose-rate exposures | 108 |

|  |  |  |
|---|---|---|
| | 4.3. Clinical implications of regeneration during fractionated radiotherapy | 124 |
| | 4.4. Residual injury and re-treatment | 130 |
| Chapter 5. | **In hindsight** | 137 |
| | 5.1. Origins (1896—1940s) | 138 |
| | 5.2. Interpretations: the time factor and power-law models (1930s to 1960s) | 148 |
| | 5.3. Interpretations: the survival-curve models (1956—1986) | 163 |
| Chapter 6. | **Radiobiological guide for radiotherapists** | 170 |
| | 6.1. Interaction of radiation with matter | 170 |
| | 6.2. Linear energy transfer (LET) | 176 |
| | 6.3. Assays of cell survival and tissue injury | 177 |
| | 6.4. Survival curves | 183 |
| | 6.5. Biological and chemical modifiers of cell survival | 189 |
| | 6.6. Cell and tissue kinetics | 200 |
| | 6.7. Radiobiology of renewing normal tissues | 204 |
| | 6.8. Radiobiology of tumours | 208 |
| | 6.9. Radiobiology of tissues and organs at long-term risk | 210 |
| | 6.10. Normal-tissue tolerance: time, dose, and fractionation | 218 |
| | 6.11. The biological hazards of irradiation | 237 |
| | 6.12. Further reading | 243 |
| Chapter 7. | **Appendix** | 245 |
| | 7.1. The time factor in radiotherapy | 245 |
| | 7.2. Repair during fractionated exposures: the IR model | 246 |
| | 7.3. Repair during continuous low-dose-rate exposures | 248 |
| | 7.4. Tissue response to fractionated or continuous irradiation | 250 |
| | 7.5. The LPL model | 251 |
| | 7.6. The time factor: slopes of isoeffect graphs | 254 |
| | 7.7. The time factor for arbitrary target-cell survival curves | 255 |
| *Glossary* | | 257 |
| *Bibliography* | | 263 |
| *Index* | | 292 |

# Foreword

In this book we describe the biological effects of fractionation of radiation dose—that is, how cells and tissues respond to a dose of radiation that is either divided into small fractions and delivered over a period of time or delivered continuously over a period of time. We give as well an early history of fractionation and the factors that influenced its development.

The first motivation for writing the book was the development in the early 1980s of some new ways of viewing fractionation. A more important reason, however, was the wish to consolidate these developments and ideas with a description of, and evidence for, a comprehensive target-cell theory of tissue responses to radiation injury. These two reasons have been closely linked in their development, but a formal treatise on the subject in monograph form is not available. Last, and not least, we wished to present a brief teaching guide for the use of clinicians that in particular would include these newer ideas, ones not featured in other teaching texts.

These goals resulted in some peculiarities of organization of chapters in the book. The primary purpose was to describe fractionation in radiotherapy—in essence, the response of normal tissues and tumours to fractionated or low-dose-rate irradiation—in the framework of target-cell theory. Therefore the book begins with a description of cell renewal, function, and death in tissues and tumours, and how these are affected by radiation injury. Then follows a collation of the evidence we could find for target-cell depletion as the primary factor determining tissue and tumour responses to irradiation. This knowledge is then applied to a treatment of the primary determinants of the time factor in radiotherapy, repair and regeneration. Finally, a historical overview is presented. This arrangement was decided on for several reasons: first, as stated above, to pursue the main purpose of the book right from the beginning. However, it will be seen that various difficulties in scheduling the appearance of topics arose, for example the presentation of target-cell theory necessitated introduction of ideas about repair before these had been formally presented in the following chapter. It also required presenting the end results of a series of historical developments before describing those developments themselves. In justification of this, we point out that a target-cell approach is central to the presentation of the chapters on repair and regeneration, and apologize for any inconsistencies of presentation that occur in the chapter justifying the use of target-cell theory. Secondly, we would point out that history may be best understood by those who have accumulated some experience in their lives with its major themes. Hence the title of the historically motivated chapter, 'In hindsight'.

The primary journal for radiotherapy and its allied disciplines up to the second world war was *Strahlentherapie*. Furthermore, one of the most influential monographs on the subject of fractionation—that of Strandqvist in 1944—was Austrian and German in its orientation. Hence a lot of the story to be told of how fractionation practice evolved during that time concerns the German and Austrian researchers and clinicians, and their very considerable contributions (in the 10 years following the discovery of X-rays, radiobiology, radiotherapy, and dosimetry had their origins in Austria). Unfortunately, however, not enough is generally said about the Scandinavians, and of the Stockholm Radiumhemmet founded by Gusta Förssell, or of the English and Americans. The purpose of the early history presented in Chapter 5 is to trace the controversies that attended radiotherapy at its birth, and which resulted finally in the triumph of fractionated over single-dose treatments. A second purpose is to outline the development of ideas about the time factor in radiotherapy.

The Radiobiological guide for radiotherapists outlined in Chapter 6 covers most of the requirements of the Royal College of Radiology (RCR) in the UK and the American College of Radiology (ACR) in the USA. Omitted were discussions of cell structure and function, biochemistry and molecular biology, damage to cell organelles, cytogenetics, and the basic principles of chemotherapy (RCR). From the ACR requirements (Davis *et al.* 1985) the following were omitted: new radiation modalities, chemotherapeutic agents, hyperthermia, and the detailed radiopathology of human tissues. However, some items are included which are not central to the theme of this book, such as the hazards of radiation. The guide is intended as a brief introduction to many of the topics, and references are made to more comprehensive books that have been written on the particular subjects.

Some of the topics in the teaching guide are presented in considerable detail, in particular the calculation of doses for practical clinical situations. A method for calculating doses based on the newer ideas developed in the main text is presented, and this is given side-by-side with the well known NSD−TDF method.

The dose unit rad appears in some of the figures that were reproduced from the literature. The rad-to-SI conversion is 100 rad = 1 Gy. Elsewhere the Roentgen exposure unit is abbreviated to R (but $r$ in Figures 5.1, 5.2, 5.5, 5.6). There is no conversion from exposure units to absorbed dose which is appropriate to all situations, but for skin the conversion is approximately 90 R per Gy.

We have benefited greatly from the advice and criticism of many of our colleagues and friends, none of whom is responsible for any inaccuracies in this book. Mr Walter Pagel did an excellent job of editing the book, but changes and additions were made afterwards. We thank Drs R. D. Hunter and L. J. Peters for helpful suggestions. In connection with the historical chapter we would like to thank Dr G. H. Fletcher who provided guidance and an overview of the subject from his many years of experience and acquaintances. Useful comments for this chapter were also received from Drs J. F. Fowler (London), D. Kogelnik (Vienna), H. Reinhold (Rotterdam), and F. Wachsmann (Munich). Drs K. K. Ang (Houston), J. V. Moore, C. S. Potten and J. Butler (Manchester) provided helpful suggestions on various aspects of both the main text and the teaching guide. Drs J. M. Wilkinson and P. C. Williams (Manchester) and L. Vanuytsel (Leuven) gave good advice for the sections on radiation physics and fractionation examples. We are grateful also to many of our colleagues for allowing us to quote results which are in papers still in the process of publication, thus enabling this book to be as up-to-date as possible.

The entire project was realized by shuffling dictation tapes, figures, etc., across the Atlantic and this was expertly managed by Ms Constance Seifert in Houston. The never-ending changes and additions were all duly registered and the whole placed in a word processor; other activities were no doubt necessary that we have no inkling of. Special thanks to Connie for having made it all work. We would also like to acknowledge the support and facilities of the Department of Biomathematics in Houston. Last, and certainly not least, we wish to thank Betsy Mims and Elizabeth Hendry for valiant help with references, editorial changes, and constant support and patience throughout this project.

HDT
JHH
October 1986

# Chapter 1
# Radiation-induced injury to tissues

There are good reasons for believing that the primary effects of radiation on tissues are cell damage and cell depopulation in renewing populations (here we exclude transient effects such as nausea and somnolence which may not result from cell death) and that the subsequent changes in function are ultimate results of damage expressed in cycling cells. These are perhaps most simply summarized by observing, first, that in general the effects produced by ionizing radiations in tissues and organs are quantitatively related to dosage, and second, that with few exceptions (specifically cells that die during interphase) it is only cells in or induced into cycle that are appreciably affected by radiation. This notion, which will be developed into the target-cell hypothesis, underlies the approach taken in this book. In broad terms, it is assumed that the intensity of an effect usually reflects the proportion of cells irreversibly damaged by radiation as a result of lesions in their replicative mechanism. Subsequently, the depopulating effect is perceived in an organ or tissue by progressive reduction in its function, unless the remainder of the regenerating cells are capable of repopulating and reconstituting the tissue. Therefore the approach to understanding the effects of ionizing radiations on tissues involves identification of target cells and emphasis on changes in tissue function as a result of their depletion. The present chapter is devoted to a survey of the patterns of cell renewal in different tissues and how they are affected by radiation injury, and to consideration of the pathogenesis of radiation-induced injury in tissues.

## 1.1. Patterns of cell renewal in tissues

It is useful to categorize tissues on the basis of whether renewal and function occur at different places in the tissue (e.g. renewal in the intestinal crypts, function on the villi), or occur in the same populations of cells (e.g. hepatocytes). Tissues in which the cell populations responsible for renewal and function are separate are designated hierarchical (type-H) tissues. For example, there is a stem-cell compartment near the base of the intestinal crypts, where pluripotent cells, the ultimate source of renewal, slowly replicate. Stem cells occasionally mature into differentiating, transit cells, which amplify cell production by division in the mid-crypt locations. These proliferate rapidly to increase cell production. Near the tops of the crypts, the amplifying cells slowly lose their proliferative potential and mature into functional villus cells. This organization of proliferation and function is depicted in Figure 1.1(a). A second category comprises tissues in which some functional cells are capable of renewal. This category has been called flexible, or type-F (Figure 1.1(b)) (Michalowski 1981). Examples include lung, liver, kidney, and spinal cord. The important distinction to be kept in mind concerning type-H and type-F tissues is that in the former, functional cells are irreversibly post-mitotic, whereas in the latter, they may retain latent radiation injury for long times until its expression at mitosis.

**Cell production**

In type-H tissues, new functional cells are produced by division, differentiation, and maturation of precursor cells. The rate of production exactly balances the rate of loss of functional cells. Negative feedback is the mechanism generally invoked to control this balance (reviewed by Lord 1986). The rate of loss of functional cells varies enormously between tissues, and even for different cell populations within a single tissue. For example, human granulocytes have a life in the blood of about

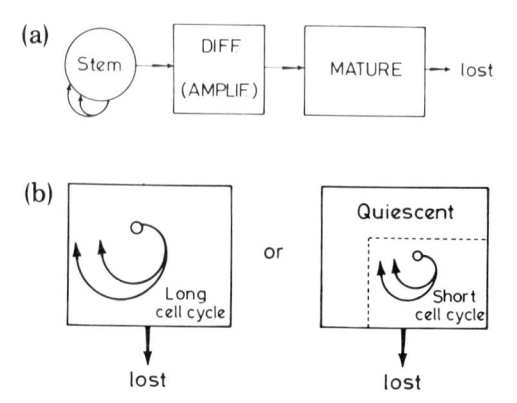

Figure 1.1. (a) Schematic representation of a type-H cell population (from Michalowski 1981). (b) Schematic representation of a type-F cell population. (Reproduced with permission of Springer-Verlag and the author.)

8 hours, whereas red blood cells have one of 120 days (i.e. about 1% are replaced per day).

The divisions of stem cells produce differentiated proliferating cells whose divisions are commonly called amplifying divisions of transit-cell populations. In general, each division amplifies the number of cells by a factor of 2 except in instances such as spermatogenesis, in which about 2/3 of spermatocytes die during normal maturation for unknown reasons, and in many tumours where there is a cell-loss factor (see below). The number of transit divisions varies markedly between tissues that have differences in the degree of specialization of functional cells in separate branches in a lineage and in the rates of production of functional cells. Studies with epithelia in the mouse have shown that there probably are up to four amplifying cell divisions in the epidermis and in the gastrointestinal mucosa (Potten 1981), whereas in haematopoietic tissues there may be six transit divisions in the granulocytic series (Hendry & Lord 1983). Similar numbers of divisions are expected to occur in man. The proliferative organizations of haematopoietic tissue, gastrointestinal mucosa, and epidermis are depicted in Figure 1.2.

Thus, the transit cells form the production factory for the functional cells. In turn, the transit-cell populations originate from other precursor cells, the stem cells. These are a minority of cells in the tissue, commonly less than 1%, and they are the ancestors of a particular lineage. Generally, they are anchored at the origin of pathways of migration of their maturing progeny (Potten and Hendry 1983a). Studies with mice have shown these cells to be either very slowly cycling or out of cycle (Potten 1986a), e.g. in haematopoietic tissue (Becker et al. 1965) or intestinal mucosa (Hendry et al. 1984). Hence, the total number of divisions of these cells during the life of an animal is low, and this minimizes the risks of inducing genetic errors during replication of the parent genome. Thus, the bulk of the divisions necessary to supply the animal continually with new functional cells is performed by the transit cells committed to a limited number of divisions. In these cells, genetic instability is of much less consequence.

Stem cells have colony-forming ability, which is the property of a cell by which it produces a family of descendants by a series of divisions. The precursor cells produced by stem cells at the origin of a branch to the lineage may also be clonogenic, depending on how many remaining divisions they are capable of. They may form macroscopic colonies visible to the eye if more than 10 divisions have been accomplished—producing more than $2^{10}$ or about 1000 cells—or microscopic colonies if many fewer divisions have been performed. In haematopoietic tissue, stem cells are colony-forming cells, as are committed precursor cells at the origin of the three main branches of

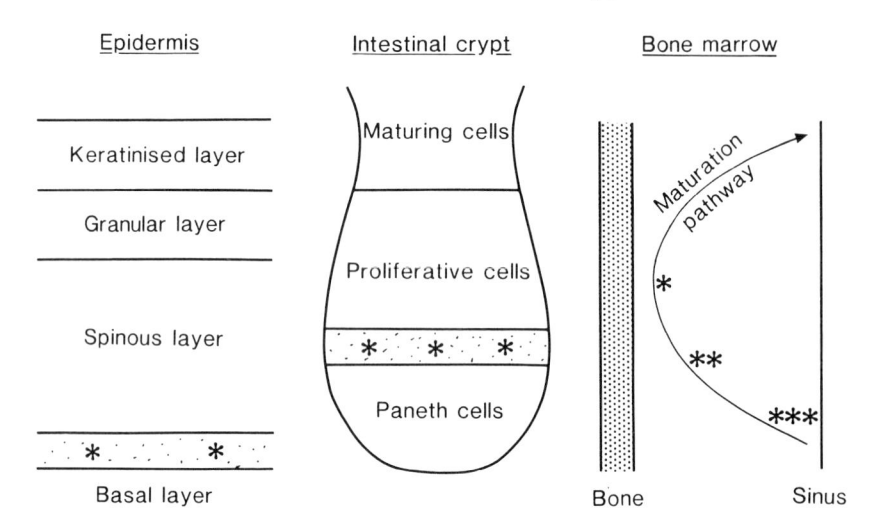

Figure 1.2. Diagrammatic representation of the proliferative organization of epidermis, crypts in the intestinal mucosa, and bone marrow. In the *epidermis*, about 1 in 10 basal cells are considered to be stem cells, with the remainder being transit cells. Proliferative activity is confined to the basal layer. Suprabasal cells are differentiated to various degrees, becoming flatter near the surface to produce flat cornified squames. In the *intestinal crypt*, the stem cells are located at the bottom of the proliferative zone which is in the middle of the crypt. The majority of the proliferative cells are transit cells, amplifying the number of cells which eventually will mature, leave the crypt, and migrate up the villus. Each villus is supplied on average by the cell output from 10 crypts. In the *bone marrow*, the stem-cell concentration is highest close to the bone surface. However, the earliest stages are found away from bone and hence it is likely that the bone surface is a site where differentiation stimuli act to produce maturing cells. The stars indicate stem cells with high self-renewal capacity.

development (granulocytic, erythrocytic, megakaryocytic). In epithelia, with only three or four transit-cell divisions, the stem cells form colonies, but the various transit cells would each form smaller and smaller colonies as their division potential diminished.

The growth fraction is defined as the proportion of cells in cycle in a population. In type-H tissues, where most cells are mature and non-cycling, the growth fraction will be small if the number of cycling cells is expressed as a proportion of the total cells present. The stem cells may be in a long cell cycle or out of cycle—the true specification is debatable (Wright & Allison 1984). The only clear case is for the dividing transit cells, where the growth fraction is obviously 1·0.

## Cell death

Cells die naturally by maturation followed by senescence. The life-time of functional cells varies enormously; it depends on whether (*a*) the particular function required of a cell is short-lived (granulocytes), (*b*) the lifetime is governed by the metabolic life of cells in fixed tissues (organs) or in migratory cell populations (red blood cells) or (c) cells are shed from a surface (epidermis, gastrointestinal tract).

The fate of dead cells varies with type of tissue. Cells abraded from the skin surface are simply shed from the body. Those cells lost from the internal surface of the alimentary canal are digested with the food if they are lost from the upper regions of the tract, and are ejected with the faeces if in the lower regions of the tract. Dead blood cells are phagocytosed by macrophages. The few cells that die in organs generally do so in a process known as apoptosis, where the nucleus of the dead cell becomes fragmented into a number of dense chromatin bodies (Kerr et al. 1972). Subsequently the bodies are engulfed by neighbouring cells. This occurs to a much larger extent in tumours (see below).

A low incidence of cell death occurs in immature normal cell populations, a phenomenon that has been described in intestine (Potten 1977; Hendry et al. 1982) and hair follicles (Potten 1985b). It is considered that apoptosis is a natural, programmed method of cell deletion, which is necessary particularly for some cells in the stem-cell region where any genetic abnormalities must be eliminated (Cairns 1975; Potten 1977).

There are two modes of cell death after cytotoxic injury, interphase death and mitotic death. The former is characteristic of certain lymphocytes (Okada 1970; Stefani et al. 1977) and serous salivary gland parenchymal cells (Sodicoff et al. 1974; El-Mofty & Kahn 1981; Stephens et al. 1986), apart from the minority immature populations described above for other tissues (apoptosis). In dividing populations, cells with damaged DNA may fail to separate at the end of mitosis into two daughter cells. This occurs predominantly in the first division after injury, but it also occurs with lower frequency in cells undergoing a second or third mitosis after a successful first mitosis following treatment. This is the most common and important form of cell death induced by radiation in tissues (Hendry and Scott, 1987). Cells which have escaped mitotic death during many divisions after irradiation are said to have retained *reproductive integrity*.

**Tumours**

A distinction must be drawn between normal tissues and tumours with respect to whether cell loss occurs in the renewing population of a tissue or in the oldest, functional, nonproliferating cells. Unperturbed adult human normal tissues exist in a steady state in which renewal and loss are exactly balanced. It is likely that no loss of proliferating cells occurs in the renewing cell populations, but rather in the oldest functional cells (e.g. abraded from the skin surface or from the internal surface of the alimentary canal). It is not known at what stage of differentiation cell loss occurs in tumours (Steel 1968, 1977).

Cell loss and cell renewal are not in balance in tumours that are in a state of growth (see section 6.8). The rate of tumour growth depends on many factors, among them the cycle time of the renewing populations and the cell-loss factor (reviewed by Denekamp & Fowler 1977). In tumours with high cell-loss factors there is no consistent relationship between cycle time and volume-doubling time (Denekamp 1970). On the other hand, when the cell-loss factor is small the tumour growth rate depends on cycle time and growth fraction, being higher when cycle times are shorter and growth fractions larger, as shown in Figure 6.18.

Since tumour response is usually judged in terms of disappearance, rather than change in 'function', it is necessary to keep in mind the distinctions between the role played by renewal and function in normal tissues versus tumours. It is interesting that tumours, although hierarchical if they retain differentiation characteristics, may be considered F-type tissues, since their 'function' is to grow, and their renewing populations are identical to those that support function.

## 1.2. Effects of radiation on cell production

Radiation injury has both transient and permanent effects on renewing populations in tissues. Mitotic delay is transient and not remembered in the progeny. This is followed in some cells by mitotic death. Further considerations are the renewal capability and cycle time of surviving cells.

### Mitotic delay

Radiation affects cell production initially by mitotic delay. The reasons for this time delay are not fully understood, but the length of the delay in the $G_2$ phase of the cell cycle is proportional to dose. For rapidly cycling populations the delay is about 1 hour per gray, and for slowly cycling cell populations it is about 1/10 of a cell cycle time for every gray (Denekamp 1975). Radiation-induced delay in more slowly proliferating cells may be even greater at the $G_1/S$ boundary than at the $G_2/M$ boundary (Nagasawa et al. 1984).

### Mitotic death

Following mitotic delay, the next effect on cell production is mitotic death of transit cells. The effect is dependent on the dose, and death can occur at any division up to about five divisions after irradiation

(Thompson & Suit 1969; Trott & Hug 1970; Joshi et al. 1982). After acute doses greater than 6 Gy the probability that a sterilized cell in culture will undergo even a single division is reduced drastically (Elkind et al. 1963; Thames et al. 1986). Hence a survival curve for total cells is asymptotic to the survival curve for colony-forming cells (Puck & Marcus 1956; Wheldon et al. 1982). However, *in vivo* it is possible that transit cells can accomplish one, and occasionally two or more, divisions even after acute doses of 10–20 Gy. These few divisions may occur because, with intestinal mucosa and epidermis, the time taken to denude the epithelium after these high doses corresponds to the time taken to lose all mature cells, including the normal number produced by transit cells (Potten 1981).

## Cycling cells

In hierarchical tissues, the stem cells are mostly out of cycle or in a long cycle, and the transit cells are in rapid cycle (although after irradiation the stem cells will come into rapid cycle as part of the regenerative response). Hence, the comparisons of sensitivity to be made are between (a) noncycling and cycling stem cells, and (b) cycling stem cells and cycling transit cells. With marrow CFU-S, cycling cells are only slightly more resistant than those in steady-state (Hendry 1973). When a cytotoxic insult has stimulated proliferation of colony-forming cells in the intestine, they are more resistant ($D_0 = 1.8$ to $2.5$ Gy) than when irradiated in the unperturbed state ($D_0 = 1.2$ Gy) (Potten & Hendry 1975). With hair follicles, there is no clear differential between the radiosensitivity ($1/D_0$) of germ cells in resting or growing follicles (Griem et al. 1979; Hendry et al. 1980). Cycling transit precursor cells in marrow vary in sensitivity, when assessed using similar colony-forming criteria. Granulocyte-macrophage colony-forming cells are slightly more resistant than cycling CFU-S, whereas the erythroid precursor cells are slightly more sensitive (reviewed by Hendry 1985a,c).

## Self-renewal of survivors

The relative probabilities of self-renewal or differentiation of surviving colony-forming cells are probably not markedly affected by acute irradiation, although few experiments have been designed to test this. The probability of self-renewal of marrow stem cells (CFU-S) was assessed by measuring the complement of CFU-S in splenic colonies derived from irradiated CFU-S (Hendry & Lord 1983). Acute doses up to 5 Gy did not significantly reduce the numbers of CFU-S per colony (or equivalently the probability of self-renewal per surviving colony-forming cell).

Any increase in the cycle time of stem cells after irradiation would tend to amplify any measured differences in renewal probabilities. This effect is probably small, because the doubling time of irradiated CFU-S populations in the sublethally irradiated mouse is similar to that of control cells grafted into a lethally irradiated mouse. Four repeated doses of 4·5 Gy (3-week intervals) reduced the renewal probability of stem cells (Xu et al. 1983), and a smaller effect was detected after four doses of 1·5 Gy (Xu et al. 1986).

Measurements of changes in self-renewal probability in surviving cells after irradiation have not been made for tissues other than bone marrow. There was a disparity in doubling times deduced for epidermal colony-forming cells by different authors (22 hours, Withers 1967a; 53 hours, Emery et al. 1970). Although the reasons for this are not known, the possibility of differences in self-renewal probability ($p$) was discussed by Withers (1967a). The values can be reconciled if $p = 0·6 - 0·65$ in the case of Emery et al. (1970), and $0·75$ in the experiments of Withers (1967a). In the former case more daughter cells would be differentiated and then would not contribute to the increase in clonogenic cell number than in the latter case.

In tumours, no measures of $p$ or of changes in $p$ have been made, but clearly these should be as important in differentiating tumours as they are in normal tissues (MacKillop et al. 1983). Long-term changes in division probability have been discussed by Beer (1979) and Seymour et al. (1986). These concern lethal mutations which are expressed after many divisions and which reduce the plating efficiency of cells maintained in culture.

**Compensatory proliferation**

Radiation-induced cell loss in mature, transit, or stem-cell populations is followed by compensatory proliferation in surviving transit and stem cells. This response is generally considered to be mediated through negative feedback control mechanisms, but these have not yet been fully elucidated in any mammalian system (Lord 1986). Compensatory proliferation begins when cell loss has reached a sufficiently high level. Surviving transit cells can contribute initially to a spurt in the production of new cells, as in the classical second abortive rise in granulocytes observed in the bone-marrow syndrome (Wald 1971). However, surviving stem cells are required to initiate a sustained recovery of all the cell types in a lineage. The rate of recovery of the stem-cell population is similar in several critical normal tissues, namely with a doubling time of about 24 hours in bone marrow (Hendry 1972), epidermis (Withers 1967a), and intestinal mucosa (Potten & Hendry 1975). In bone marrow this doubling time reflects a cell-cycle time as low as 6 hours with a concomitant 40% loss of stem cells to differentiation

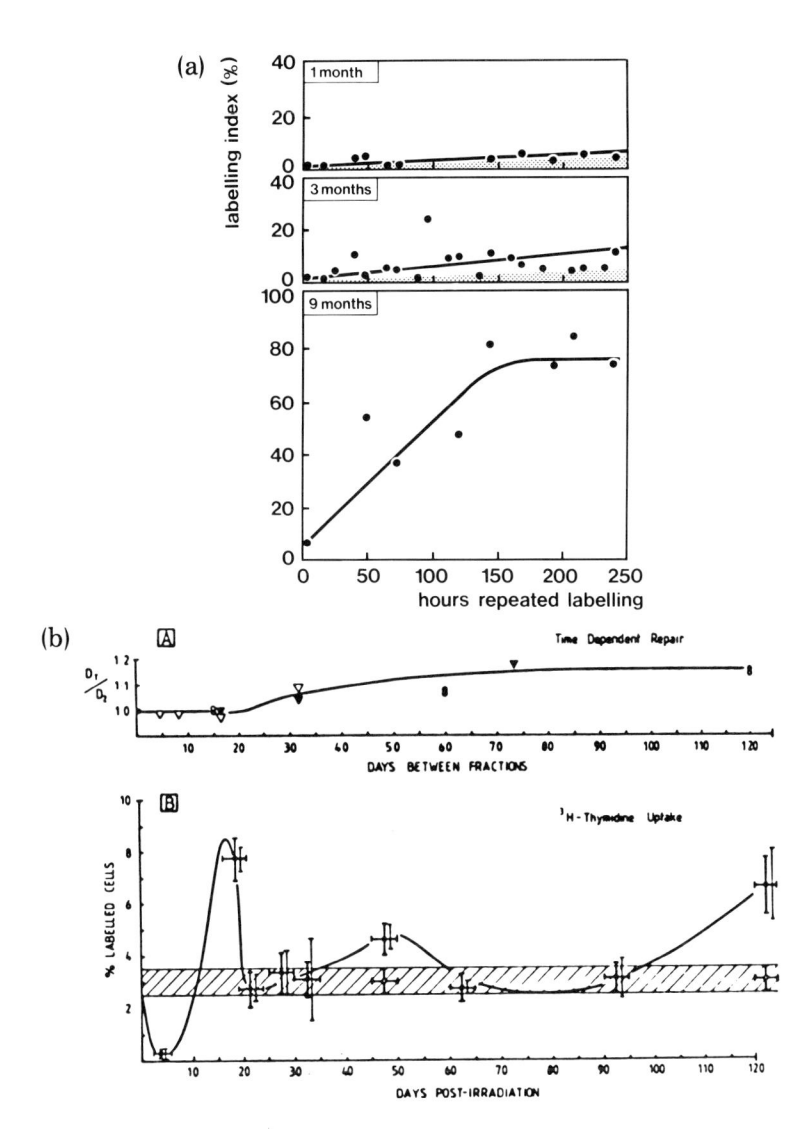

Figure 1.3. (a) Continuous labelling data for mouse bladder epithelium at 1 to 9 months after irradiation with 25 Gy electrons (from Stewart 1986). The LI is plotted as a function of time of exposure to [$^3$H]-TdR. Hatched areas indicate the very low rate of uptake of [$^3$H]-TdR in controls (reproduced with permission of Macmillan Press Ltd and the author).
(b) (A) The ratio ($D_T/D_2$) of the doses needed to cause myelopathy in 50% of rats when the dose is given in two halves separated by various times ($D_T$) to the dose when separated by one day ($D_2$) shown in relation to the time between the dose fractions (from Hornsey et al. 1981). Cervical cord, neutrons (open circles), lumbar cord, neutrons (closed circles); cervical cord, X-rays (open triangles); lumbar cord, X-rays (closed triangles).
(B) The percentage of neuroglial cells in the white matter of the cervical cord labelled in five-day periods with tritiated thymidine at various times after 20 Gy X-rays. Horizontal bars represent the five-day period over which the animals were labelled with tritiated thymidine. Open symbols are for control mice, closed symbols for irradiated mice. The hatched area represents the range of control values. (Reproduced with permission of The British Institute of Radiology and the authors.)

pathways at each division (Lajtha et al. 1971). The cells differentiate into committed lines of development, and there is often an overshoot in both maturing and mature cells because of extra divisions in the transit-cell populations. This is noted, for example, in mouse granulocyte—macrophage precursor cells in the expandable spleen (Testa et al. 1974) and in the intestinal crypt (Potten & Hendry 1975; Hagemann 1976). However, there is no convincing evidence for an overshoot in the stem-cell population in any tissue, and more likely it approaches normal or slightly subnormal levels. Priming doses of radiation can make animals more resistant to subsequent doses, for example in mice (Porteous & Lajtha 1966) and in sheep (Hanks et al. 1966). Although the reasons for this are unknown, it is possible that there are contributions from overshoots in transit cells and possibly from the slightly greater resistance of regenerating rather than unperturbed stem cells.

Compensatory proliferation in late-responding tissues occurs when the slow rate of cell turnover has sufficiently expressed the latent genetic injury to stimulate a regenerative response. This is assumed to occur in conditionally-renewing tissues, e.g. liver and kidney, but not in irreversibly postmitotic cells such as neurons. The former are tissues that can be stimulated artificially into proliferation by cell depletion resulting from surgical removal or cytotoxic injury. This stimulation occurs in e.g. bladder (Stewart et al. 1980; Stewart 1986), spinal cord (Hornsey et al. 1981, 1983), and lung (Coggle 1987).

There may even be an accelerated expression of injury if the cells brought into the division cycle, which then die when they attempt to divide, initiate a further increase in the number of cells induced to proliferate and thereby to express their latent, lethal injury (Michalowski 1981). This possibility, termed an 'avalanche', has not yet been clearly demonstrated, e.g. by measurement of significant curvature in (flash) labelling index versus time data, reaching high levels ($\geqslant 50\%$ L.I.) when all cells are in rapid cycle.

## 1.3. Pathogenesis

The pathogenesis of radiation-induced injury to tissues may be considered in terms of the preceding. The first consideration is given to the identification of renewing populations within tissues, and the second to manifestation of radiation injury, identified by nature of histological change as well as length of the latency observed, particularly in relationship to the turnover times of the identified renewing populations.

This brings in the concept of target cells for radiation-induced tissue injury:

*A target cell is a renewing cell whose death following irradiation contributes to a reduction in tissue function.* Assays of tissue injury may include somewhat arbitrary criteria, and as these change so also does the specification of the target-cell population. Moreover, stem cells and renewing transit cells may both be considered target-cell populations, depending largely on the time of assay (e.g. transit-cell renewal may sustain function for a sufficient time to allow stem-cell regeneration which is needed for long-term recovery). Specific functions in tissues are dependent on particular renewing populations,

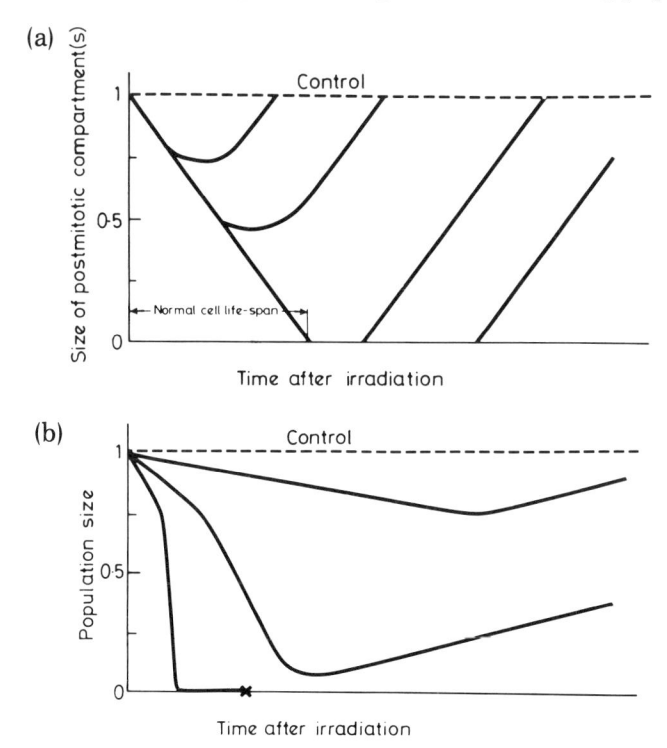

Figure 1.4. (a) Theoretical response of a type-H cell population to a range of single doses of ionizing radiation (from Michalowski 1981). During the period of zero input to the mature compartment of newly born mature cells, the total number of these cells declines linearly at a rate equal to that characteristic of steady-state conditions of the tissue concerned. The onset of complete depletion occurs at a time equal to normal mature-cell longevity. Recuperation sets in later the higher the dose.

(b) Theoretical response of a type-F cell population to a range of single doses of ionizing radiation. The first, slower phase of depopulation is followed by the 'avalanche', if the dose is large enough. The overall rate of depletion is inversely related to dose, the more severe damage developing earlier. (Reproduced with permission of Springer-Verlag and the author.)

and hence target-cell populations for various functions may be different. Lastly, it should be noted that certain types of nondividing, mature cells (e.g. certain lymphocytes and serous salivary parenchyma) undergo interphase death and these are target cells although they are nonrenewing.

Relationships between target-cell depletion, dose, and expression of tissue injury are shown in Figure 1.4 for both type-H and type-F tissues. The latency interval before tissue dysfunction or death is a function of the life span of the mature cells in a tissue (apart from, notably, small lymphocytes, which are a radiosensitive mature cell population). The latency interval for a given response will reflect the time taken to reach a certain level of depletion of functional cells. The tissues in which the life span of functional cells is short, e.g. intestinal mucosa, will demonstrate injury within a few days. In contrast, anaemia in the short term is seen only when there are haemorrhages, because of the long life (about

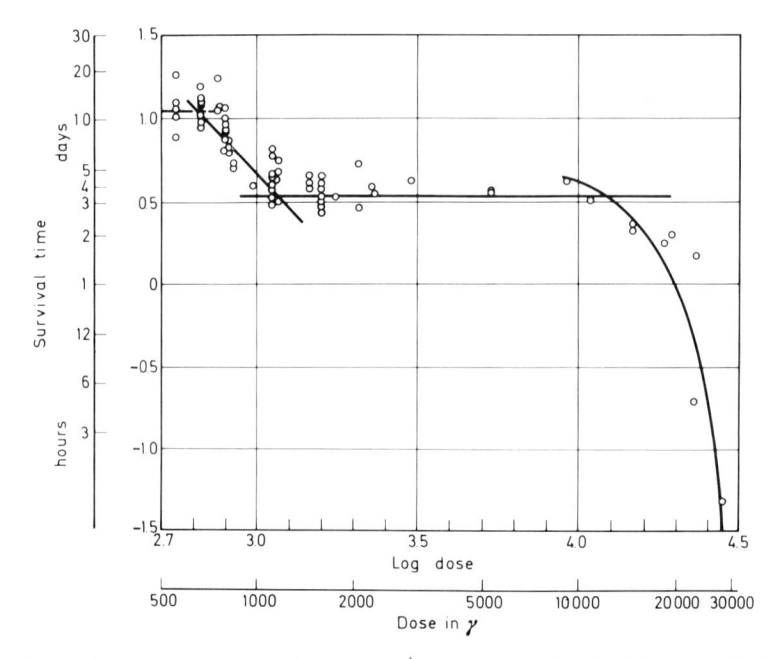

Figure 1.5. Relationship between the mean survival time of whole-body-irradiated mice and the dose of gamma-rays (from Quastler (1945) and Michalowski (1981)). The first plateau at 11 days (doses of less than 750 R) is set by fatal bone-marrow insufficiency (R = röntgen unit of exposure). With higher doses (up to 1000 R), increasing relative probability of occurrence of the intestinal syndrome gradually reduces the value to 3·3 days. Further dose increments are ineffective in reducing the survival time, until with more than 10 000 R animals die of the CNS syndrome whose time-course is apparently dose-dependent (Reproduced with permission of Springer-Verlag and the author.) $\gamma = R$.

4 months in man) of red blood cells. Because of the radioresistance of most mature cell types in contrast to the radiosensitivity of stem cells and transit cells in type-H tissues, the latency interval with increasing severity of response will be dose dependent after doses low enough for sufficient stem cells to survive to mount a regenerative response. However, after high doses the stem-cell compartment is ablated, and the latency interval will be independent of dose and the response will be similar, namely tissue failure. These relationships are illustrated in Figure 1.5, which shows the survival time of whole-body-irradiated mice after different doses.

The plateau in survival time following the intestinal syndrome extended from about 15 to 100 Gy. The tendency towards a longer latency interval below about 12 Gy could have been due to an abortive regenerative response in the mucosa sufficient to prolong the life of the animals by a day or two after the lower doses, but not after higher doses, or a contribution from (abortive) granulocyte production helping to counteract infections after the lower doses.

In F-type tissues, the mature cells are gradually depleted according to the naturally slow rate of cell turnover. The rate of depletion will be dose dependent because the proportion of cells capable of division is proportional to dose. Hence the latency time to a given level of depletion will also be dose dependent. However, after very high doses virtually all cells will be prevented from successful division, and in this case latency intervals will be dose independent. This will produce a biphasic curve of latency interval against dose, as evidenced in Figure 1.6. for lung.

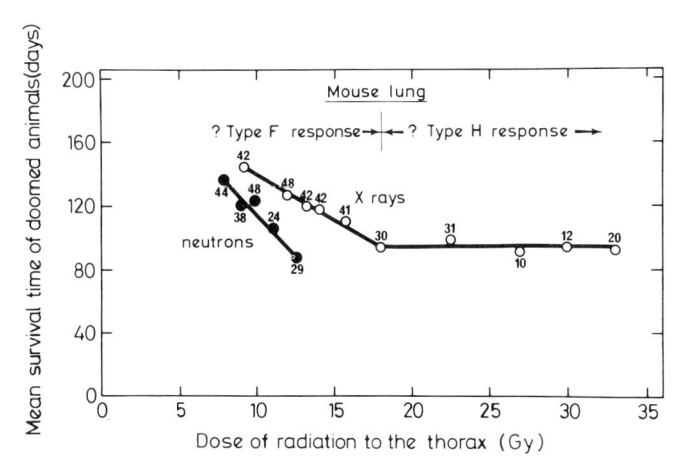

Figure 1.6. Mean survival time of mice dying from lung damage as a function of dose delivered to the thorax (from Michalowski 1981). The numbers refer to the number of animals in each dose group. (Reproduced with permission of Springer-Verlag and the author.)

In the following we will consider selected hierarchical tissues that are important clinically and for which the latency, dose−response, and fractionation relationships can be interpreted on a target-cell basis. For flexible tissues, examples are chosen on the basis of their clinical relevance and of the amount of information available concerning these relationships. Target-cell interpretations for injury in these tissues are more speculative than in hierarchical tissues, but the same framework is employed for simplicity.

**Bone marrow**

The causes of death from the bone-marrow syndrome are granulocytopenia, thrombocytopenia, and lymphopenia, which occur with different degrees of severity among species (Bond et al. 1965). Granulocytopenia is the prime cause in many species, inducing an inability to counteract infections. Granulocytes are produced from precursor cells in the marrow, and these in turn originate from stem cells in the marrow. After irradiation it is likely that divisions of the precursor cells help maintain the population of granulocytes, which may prevent the animal's dying before regeneration of the stem cells produces sustained recovery in the precursor cell population (Tannock 1986). However, although the target cells for acute effects after irradiation may be the granulocytic precursor cells, it is the stem cells that are the target cells for long-term recovery.

Most species that die from the bone-marrow syndrome do so within 30 days. Man is an exception, with some deaths occurring up to 40 to 50 days after irradiation (Bond et al. 1965). The syndrome occurs after doses between 2 and 10 Gy, depending on species. The dose to produce 50% deaths within 30 days (the LD50/30) is between 2·5 and 6 Gy marrow dose for many large species, e.g. dog, goat, sheep, pig, and monkey. For mice and rats the LD50/30 is generally higher: 6−9 Gy. The LD50/60 for man is generally considered to be between 3 and 6 Gy marrow dose, with a likely mean value of 4·5 Gy (Mole 1984). The syndrome can be treated by conventional supportive measures including antibiotics and barrier nursing, and by infusions of blood cells or marrow cells. Infusions of blood cells will help counteract infections and haemorrhages to allow natural recovery of endogenous marrow. Transplants of marrow, preferably isogeneic, assist in persistent marrow recovery.

At long times after irradiation marrow aplasia may develop (see, for example, Knospe 1966). These late effects are probably a combination of stromal injury expressed gradually and chronic stem-cell depletion.

For further discussion see the reviews by Hendry & Lord (1983), Testa et al. (1985), and Hendry (1985a).

## Gut

There is a prodromal phase which consists variously of stomach sickness and neuromuscular disturbances, depending on the dose. This phase may progress to the gastrointestinal (GI) syndrome, where death is due to loss of fluid, electrolytes, and protein from the denuded alimentary canal, together with infection and haemorrhages that are exacerbated by granulocytopenia and thrombocytopenia.

It is highly likely that the target cells for the radiation-induced GI syndrome are the stem cells and the transit cells of the intestinal crypts. The life of a new-born cell in the crypts of the intestine is about 3—4 days, after which it is shed from the villus. If the supply of new transit cells is cut off by radiation the crypt shrinks in size first, as transit cells continue a few cell divisions to maintain some cell output for the villus. The villus then shrinks and eventually, if the dose is high enough, the intestine will be denuded. There is then a literal 'life and death' race between the developing GI syndrome and compensatory regeneration. The GI tract possesses an astonishing ability to regenerate. At the $LD_{50}$, about half the crypts will be totally destroyed, while in the remaining half each crypt will contain on average near to 1 surviving clonogenic cell. Nonetheless, half the animals survive the syndrome. The time of death corresponds to the time taken to denude the villous epithelium, which consists of those functional cells present at the time of irradiation together with those produced after irradiation by transit cells completing some of their few divisions (Potten 1981). This correlation is seen particularly well using germ-free mice, which have more slowly cycling intestinal cells, longer-lived villus cells, and a correspondingly longer latency interval before death (Tsubouchi & Matsuzawa 1973).

Death occurs in most species between 3 and 10 days after doses from 10 to 50 Gy. The LD50/7 for conventionally housed mice is about 11 Gy, and other species probably do not differ by more than a few gray from this. It varies with the type and level of bacterial flora. Higher doses produce the same signs of injury and the same latency intervals (see Figure 1.5), although there are more severe and earlier prodromal responses.

The effects can be alleviated using fluid and antibiotic infusions, which may allow sufficient regeneration of the mucosa to prevent death. However, there is no cure for this syndrome after high doses because intestinal progenitor cells cannot yet be successfully transplanted.

Late effects in the gut include strictures and stenosis (Geraci *et al.* 1974, 1977; Terry *et al.* 1983; Terry & Denekamp 1984; Breiter & Trott 1986). As in the case of bone marrow, these effects may be due to a combination of chronic stem-cell depletion, slowly developing stromal damage, and scarring from acute denudation.

Further discussion can be found in the reviews by Potten and Hendry (1983a) and Michalowski & Hornsey (1986).

**Skin**

The first sign of radiation injury in the skin is erythema. There is an acute erythema that is dose dependent above a threshold of about 5 Gy and appears within a few hours of acute exposure. A target cell has not been identified for erythema, which appears to be related to a vascular response. This initial erythema disappears, but reappears after about one week (longer in humans) as a more sustained response just before the epidermis shows signs of denudation. The denudation results from continued loss of mature cells from the surface with a lack of production of new cells from precursor cells in the basal layer. The denudation is characteristic of a type-H tissue, and the severity of response is dose and time dependent until the dose is high enough to result in total sterilization of all basal cells. In this case, after doses ranging from 20 to 40 Gy, the time to denude the epithelium to various levels is similar (Potten 1981). The severity of the effects is dependent on the area of skin and site irradiated, and the reason for this is not known. However, recent data indicate that this field-size effect is also observed for the survival of epidermal clonogens (Chen & Hendry 1986b).

After doses that allow healing of the epidermis from regenerating stem cells together with migration from the unirradiated margins, there are later responses. These may be due either to long-term ulceration arising from severe acute desquamation or to injury in the dermal components and other underlying tissues. There is a phase of dermal erythema and then fibrotic reactions with deposition of collagen.

Target-cell populations for these long-term stromal injuries are in general unknown (except those for injuries arising as a consequence of severe acute damage). It is likely that the vasculature is involved to some extent (Hopewell 1980), for example in telangiectatic reactions (Turesson & Notter 1984a, b) and arterial occlusions causing ischaemic necrosis (Hendry 1987). There are other late effects, such as contraction (Hayashi & Suit 1972) and induration. A postulated mechanism for these effects is imbalance of collagen production and resorption on account of radiation-induced loss of fibroblasts (Rantanen 1973).

Skin injury has been reviewed by Hopewell (1980), Potten (1985a; 1986), and Jammet et al. (1986).

The tissues we have discussed so far are generally associated with acute radiation effects, and are hierarchical in their proliferative organization. We move now to a consideration of some late-responding tissues in which cell renewal is very slow. These may be thought of as type-F tissues (Figure 1.1(b)), in which functional cells are also capable of renewal. We will consider lung and spinal cord.

## Lung

The earliest phase of radiation-induced lung injury after a high dose is exudative, resulting from early permeability changes in the alveolar walls and leading to an inflammatory protein-rich exudate up to about one month after irradiation. This phase is unlikely to play a dominant role in the development of radiation pneumonitis, which occurs most often three to six months after irradiation. Pneumonitis is associated with histopathologic phenomena characterized by the collapse of osmotic equilibrium at the alveolocapillary interfaces, resulting in alveolar instability with atelectasis and a passage of blood transudates and haemorrhage into the alveolar lumen. These phenomena can in turn be interpreted as results of the loss of two critical elements of lung function, namely production of alveolar surfactant and barrier activity.

The most likely candidates for target cells whose depletion results in radiation-induced pneumonitis are the type-2 alveolar cells and endothelial cells. The endothelial cells form a barrier that prevents leakage of water and macromolecules into the interstitium. In this picture, the high turnover rate of lung alveolar cells serves respiratory function by providing a constant supply of surfactant, the entire cell disintegrating to liberate the surfactant. Ionizing radiation acts to reduce drastically the supply of these cells and thus to undermine osmotic balance in the lung.

The turnover rates of alveolar cells have been studied using colchicine arrest to measure the rate at which cells entered mitosis within a 24-hour period (Bertalanffy & Leblond 1953) and using tritiated-thymidine labelling (Spencer & Shorter 1962). The turnover rates of approximately one to four weeks correlate reasonably well with the times at which cell loss leading ultimately to pneumonitis might be expected to begin.

Animals surviving the pneumonitis phase usually undergo a second phase of injury, known as radiation fibrosis of the lung, which can result in lung failure and death. Damage to alveolar walls (possibly endothelial cells) produces reactive inflammatory changes and transudation of fibrin and other serum proteins into the wall and alveolar lumen. This fibrin may become organized and result in an abnormal condition of the reticulo-elastic skeleton that adversely affects the mechanisms of respiration. These pleural effusions, for which the target-cell population is unknown, can also result in death (Down *et al.* 1984). The delicate reticulum of the normal lung changes to produce a 'proliferation' of reticulum fibres, the latter being more numerous and thickened. The severity of change at this stage is dose dependent, ranging from focal patchy consolidative changes to confluent consolidation of lung tissue.

Table 1.1. Radiation-induced lesions in the mouse lung

| Parameter | Pneumonitis | Late lung injury |
| --- | --- | --- |
| Dose range (single doses) | 10–15 Gy | 10–13 Gy |
| Latent period | Inversely related to dose (6 → 3 months) | Inversely related to dose (12 → 6 months) |
| Repopulation | Not observed for intervals ⩽ 4 months | Not known |

Taken from Coultas (1984) and Travis & Tucker (1986).

In this reparative phase, many cell activities appear devoted to the organization of dead cells and inflammatory exudates, with a progressive fibrosis occurring in which the delicate reticulin-elastic framework becomes replaced by cicatricial (collagenized and later ossified) tissues, with concomitant increase in avascularity (van den Brenk 1971). Relationships of dose and effect are illustrated in Table 1.1.

The threshold dose for pneumonitis is about 10 Gy to the lung in mice, and about 7·5 Gy in man (Figure 1.7). In man, the dose to lung tissue giving pneumonitis in 5% of cases is about 8·2 Gy, and in 50% of cases is about 9·5 Gy (van Dyke et al. 1981). These doses were deduced from results of hemi-body or whole-body treatment of leukemia prior to marrow transplantation. In 52 patients who showed signs of pneumonitis, it developed between one and seven months in 90% of them (mean = 15 weeks). The time of onset was not significantly dose

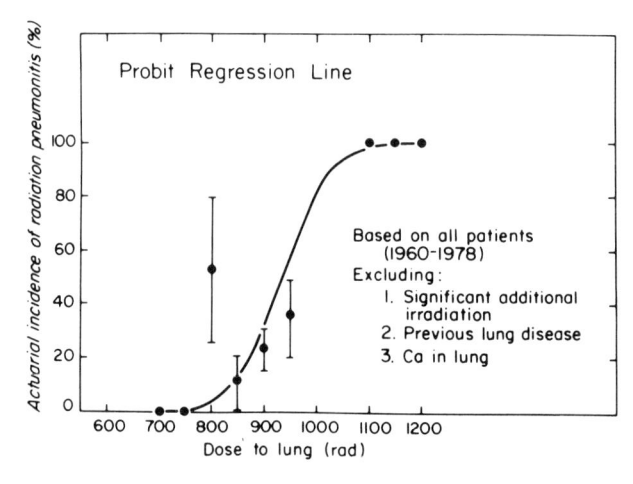

Figure 1.7. Sigmoidal complications curve for patients irradiated to the lung using single doses. (From van Dyke et al. 1981; reproduced with permission of Pergamon Journals Ltd and the authors.)

dependent between 6·5 Gy and 12·5 Gy, but this may reflect the small number of patients irradiated at each dose level.

Experimental data concerning dose-fractionation effects show that the $\alpha/\beta$ ratio (see Sections 3.3 and 6.10) has a value of 3−6 Gy for pneumonitis, and a value at the lower end of this range for the later response. Radiation-induced lung injury has been reviewed by van den Brenk (1971), in the UNSCEAR report (1982), and by Travis & Tucker (1986).

## Spinal cord

The effects of irradiation on the cord are manifest as paralysis of the limbs after a considerable delay (at least four months), a feature that has prompted a great deal of interest in this injury. In most reports on human radiation myelopathy it has been concluded that the lesions were of vascular origin (Jellinger & Sturm 1971), although others have felt that vascular lesions were secondary to white matter necrosis (Zeman 1971). It can be said with some certainty only that late functional damage to the spinal cord probably does not result from direct effects on the neurons, as deduced from morphologic studies. Instead, the most

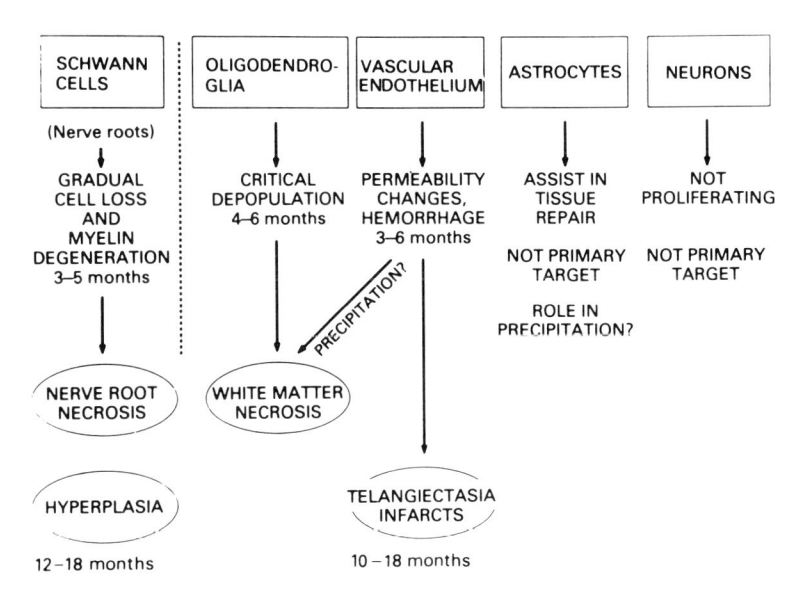

Figure 1.8. A schematic representation of the major cell types in the CNS, and their assumed participation in the development of different types of radiation-induced lesions (from van der Kogel 1986). Schwann cells (on the left) are not part of the CNS, but are the primary parenchymal cells in the spinal nerve roots (Reproduced with permission of Macmillan Press Ltd and the author.)

likely targets are (a) glial cell populations and (b) endothelial cell populations (Figure 1.8).

Whether glial or endothelial cells are the most likely targets depends on dose and latency period. After doses in the range 20–40 Gy, and with a latent period less than 210 days (van der Kogel 1980), delayed radionecrosis in the rat occurs both in the brain and the spinal cord and has a predilection for white matter. This is manifest as segmental demyelination, a direct expression of glial cell damage. It occurs as early as two weeks after doses in this range and is accompanied in humans by Lhermitte's sign of electrical paresthesias after cord irradiation or a somnolence syndrome after brain irradiation.

With increasing doses the latent period decreases, and vascular damage becomes more pronounced (van der Kogel 1986). Possible target-cell populations for CNS injury are shown in Figure 1.9, and these are illustrated in Table 1.2.

In the lumbar cord, nerve-root necrosis occurs at 5–8 months due to the gradual depletion of Schwann cells. The latter are not part of the CNS, but are the primary parenchymal cells of the nerve roots.

A different type of vascular damage that is not associated with white-matter necrosis is observed in the rat after very long time intervals and after lower single doses. For doses less than 20 Gy, and with a latency period of 200 to 500 days (van der Kogel 1980), variable

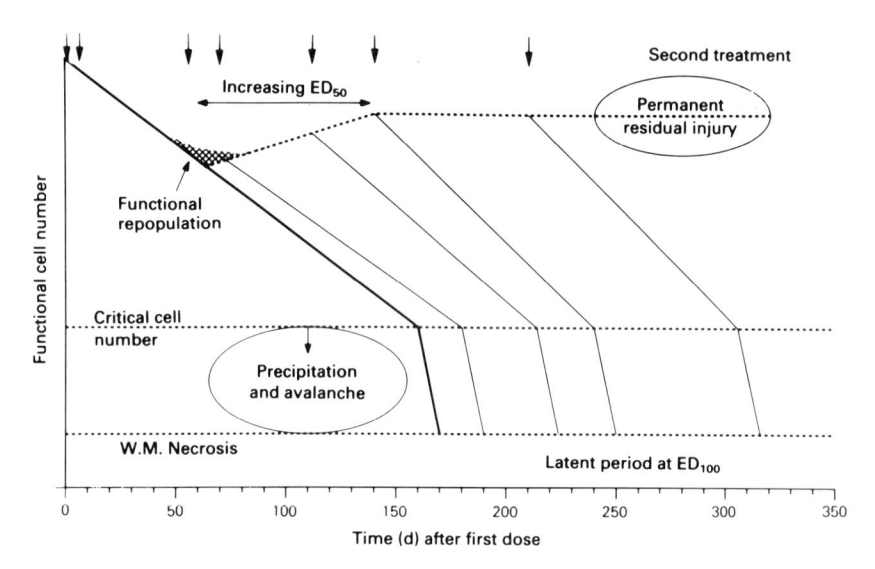

Figure 1.9. Schematic representation of a model for the development of white-matter necrosis in the cervical spinal cord, as derived from results of split-dose treatments (from van der Kogel 1986). The time of the second treatment is indicated on the upper x-axis. W.M. = white matter. d = days. (Reproduced with permission of Macmillan Press Ltd and the author.)

Table 1.2. **Characteristics of different types of delayed radiation damage in the rat spinal cord**

|  | Cervical, early delayed damage | Cervical, late delayed damage | Lumbar, progressive radiculopathy |
|---|---|---|---|
| Type of lesion | white-matter necrosis | telangiectasia, haemorrhage | nerve-root necrosis |
| Possible target cell | oligodendrocyte | vascular endothelium | Schwann cell |
| Dose level (single dose) | $\geqslant 20$ Gy | ~15−20 Gy | $\geqslant 20$ Gy |
| Latent period | ~6 months | 8−18 months | ~5 months |
| Repair $(D_2-D_1)$ | 8 Gy | 5·5 Gy | 7·5 Gy |
| Start of regeneration after irradiation | 8−10 weeks | 16−20 weeks | 1−4 weeks |

From van der Kogel (1983).

lesions are observed, from telangiectasia and petechial haemorrhage to extensive haemorrhagic infarcts in acutely paralysed rats. A similar distinction between dose and latency interval was observed in the rat brain (Hopewell & Wright 1970). Sudden death after 20−30 Gy was due to vascular damage, while glial-cell depletion led to white-matter necrosis after doses of 30−40 Gy.

Van der Kogel (1986) has adopted the following model of the response of the spinal cord. Within a few weeks of irradiation demyelination is observed after doses as low as 5 Gy, as a direct result of the loss of glial cells and with increasing frequency as a function of dose. After 2−3 months, the accumulated damage is sufficient to stimulate repopulation by oligodendrocytes (Figure 1.9). If this proliferating pool cannot compensate for the loss of functional cells, a critical number of glial cells will be reached and tissue breakdown may occur rapidly. At this point it is possible that the other target cells (e.g. endothelial) may play a role in precipitating the injury. At doses too low to effect the reduction of glial cells to this critical level, the possibility of radiomyelitis from vascular injury arises. Here the course would follow that expected from progressive injury expressed because of depletion of endothelial-cell populations.

There are many other tissues of clinical importance where the pathogenesis is understood to various degrees, for example, kidney and eye. The reader is referred to the following texts for further information: Casarett (1981); Annex J in UNSCEAR (1982), Potten & Hendry (1983b); and Proceedings of the 12th L. H. Gray Conference (1986).

# Chapter 2
# Evidence for target-cell depletion as the determinant of tissue response

The target-cell hypothesis may be formulated as follows:

> The responses of tissues to irradiation are quantitatively related to dosage. The increase in response will reflect the increase in the number of cells affected, primarily regarding their replicative ability. The important cells in the tissue regarding this endpoint may be a small proportion of the cells, as in type-H tissues, or the majority of cells, as in type-F tissues. In both cases those cells capable of replication and regeneration of the tissue are the *target cells*. The effects on tissue response of alterations in radiation quality or distribution of dose in time can be described in terms of alterations in survival probability of the target cells. (Modified from van den Brenk 1971.)

In type-H tissues, lifesaving or tissue-rescuing cells are generally the precursor cells of the mature functional cells. The latter are radioresistant in most tissues (notable exceptions are lymphocytes and salivary-gland parenchymal cells). The precursor cells are a minority population, and they vary in radiosensitivity depending partly on their division capabilities. In F-type tissues, on the other hand, the precursor cells may be considered the functional cells and would therefore constitute a majority. Cells with the greatest division capacity, the stem cells and their immediate daughters, e.g. those in haematopoietic tissue, are the most sensitive with respect to retaining *reproductive integrity* (escaping mitotic death through multiple divisions).

In the following, the responses of tissues will be interpreted on the basis of depletion of a target-cell population. Of course there are many other complications and modifying factors, such as physiological load on the tissue, concurrent disease conditions, and age of the animal. Let it be made clear, then, that the purpose of the present discussion is to organize the available evidence for a *direct* influence of target-cell depletion on the incidence of tissue failure, functional modification, or other injury. The issue is not whether the expression of injury can be modified, e.g. by the physiological demand placed on a tissue (it can), but rather whether the observed effects can be described on a cellular basis, for whatever set of ancillary influences. The evidence to be put forth is perforce of the necessary, but not sufficient, type. It comprises three types: (1) the numerical equivalance of $D_0$ values derived from the functional response of the tissues as opposed to those values measured for their renewing populations of cells, (2) the equivalence of clonogen survival at tissue-isoeffect doses after altered fractionation and dose rate, and (3) the limiting slopes of isoeffect graphs for tissue response to fractionated and continuous exposures as opposed to those deduced from target-cell models.

## 2.1. $D_0$ values: functional or in situ colony assays

Hornsey (1973a,b) measured crypt-cell survival at doses isoeffective for animal lethality after altered LET or oxygen status. As may be seen from Figure 2.1, the changes in the LD50/5 corresponded closely to the changes in survival as measured by the microcolony assay of crypt-cell survival at 0·01 surviving fraction. This confirmed the close relationship between death from the acute intestinal syndrome and epithelial damage in the small intestine: the same level of cell survival resulted in 50% animal survival when irradiated under different conditions of oxygenation or with different qualities of radiation.

It can be seen that the changes in slopes of the cell-survival and dose−incidence curves in Figure 2.1 are related. Indeed, the steepness of dose−incidence curves should permit in principle the calculation of absolute dose−response parameters for putative clonogens whose depletion results in normal tissue injury or in tumour cure (Munro & Gilbert 1961; Suit et al. 1964; Robinson 1968; Gilbert 1969; Andrews 1978; Wheldon et al. 1977; Withers & Peters 1980; Hendry et al. 1983b; Hendry & Moore 1985). When these can be compared with parameters derived from *in situ* colony survival, a direct plausibility test of the target-cell hypothesis is possible. In this first section emphasis will be on comparisons of slope and on responses to single doses. The ensuing sections will consider evidence for the proposition that target-cell survival is the same at tissue isoeffect doses that change because of altered fractionation or dose rate.

**Sensitivity *in situ***

The dose-incidence curve for tissue failure (or other specified level of tissue injury such as animal death) is generally sigmoid. There is a

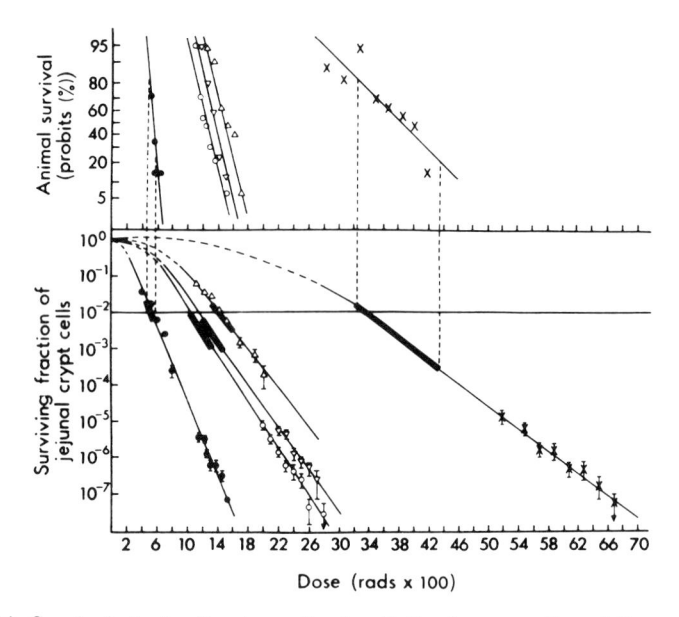

Figure 2.1. Survival of mice five days after irradiation (upper section of diagram) matched with survival curves for jejunal crypt cells (lower section) (from Alper 1973). The curves show, from left to right, the results of mice breathing oxygen while irradiated with: neutrons (closed circles); electrons, 60 Gy/min (open circles); electrons, 500 cGy/min (inverted triangles); X-rays, 7 MV, 100 cGy/min (triangles). At the right, the curves with the symbol × relate to mice breathing nitrogen while irradiated with electrons, 150 Gy/min.

The thickened sections of the curves depicting crypt-cell survival correspond with dose ranges within which animal deaths range from 20% to 80% as shown by two pairs of vertical dotted lines. For all conditions, animal deaths started to occur at the doses for which cell survival was near $10^{-2}$. A horizontal line has been drawn across the diagram at that level. Vertical bars in the lower section represent $\pm 1$ S.E.M. (Reproduced by permission of the British Council and Drs. S. Hornsey and T. Alper).

threshold region of dose where the effects increase in severity but are not too threatening to tissue function, followed by a steeply rising incidence of tissue failure with increasing dose, tending toward a plateau of 100% failure. The shape of the curve for increasing incidence with increasing dose is shown in Figure 2.2(a). The curve can be linearized by an appropriate transformation of the probability scale (Fig. 2.2(b)), which is important in its own right and which we next consider in more detail.

The slope of the probability curve describes the heterogeneity between responders as a function of dose. If there were no variation between responders, the slope would be infinitely steep, and at one dose there would be no response but at a slightly higher dose all samples would have responded. However, in practice this never happens, since there is always some heterogeneity. There are statistical and biological reasons for this variation.

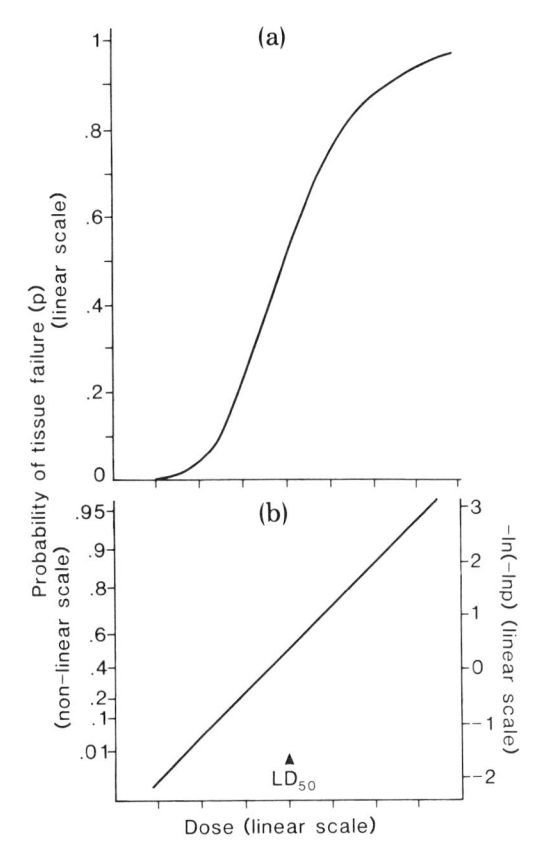

**Figure 2.2.** (a) Sigmoid relationship between the probability of tissue failure and the dose. The sigmoid curve is transformed into a linear relationship (b) by changing the scale on the y-axis (see text).

Possible biological sources of variation that can modify the shape of the dose-incidence curve include the following (Hendry & Moore 1985b): (1) variations in $N$ or $D_0$ among the samples irradiated, (2) the presence of a resistant subpopulation of cells, e.g. cells in late S phase, or hypoxic cells, which form the majority of the surviving target-cell population in the dose range where tissue failure occurs after single doses, and (3) the presence of two target-cell populations, e.g. parenchymal and vascular, that fail over ranges of dose that overlap. Possibilities (1) and (2) would make the curve shallower, but possibility (3) would steepen it.

However, the primary cause of this variation in radiation response is the random nature of dose deposition, as illustrated in Figure 2.3. Randomness is of great importance in appreciating the form of the dose–survival relationship, which is essentially exponential. This may be understood by a simplified, intuitive argument as follows.

26        *Fractionation in Radiotherapy*

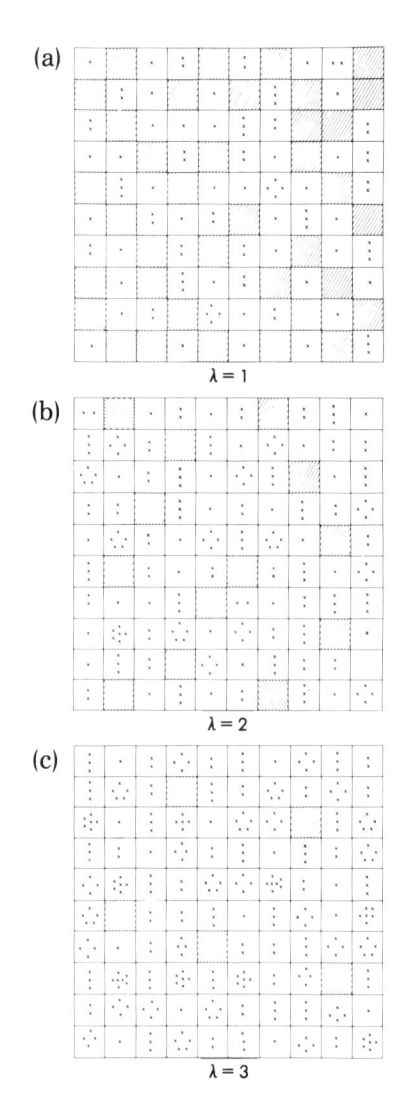

(a) $\lambda = 1$

(b) $\lambda = 2$

(c) $\lambda = 3$

Figure 2.3. Panels illustrating the random distribution in 100 equal-sized targets (small squares) of 100, 200, or 300 hits (×'s) (from Withers & Peters 1980). The probability that any one of the 100 targets will not be struck when 100 hits are delivered randomly is $e^{-1}$ or 37%. Thus, when an average of 1 lethal hit per target is delivered in a random fashion (a), 37% of the targets will 'survive'. The same proportionate reduction in survival applies for each equal increment in the number of hits: 200 hits (b) would result in a probability of survival of $e^{-2}$ (or $0 \cdot 37 \times 0 \cdot 37$), and even after 300 hits are delivered (c), there is still a chance $e^{-3} = 5\%$ that any one target will 'survive'. This proportionate, or geometric, decrement in survival may be plotted as a straight line on semilogarithmic coordinates (Figure 2.4). (Reproduced by permission of Lea & Febiger and the authors.)

Suppose we call the dose necessary to deliver *one lethal event per cell* (Figure 2.3a) $D_0$, so that after a dose $D$ the number of lethal events per cell is $D/D_0$. In Figure 2.3(c), for example, a dose $3D_0$ has been absorbed, there is an average of 3 lethal events per cell, and fewer cells (shaded squares) remain free of lethal events than after smaller doses (a) and (b). Now if there is a large number $\nu$ (100 in Figure 2.3) of target cells, the chance of getting a lethal event in a given cell equals the average number of such events per cell divided by the number of cells, i.e. $(D/D_0)/\nu$. Therefore, the likelihood of *not* getting a lethal event in a given cell is $1 - [(D/D_0)/\nu]$. To get the *surviving fraction* (s.f) of cells, i.e. *the proportion of cells with no lethal events*, we simply multiply the probability of no lethal event for a given cell times itself $\nu$ times: $(1 - (D/D_0)/\nu).(1 - (D/D_0)/\nu)...(\nu \text{ times})...(1 - (D/D_0)/\nu)$. This is the $\nu$th power of $(1 - (D/D_0)/\nu)$, which for large $\nu$ is closely approximated by an exponential:

$$\text{s.f.} = [1 - (D/D_0)/\nu]^\nu \simeq e^{-D/D_0} \qquad (2.1)$$

The form of this simple exponential survival curve is illustrated in Figure 2.4. Note that as a consequence of randomness of dose deposition, the same proportion, not the same number, of cells is killed with a given increment of dose. Thus the dose $D_0$ reduces survival to 37% ($e^{-1}$); in other words, 63% of the cells have one or more lethal events (cf. Figure 2.3(a)). This is true at any point on the curve: the dose increment $D_0$ reduces survival to 37% of its previous value (B to A, Figure 2.4).

The same reasoning can be applied to dose−incidence curves for tissue failure. It is not unreasonable to think that tissues may be rescued from failure by a death-preventing or tissue-rescuing unit (TRU) (Hendry et al., 1983b; Hendry & Thames 1986). If the units are inactivated at random, the number of viable TRUs after a dose $D$ can be described by $K.\exp(-D/D_0)$, assuming exponential survival and an initial number $K$ of TRUs. Note that $D_0$ refers to inactivation of TRUs, not cells. Otherwise this is analogous to cell-survival theory, and by analogy with this theory, in which the probability of no lethal events in a cell (with the average number per cell given by $D/D_0$) is $\exp(-D/D_0)$, the probability of no TRUs surviving given an average number $K.\exp(-D/D_0)$ is

$$\text{probability of tissue failure} = \exp[-K \exp(-D/D_0)] \qquad (2.2)$$

This expression, known as a Poisson model, gives a sigmoid dose−incidence curve (Figure 2.2(a)). We may now define the $D_0$ for tissue failure by transforming the probability scale as a function of dose. The Poisson model (equation (2.2)) is linearized by taking logs twice; if we denote the probability of tissue failure by $p$, then $-\ln p = K \exp(-D/D_0)$,

28                    *Fractionation in Radiotherapy*

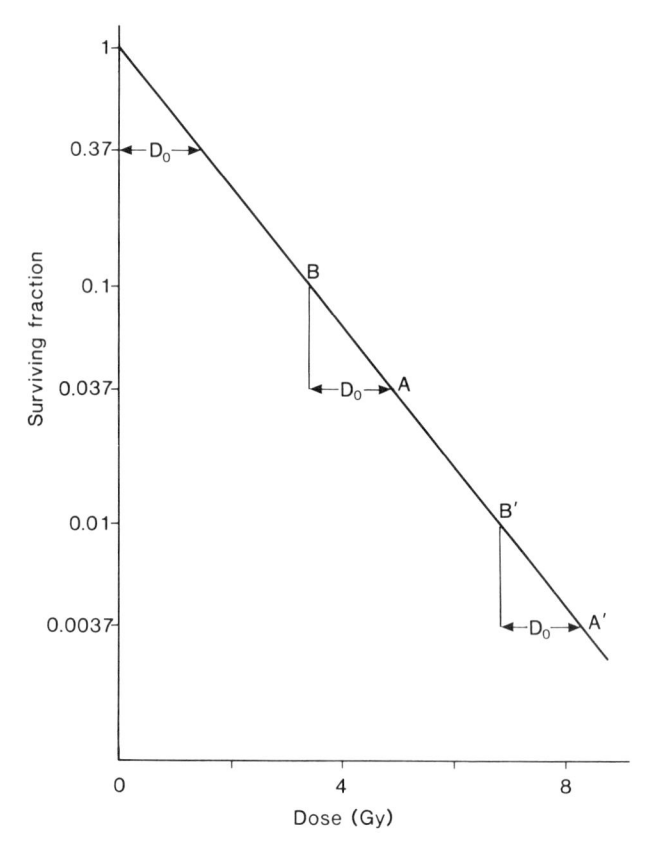

Figure 2.4. An exponential survival curve. The $D_0$ is the dose which reduces survival to 37% of the previous value, i.e. from B to A or B' to A'. Thus $D_0$ is the dose required for an average of one lethal lesion per cell (Figure 2.3a).

and

$$-\ln(-\ln p) = D/D_0 - \ln K \tag{2.3}$$

This linearizing of the sigmoid curve is illustrated in Figure 2.2, which shows a dose–incidence curve in the sigmoid (*a*) and double-log (*b*) forms. Over the common range of measurement of incidences from 5% to 95%, the double-log transformation is very similar to the probit transformation (Lange and Gilbert 1968).

In hierarchical tissues, the TRU would be composed of a certain number of clonogenic cells, capable of producing a life-saving number of mature cells. In these cases the number of rescuing units in a tissue, $K$, is proportional to the number of rescuing cells, $k$(cells), i.e. $K = C.k$(cells), and the number of viable TRUs after a dose $D$ will be given by, for example, $C.k\,(\text{cells}).N.\exp(-D/D_0)$ where $D_0$ describes the sensitivity of the rescuing *cells* and $N$ is their extrapolation number (Section 6.4). Thus,

$$-\ln(-\ln p) = D/D_0 - \ln C.k\,(\text{cells}).N \qquad (2.4)$$

Hence, *on the target-cell hypothesis the same $D_0$ would be measured for the response of target cells and for tissue failure caused by their depletion.* There is at least one caveat which should be noted: if the probability of repopulation by a single cell was dependent on the number of surviving cells, the observed $D_0$ for tissue failure would be steeper than the $D_0$ for the target-cells (Hendry, 1985b; Withers et al. 1986).

This hypothesis has been tested in three normal mammalian tissues, all hierarchical in structure and all responding acutely after irradiation, namely bone marrow (Robinson 1968; Hendry & Moore 1985a), intestinal mucosa (Hendry et al. 1983b), and epidermis (Hendry 1984b). In all of these, colony techniques can be used to measure $D_0$, which can be compared with values of $D_0$ deduced from the linearized dose–incidence curve for tissue failure (equation (2.3)) as described above. It is important to compare measurements of colony survival and tissue survival over similar ranges of dose whenever possible because of the possibility of the survival curve bending more than predicted by an exponential decline. Also, it is better to use a colony assay *in situ*, rather than after transplantation, in order truly to represent the survival of colony-forming cells in the irradiated environment. Potential difficulties with transplantation assays are the selection of a more easily transplantable subpopulation of cells and changes in repair capacity that modify survival, particularly dose-modifying changes that change $D_0$.

No direct comparisons of sensitivity deduced from lethality data or measured for clonogens in normal tissues are yet available for species other than mouse.

**Bone marrow**

On the basis of the slope of the lethality curves, the corresponding value of $D_0$ for the target cells was deduced to be approximately $0\cdot 6\,\text{Gy}$ (Robinson 1968). This was less than the $D_0$ value of $0\cdot 95\,\text{Gy}$ gamma-rays for the stem cells, measured by Till & McCulloch (1961) using a colony assay. However, the latter value was the average value of the slope over the dose range $0-5\,\text{Gy}$ (allowing a small shoulder), in contrast to the measurement of slope of the lethality curve over the higher dose range of $7-10\,\text{Gy}$, where the appropriate $D_0$ could be lower if the survival curve for target cells were bending faster than an exponential. A detailed survival curve for marrow stem cells (Hendry 1979a) showed that at doses near 6 Gy gamma-rays the $D_0$ could be as low as 0·65 Gy, approximately the same as the value expected at slightly higher doses from the analysis of the LD50/30 data. A recent analysis of three other sets of LD50/30 data, where orthovoltage X-rays were used, resulted in a low estimate of $D_0$, 0·57 ± 0·10 Gy (Hendry & Moore 1985a).

Curvature in the survival curve using high dose rates can be confirmed using low dose rates. The value of $D_0$ should increase with decreasing dose rate to reflect (in the limit) the initial slope of the target-cell survival curve, if there is no repopulation during the irradiation period and if postirradiation repair processes are complete. An analysis of nine lethality curves in the literature, where dose rates were between 1 and 3 cGy per minute, resulted in a mean $D_0$ for five series using X-rays of 1·14 ± 0·40 Gy, and for four series using gamma-rays it was 1·73 ± 0·43 Gy (Hendry & Moore 1985a). The latter value is higher than the mean $D_0$ value of 1·0 Gy from four reports in the literature for CFU-S using gamma-rays at dose rates between 0·7 and 0·9 Gy per minute (reviewed by Hendry & Lord 1983). However, one of the estimates from the sample with the mean of 1·73 Gy was unusually high at 3·46 Gy, and if it is excluded, the mean of the three remaining $D_0$ values is 1·15 Gy. The latter value would then be similar to the mean $D_0$ value of 1·0 Gy for stem cells using low dose rates.

This analysis demonstrated how the relevant $D_0$ for the target cells increased from about 0·65 Gy to 1·0 Gy with a decrease in dose rate, in line with the increase in $D_0$ from about 0·6 Gy to 1·15 Gy, deduced from LD50/30 data, as expected from the target-cell hypothesis. However, there is still the possibility that an important transit-cell population, for example the granulocyte-macrophage colony-forming cells (GM−CFC), forms the target-cell population, as suggested by Tannock (1986). In this event, the surviving GM−CFC could be producing granulocytes to counteract infections for a sufficient time to allow regeneration of the stem-cell population and its progeny. This could be pertinent in the present context because of the similarity in the $D_0$ value of 1·9 Gy for GM−CFC using a low dose rate (0·05 Gy per minute: Testa et al. 1974) and the above value of 1·73 Gy deduced for all four sets of LD50/30 data. However, this state of affairs is not consistent with previous data at high dose rate, where the $D_0$ for GM−CFC is 1·79 ± 0·10 Gy gamma rays (the mean of values reviewed by Hendry and Lord 1983) compared with the $D_0$ of about 0·6 Gy deduced for the target cells from LD50/30 data. Caution must be introduced into these comparisons because of the variation in the $D_0$ of GM−CFC under different growth conditions (Testa et al. 1974; Broxmeyer et al. 1976), and recent reports of a much lower $D_0$, 0·7 Gy, for GM−CFC in the mouse (Peacock et al. 1986).

Also, it should be noted that target-cell sensitivity was assessed by a transplantation assay (stem cells) or in culture (GM−CFC), and it can be questioned whether these measurements reflect radiosensitivity *in situ*. When colonies from regenerating marrow were counted *in situ* in various bones in the mouse, survival after doses between 5 and 7 Gy acute gamma rays was characterized by a $D_0$ of $0 \cdot 91 \pm 0 \cdot 09$ Gy, and in the ribs by a $D_0$ of $1 \cdot 08$ Gy (Hendry *et al.* 1986). If the survival curve was gently bending between these doses of 5 to 7 Gy, the $D_0$ values might have been less at higher doses around the LD50/30. Indeed the values $0 \cdot 91 - 1 \cdot 08$ Gy were higher than those that would be expected (of $60-70$ cGy) if these regenerating cells represented the target cells for LD50/30. Even without this extrapolation the correlation is better than if the GM−CFC were concluded to be the target cells, since for these the $D_0$ values have been reported up to $1 \cdot 8$ Gy. Nonetheless, it is likely that GM−CFC play an important role in animal survival. This remains to be tested experimentally, for example by transfusing sorted subpopulations of marrow cells into mice immediately after doses just above the LD50/30 and measuring their effectiveness for rescue.

Thus, the simplest and most useful interpretation is that haematopoietic stem cells, or another closely related cell population with very similar radiosensitivity, form the true target-cell population for the bone marrow syndrome in the mouse.

Dose−response curves for different species have been considered. Mole (1984) and Baverstock *et al.* (1985) analysed data in the literature for various species of large animal, namely monkey, pig, goat, sheep and donkey. We have reanalysed these data by pooling results from different

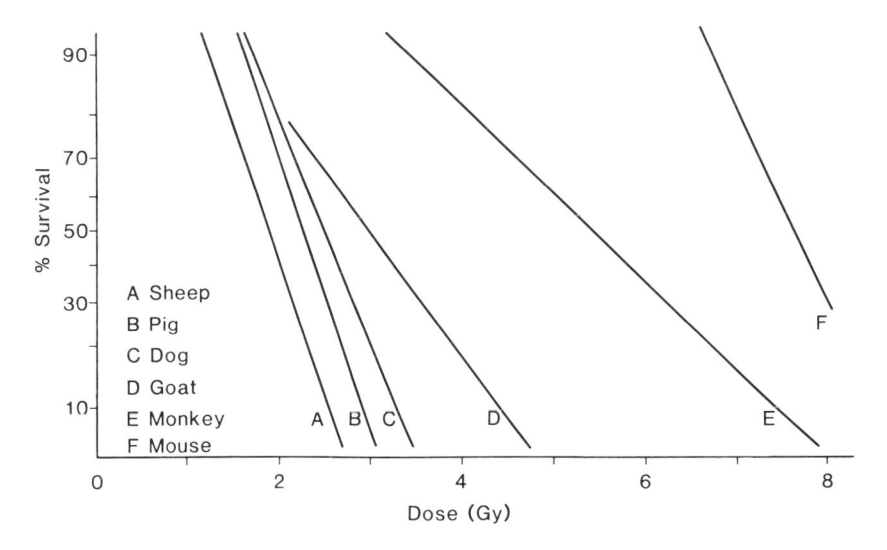

Figure 2.5. Dose−response curves for marrow failure in different species, plotted on a probability scale of response.

experimenters for each species and normalizing the doses to a common LD37 among experiments. This assumes that the differences between experiments relate to dose-modifying factors such as dose rate and radiation qualities. The mean dose−response curves obtained in this way for each species are shown in Figure 2.5.

For the large animals the sensitivity (slope) is higher in general for those species that show the lowest values of LD50/30 (dog, pig, and sheep). This is the opposite of what would be expected on the target-cell hypothesis if the same target-cell survival curve was applicable to all these species and was gently curving, and if the reason for the displacements was the different levels of target-cell depletion tolerable by different species. The higher sensitivity deduced from lethality data for the dog is supported by measurements of cell sensitivity, where the $D_0$ for GM−CFC is low (0·50 Gy: Nothdurft et al. 1983). Hence differences in cell sensitivity between species may be an important factor in these comparisons.

**Intestine**

A comparison of the sensitivity of target cells for intestinal failure in mice (LD50/7), and of microcolony-forming cells *in situ* was made by Hendry et al. (1983b). This comparison of slopes is to be distinguished from Hornsey's (1973) comparison of cell survival at the LD50/5 under different oxygenation and LET conditions (cf. Figure 2.1).

In the intestine, the mucosa is folded into a large number of crypts ($\sim 10^6$ in mice). Hence death from the GI syndrome can be prevented by a certain minimum number of surviving crypts, which would comprise one TRU. (This number of crypts could be determined histologically, for example by counting the number of crypts in mice which had just died, and in those which had survived. The number required for rescue would be just above the borderline between the two ranges of counts.) After high doses, where crypts regenerate from only single surviving clonogens, the $D_0$ for the TRU would be equal to the $D_0$ not only for the clonogens but also the crypts. Also, a TRU in the intestine could be equated with either a number of crypts or a number of clonogens. At lower doses where there is a multiplicity of clonogens in surviving crypts, the dose−survival curve for crypts will be less steep than that for single clonogens, and a Poisson correction can be made to the crypt data to take this effect into account (Withers & Elkind 1970).

The $D_0$ for the target cells for lethality was $1 \cdot 25 \pm 0 \cdot 22$ Gy, very similar to the value $1 \cdot 23 \pm 0 \cdot 08$ Gy for microcolony-forming cells (Figure 2.6(*b*)). These similarities present good evidence for the applicability of the target-cell hypothesis for intestinal failure, in particular as

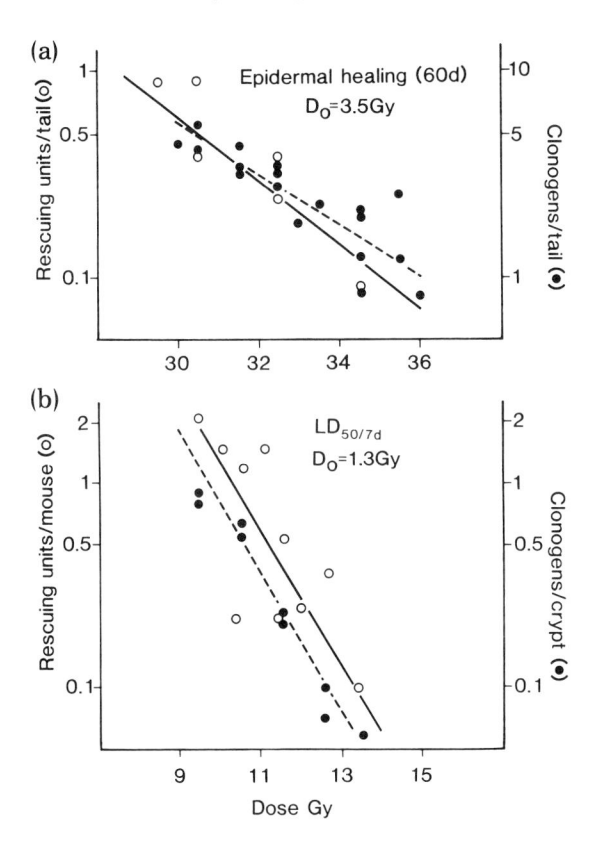

Figure 2.6. Correspondence between $D_0$ for target-cell killing and $D_0$ for depletion of TRUs: (a) epidermis; (b) intestine.

the conditions were met for (a) an assessment of cell sensitivity *in situ* and (b) measurement over the same range of doses in both systems.

Clearly there are many factors that contribute to the intestinal syndrome, such as the content of bacterial flora and the lack of granulocytes, but these are likely to be dose-independent factors over the range of doses under consideration (9–14 Gy). Hence, they would be expected to change the position of the curve, but not its slope. The deduced $D_0$ reflects largely the depletion of target cells, each of which can colonize and contribute to the renewal of the intestinal mucosa.

### Skin

Severe desquamation of the epidermis can lead to skin necrosis if regeneration from colony-forming cells in the basal layer is insufficient for re-epithelialization and healing. A comparison of the $D_0$ deduced for

34     *Fractionation in Radiotherapy*

healing (2·8 ± 0·5 Gy) with that measured for colony-forming cells (3·5 ± 0·5 Gy) was made by Hendry (1984b) using mouse tail epidermis (Figure 2.6(a)). A problem in making this comparison was choosing the criterion for healed or unhealed epidermis, since this choice affected the deduced $D_0$. The closest numerical equivalence of $D_0$ values was achieved when healing was classified as a stage reached by 9 weeks after irradiation, at which time there was at most a small erythematous or thin epidermal region remaining (Figure 2.7). The $D_0$ value deduced from

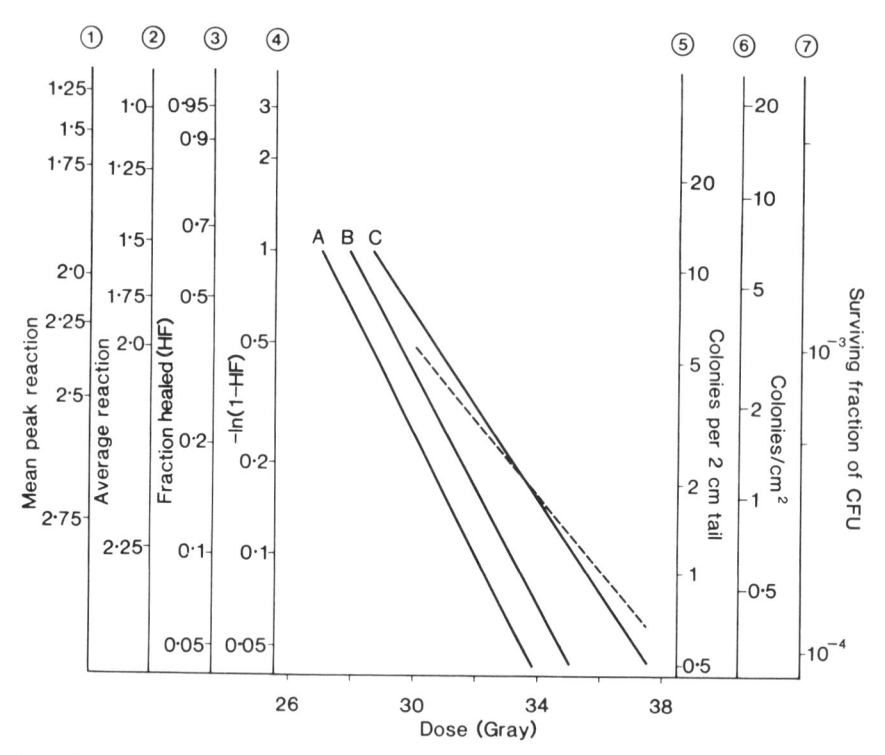

Figure 2.7. Correlation between dose—response curves in mice for skin reactions, proportions of tails healed, and macrocolony number (from Hendry 1984b). A 3-cm length of tail was irradiated, and colonies were counted in the central 2-cm portion. Ordinate 4 shows the double log transformation of the probabilities of healing (HF) where $-\ln(1 - \text{HF})$ is plotted on a log scale. Ordinate 3 shows values of (HF) corresponding to the values on ordinate 4. The values for the mean peak reaction (ordinate 1) and average reaction (between 3 and 6 weeks after irradiation, ordinate 2) were put on arbitrary scales with the values corresponding to particular values of (HF) at each dose. The lines A, B and C are transformed values of HF according to ordinate 4 using different criteria for scoring healing; A = tails with reactions at most slightly different from normal, designated 'healed'; B = at most, patches of thin epidermis with slight reddening; C = at most patches of persistent erythema with marked thinning of the epidermis. Dashed line and ordinates 5 and 6, macrocolony survival curve positioned to cross mid-way line C. Ordinate 7, surviving fraction of clonogens deduced from split-dose experiments. (Reproduced with permission of the British Institute of Radiology.)

the healing data decreased when the criterion was made stricter to exclude small erythematous regions of epidermis, which may reflect a dose-dependent production of smaller colonies that were less effective in colonizing the epidermis.

## Tumours

In theory, the comparison of dose-cure curves for tumours with survival curves for tumour colony-forming cells should be a more valid test of the target-cell hypothesis than analyses for many normal tissues. This assertion is founded on the belief that tumours can recur from a single cell, whereas intact networks of cells may be necessary for rescue of some nonhierarchical normal tissues (see below). There are, however, difficulties with tumour data, for example the nonlinearity for transplantation 'takes' of some tumours in mice (Porter et al. 1973). An immunogenic, cytotoxic effect on the clonogens would be consistent with this nonlinearity. Changes in the slope of the dose−cure curve in hosts with different immune statuses have been reported by Suit (1984), and this would be expected if the toxic effect acted on a fixed *number* of target cells after all radiation doses, not a certain *proportion* of cells. Also, comparisons for tumours are more difficult because of the variations in tumour size, which will lessen the slope. This is in contrast to the homogeneity of multicellular structures in normal tissues, e.g. intestinal crypts and tubules in kidney and testis.

There is a scarcity of assays for tumour colony-forming cells *in situ*. Only two such assays have been described (Marsden et al. 1980; Kummermehr 1985), and neither has been used to test the target-cell hypothesis in terms of slopes of cell-survival curves versus slopes of dose−cure curves. Conventional assays *in vitro* for colony-forming cells are known to be subject to dose-dependent effects related to cell contact or repair of potentially lethal damage. A relatively 'clean' comparison of slopes for cells and tumours was described by Moore & Hendry (1984), using data for the sterilization *in vitro* of tumour spheroids and for cell survival measured *in vitro* from the disaggregated spheroids. In the two cell lines examined, one gave good agreement between slopes, and in the other the slope was higher for colony-forming cells than deduced for the repopulating cells by a factor of 1·4 to 1·5. A further analysis, using data for four other cell lines, showed quite good agreement between the two determinations of slope (Moore et al. 1987). There is thus evidence for and against the applicability of the target-cell hypothesis to the cure of tumours, as was originally discussed by Munro & Gilbert (1961), and later by Wheldon et al. (1977), Andrews (1978), and Withers & Peters (1980).

The study of experimental tumours in animals is beset by inherent problems of inhomogeneity and of suitability of assays as described above, and this is even more true for human tumours. Nonetheless, the analysis of dose−cure curves provides a lower limit to the slope of the relevant target-cell population, if there is heterogeneity in the group of tumours under consideration. Some of the dose−cure curves in the literature (collated by Moore et al. 1983 and Mijnheer et al. 1987) are indeed quite steep. One of the steepest and probably an exception to the general rule is that reported by Stewart & Jackson (1975) for the recurrence of T3 laryngeal carcinoma. The failure rate fell from 65% to 35% when the dose in 15 fractions was increased from 52·5 Gy to 57·5 Gy. This would be expected if the $D_0$ for the target cells was about 5 Gy at the mean dose per fraction of 3·7 Gy (Hendry & Moore 1985b). This value of $D_0$ is at the upper end of the range of values that can be calculated for many examples of single cells *in vitro* (Proceedings of 6th L.H. Gray Conference 1975). Hence, the data of Stewart & Jackson (1975) are compatible with the target-cell hypothesis, bearing in mind the probable heterogeneity among tumours.

Other reported dose−cure curves for human tumours generally have shallower slopes, e. g. those described by Thames et al. (1980) where the deduced $D_0$ was 10−50 Gy for various stages of head and neck cancer. The treatments were given with fraction sizes close to 2 Gy, and the $D_0$s

Table 2.1. Comparison of $D_0$ values deduced from dose−incidence and colony assays

| Tissue | $D_0$ from dose− incidence curve (Gy) | $D_0$ for colony- forming cells (Gy) | Reference |
|---|---|---|---|
| Intestine | 1·3 ± 0·2 | 1·2 ± 0·1 | Hendry et al. (1983b) |
| Epidermis | 2·8 ± 0·5 | 3·5 ± 0·5 | Hendry (1984b) |
| Marrow | 0·6 ± 0·1 (X, >50 cGy/min) 1·1 ± 0·4 (X, 1−3 cGy/min) 1·2 (γ, 1−3 cGy/min) | 0·7 ± 0·09 — 1·0 | Hendry and Moore (1985) |
| Tumour spheroids | (Na11) 1·3 ± 0·7 (V79−171 3·8 ± 0·5 at day 8) (V79−171 4·3 ± 0·3 at day 21) | 1·1 ± 0·1 2·6 ± 0·1 3·1 ± 0·1 | Moore and Hendry (1984) |
| | (VN) 0·99 ± 0·03 (VE) 1·00 ± 0·05 (MF) 0·84 ± 0·10 (GE) 0·81 ± 0·03 | 0·78 ± 0·12 0·90 ± 0·05 0·92 ± 0·02 1·13 ± 0·07 | Moore et al. (1987) |

X = X-rays
γ = γ-rays

Table 2.2. *K* values reported for different tissues

| Tissue | K(TRU) | TRU content | Reference |
|---|---|---|---|
| Planaria | 5·3 | $2·7 \times 10^4$ neoblasts | Lange & Gilbert (1968) |
| Mouse intestine | 1·5 (crypts) | $5 \times 10^5$ crypts | Hendry et al. (1983) |
|  | 45 (clonogens) | $1·5 \times 10^7$ clonogens |  |
| Mouse bone marrow | $10^4$ | 100 CFC-S | Hendry & Moore (1985) |
| Mouse tail epidermis | 450 cm$^{-2}$ | 9 clonogens | Hendry (1984b) |
| Tumour spheroids |  |  |  |
| Nall | 232 ± 235 | 1·6 cells[a] | Moore & Hendry (1984) |
| 8-day V79 | 98 ± 29 | 78 cells[a] |  |
| 21-day V79 | 350 ± 93 | 88 cells[a] |  |
| Mouse lung | $10^2$ | — | Hendry & Moore (1985) |
|  | $(4-27) \times 10^3$ | — | Thames et al. (1986b) |
|  | $10^3 - 10^5$ | $10-10^3$ Type II cells | Travis & Tucker (1986) |
| Mouse oesophagus | $10^2$ | — | Hendry & Moore (1985) |

[a]Morphologically viable cells.
From Hendry and Thames (1986)

thus reflect the 'slope of the chord' (see Figure 3.1). On the other hand, constant numbers of fractions were used in the series reported by Stewart & Jackson (1975), so that the $D_0$s reflect the 'slope of the tangent' (Figure 3.10). The latter are expected to be steeper than the former.

A comparison of $D_0$ values for target cells deduced from dose–incidence curves or measured by colony techniques is given in Table 2.1.

Reported values for the number and content of TRU in various tissues are shown in Table 2.2. This serves to emphasize the reasonableness of some of the values, e.g. for bone marrow, the interestingly low and variable number of repopulating cells in tumour spheroids, and the variability in the number of TRU calculated for lung. Further values for *K* are quoted in Table 3.2, calculated from fractionation data with early- and late-responding tissues.

## Other tissues

Dose–incidence curves for other tissues can be analysed to deduce sensitivity parameters for TRU, but in F-type tissues the underlying pathogenesis is largely unknown. Hence in these cases, although attempts can be made to equate the TRU with a number of independent subunits, e.g. nephrons and lung acini, the assumption of independent survival of target cells, each capable of regenerating a subunit, may not be true and cannot yet be tested experimentally. There are insufficient data on the dose–incidence curves for single doses to perform the same analyses as described above for marrow, intestine, and skin. Therefore the dose−incidence curves for various fractionation schedules including single doses were analysed together. A discussion of these data in terms of the number and sensitivity of TRU can be found in Section 3.3.

This section was concerned with single doses of radiation and whether the steepness of dose−incidence curves for tissue responses corresponded to those that could be deduced from appropriate colony assays. In general the finding was that the steepness of the incidence curve for tissue failure closely corresponded to the $D_0$ that could be deduced from colony assays for hierarchical tissues. In the following sections we consider the evidence for the target-cell hypothesis that can be gleaned from the response to altered fractionation or dose rate, based on data for both clonogen survival and tissue-isoeffect doses.

## 2.2. Altered fractionation and dose rate

The split-dose studies of Elkind & Sutton (1959), the first to point toward rapid recovery processes in mammalian cells, showed that the response to a second dose of radiation closely resembled the response to the first dose after a sufficient time had elapsed. In other words, memory of the previous dose was lost, and the dose in two fractions required for a specified level of cell killing was higher than the biologically equivalent single dose, if time for Elkind recovery was allowed between the two doses. According to the target-cell hypothesis a similar phenomenon should be observed with tissues exposed to single or split doses. With a view to making such a comparison, Withers & Elkind (1969) determined the LD50/5 for whole-abdomen exposures using single or split doses. Survival curves were determined using a macrocolony technique (Withers & Elkind 1968), and extrapolated back to the LD50/5 for a single dose (10·6 Gy). As shown in Figure 2.8, the calculated survival ratios for split doses given at 4-, 8-, and 24-hour intervals were equal at the LD50/5 doses (vertical arrows) for single doses and for split doses separated by these intervals.

Similar comparisons are possible with more than two fractions. Elkind & Sutton (1960) showed that the initial shoulder could be reconstructed after repeated doses in experiments in which five fractions of 5·05 Gy were separated by 22-hour intervals. As indicated in Figure 2.9, the response was exponential when measured along the chord, in agreement with an equal decrement in log survival with each dose. Clearly the slope of this exponential response depended on the size of dose per fraction: a steeper slope resulted from repeated 6·32 Gy doses.

Some results diverge from the simple picture of equal cell kill after each of repeated equal doses. McNally & de Ronde (1976) found that when tumour cells *in vitro* were exposed to more than five fractions, there was a progressive loss of repair capacity and a bending downward away from the expected exponential curve describing response to fractionated doses (Figure 2.10). Loss of repair capacity was also noted by Zeman & Bedford (1985).

On the other hand, it was shown with hepatocytes *in vivo* that an equal cell kill occurred for as many as 70 fractions, each of 1 Gy (Fisher & Hendry 1986). Similarly, the equal-effect-per-fraction hypothesis could not be rejected in studies of the response measured by *in vivo* colony assay of regenerative populations in the testis (Thames & Withers 1980), jejunum (Thames *et al.* 1981), and colon (Tucker *et al.* 1983).

Although no definite conclusions may be drawn from these conflicting

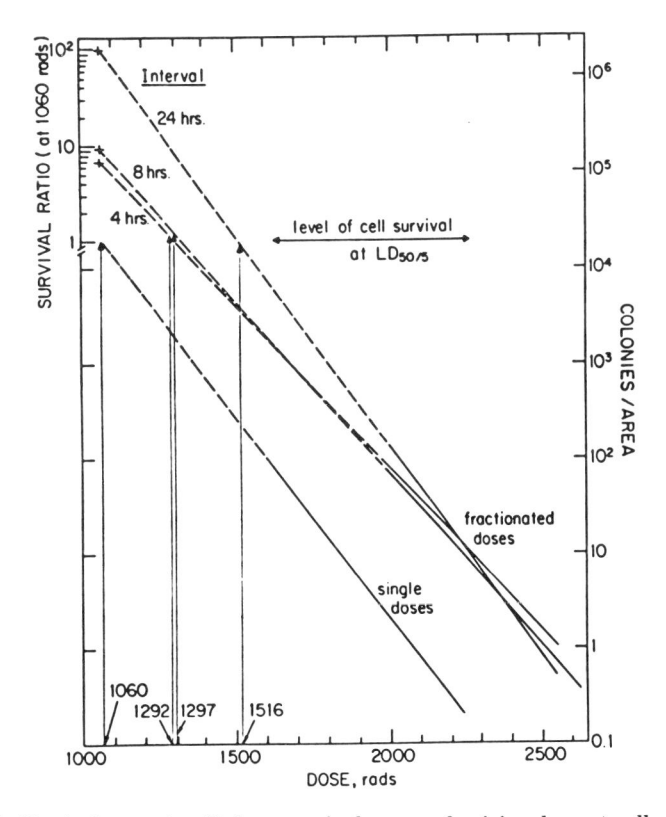

Figure 2.8. Single-dose and split-dose survival curves for jejunal crypt cells determined from macrocolony assay (from Withers & Elkind 1969). The curves have been extrapolated back to the 10·6 Gy ordinate. The mean survival ratios at 10·6 Gy are 6·7, 9·4, and 92 for the 4-, 8-, and 24-hour fractionation intervals. The LD50/5 values for single doses and for 4-, 8-, and 24-hour split doses are marked by vertical arrows. All arrows intersect their corresponding cell survival curves at a constant level of about 20 000 survivors per 2-cm length of jejunum. (Reproduced with permission of Academic Press Inc and the authors.)

40                  *Fractionation in Radiotherapy*

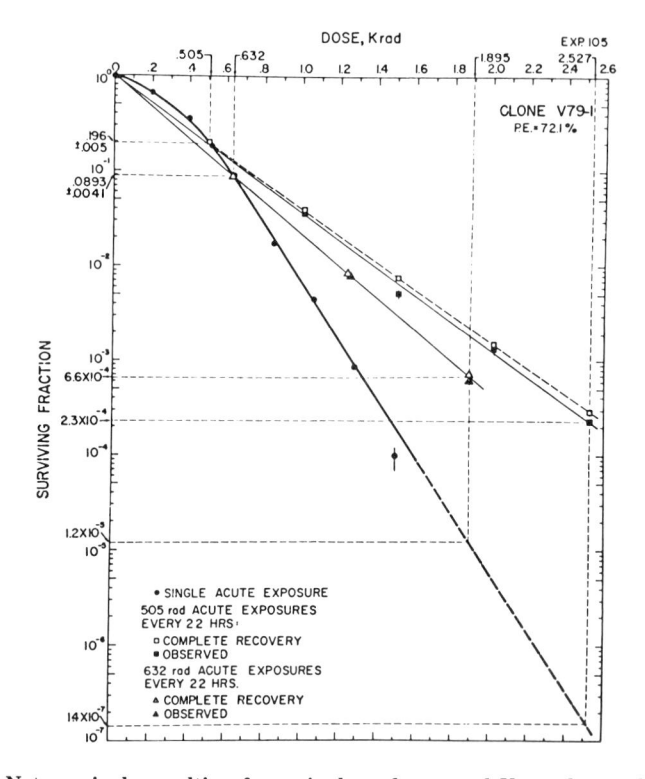

Figure 2.9. Net survivals resulting from single and repeated X-ray doses: closed circles, single exposure; closed squares, 5·05 Gy exposures separated by 22 hours; closed triangles, 6·32 Gy exposures separated by 22 hours (from Elkind & Sutton 1960). The open squares and triangles show the theoretical survivals expected from repeated 5·05 Gy and 6·32 Gy doses respectively (see text). Standard errors are omitted unless larger than the points plotted. This figure is presented as an illustration of the expected log-linear response to multiple equal fractions, it cannot be excluded that the results were influenced by proliferation of survivors. (Reproduced with permission of Academic Press Inc. and the authors.)

results (*in vitro* vs. *in vivo*), it is likely that the response of target-cell populations in tissues to fractionated doses is characterized by approximately equal proportions of cell killing after repeated, equal-dose fractions. In any event, one would predict an increasing dose for a given level of tissue reaction as the number of fractions increases, even when the multifraction response departs from the expected log-linear one. This expectation is borne out in most tissues that have been assayed under these conditions.

The target-cell hypothesis can be tested in the setting of tissue responses to altered fractionation or dose rate, by comparing not the slopes but rather the level of target-cell survival after isoeffective doses under different fractionation regimens or dose rates. The aim is to make

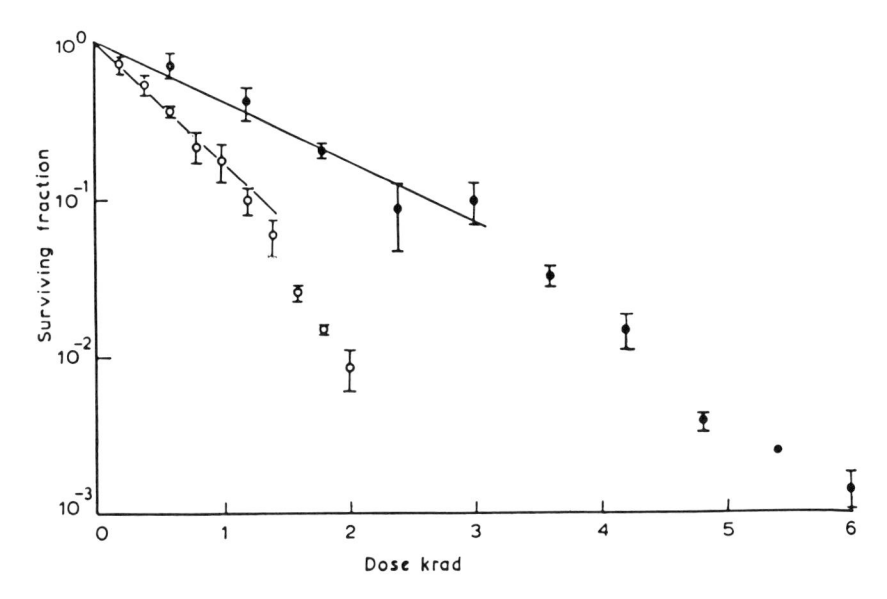

Figure 2.10. Fractionated-dose survival curves for 2 Gy per fraction, aerobic (open circles) and 6 Gy per fraction, hypoxic (closed circles), corrected for recovery from potentially lethal damage (from McNally & de Ronde 1976). The points and error bars are the means and standard deviations of the means of three experiments. (Reproduced with permission of Taylor & Francis, Ltd. and the authors.)

a comparison similar to that shown in Figure 2.8. There are four tissues where such comparisons can be made—testis, bone marrow, gut, and epidermis.

## Testis

Both colony survival and functional assays are available for the testis (Withers & Mason 1974; Lu et al. 1980). Fertility of the male mouse depends on a broad range of factors: quantity and quality of sperm produced and the ability to deliver the sperm to the ovum, which depends in turn on androgen-stimulated processes of sexual behaviour. Radiation-induced sterility can last for over 200 days in the mouse; stem-cell survival is an important determinant of its duration. Figure 2.11 shows the close correlation between duration of sterility and surviving spermatogenic stem cells, for single and fractionated doses of gamma rays, neutrons, and gamma rays with the radioprotector WR-2721. Without regard to fractionation or quality of radiation, sterility resulted when stem-cell survival was reduced to less than $0 \cdot 2$ stem cells per tubule cross-section (Meistrich 1986). This example is of particular historical significance, since it was the comparative responses

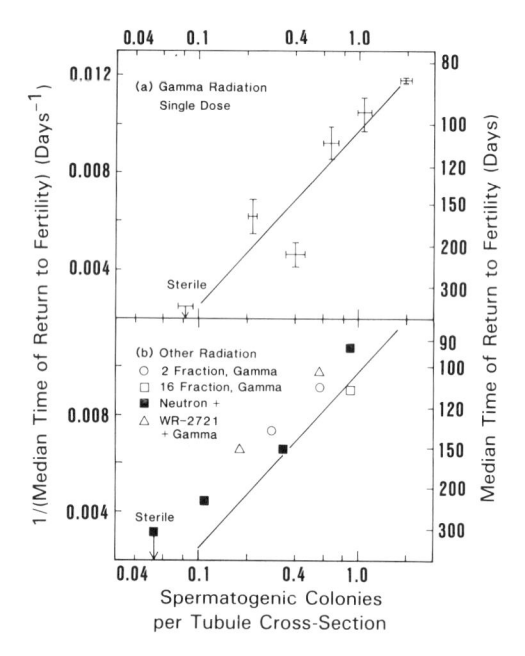

Figure 2.11. Relationship between time of recovery of fertility and testicular stem-cell survival (from Meistrich 1986). The time of recovery of fertility is plotted as the reciprocal of the median time after treatment at which fertility is regained (left ordinate); the corresponding actual numbers of days are also indicated (right ordinate). Each point represents one dose level of radiation. The points for more highly sterilizing treatments, in which half of the animals did not regain fertility, are plotted at the time the fertility testing was terminated. (a) Single-dose gamma-radiation (dose range to mice regaining fertility, 6–10 Gy): error bars represent between-experiment standard errors with one exception, in which the within-experiment standard error is used. The regression line has a correlation coefficient of 0·89. (b) Other radiation protocols: 2 fractions of gamma-radiation 24 h apart (dose range/fraction 4–5 Gy); 16 fractions of gamma-radiation, 4h apart (dose/fraction 0·64 Gy); neutron radiation from M.D. Anderson Hospital cyclotron (dose range, 3–5 Gy); gamma-radiation (dose range, 10·5–13·5 Gy) given 15 minutes after WR-2721 at 400 mg/kg. The regression line for single dose gamma-radiation is shown for comparison. (Reproduced with permission of Macmillan Press Ltd and the author.)

of the testicle as opposed to skin that led Regaud & Ferroux (1927) to postulate an advantage for fractionated irradiation over single doses in achieving tumour cure with moderate normal tissue reactions (see Chapter 5).

**Bone marrow**

Puro & Clark (1972) studied the response of mice to whole-body exposures of X-rays delivered at dose rates of 2·86 to 105 cGy/min and found that the LD50/30 increased with decreasing dose rate. Parallel studies were conducted of the effect of variation of exposure rate on

Table 2.3. Survival of Haematopoietic Stem Cells at the LD50/30

| Dose rate (Gy/min) | LD50/30 (Gy) | Number of endogenous spleen colonies at LD50/30 | Surviving fraction of transplanted bone marrow cells $(\times 10^4)$ at LD50/30 |
| --- | --- | --- | --- |
| 1·05 | 6·56 | 0·24 | 2·4 |
| 0·116 | 7·85 | 0·16 | 0·9 |
| 0·0537 | 8·20 | 0·34 | 1·1 |
| 0·02986 | 8·69 | 0·29 | 1·9 |

From Puro & Clark (1972)

haematopoietic stem-cell survival. Cells obtained from the femoral marrow of mice were transplanted into irradiated recipient mice and subsequently irradiated within the recipients. Lower exposure rates were clearly less efficient at killing colony-forming units (CFU-S) for doses above 2 Gy, but not for low doses. The lesser efficiency also was seen using the endogenous spleen-colony assay, after doses approaching LD50/30.

The predicted values of CFU-S survival at the LD50/30 doses, obtained by linear extrapolation of the transplantation-assay survival curves, were approximately the same for each dose rate (Table 2.3). Moreover, the results of the endogenous spleen-colony experiments indicated that CFU-S survival was exponential in the region of the LD50/30 doses, and the number of spleen colonies at the LD50/30 could be obtained by extrapolation. As shown in Table 2.3, no systematic differences in CFU-S survival at the LD50/30 doses were evident. The level of CFU-S survival of about $10^{-4}$ at LD50/30 was of the same order as deduced by others (Robinson 1968; Hendry & Moore 1985). Hence the changes in LD50/30 with changing dose rate occurred in a manner predicted from the changing response of the target cells, the CFU-S.

As indicated in Section 2.1, the survival curve probably bends down at high doses in the LD50/30 range but is virtually exponential at doses much lower than this. Hence dose-rate effects will not be clearly apparent over the dose range commonly used to measure CFU-S survival curves—up to only about 5 Gy using the transplantation technique. This is the consensus in the literature (reviewed by Hendry & Lord 1983). Also, this was the finding invoked by Krebs & Jones (1972) to postulate a lack of correlation between CFU-S survival and LD50/30. Higher doses are needed to demonstrate clear dose-rate effects, as observed by Puro & Clark (1972) using the endogenous spleen colony technique.

## Gut

Krebs & Leong (1970) studied in detail the influence of the dose rate of

$^{60}$Co gamma-rays and 250 kVp X-rays on the LD50 in mice that died from gastrointestinal injury. They did not conduct parallel studies of crypt-cell survival (the assay was probably unknown at the time), so there was no direct comparison of cell survival at different LD50 doses. Subsequently, however, the influence of dose rate of $^{60}$Co gamma-rays on crypt-cell survival has been studied by various authors. The changes in dose versus dose rate are summarized in Figure 2.12, where the isoeffect was either LD50/7 or the level of crypt survival at about LD50/7 using high dose rates (about 50 crypts per circumference). It is clear that similar changes in dose are seen for both endpoints over two orders of magnitude change in dose rate.

A similar comparison of endpoints can be made for the response to split doses. There was a close correspondence between target-cell killing and animal lethality from the GI syndrome (Figure 2.8) in the experiments of Withers & Elkind (1969). This showed a correspondence in the effect of Elkind repair. The comparison can be extended, however, to situations in which regeneration of survivors influenced the results.

A summary of data in the literature is shown in Figure 2.13. The ratio of total doses given either as a single dose ($D_1$) or as two doses ($D_2$) separated by various intervals of time is similar when $D_1$ is of the same order for both endpoints. This is the case for intervals ranging from a

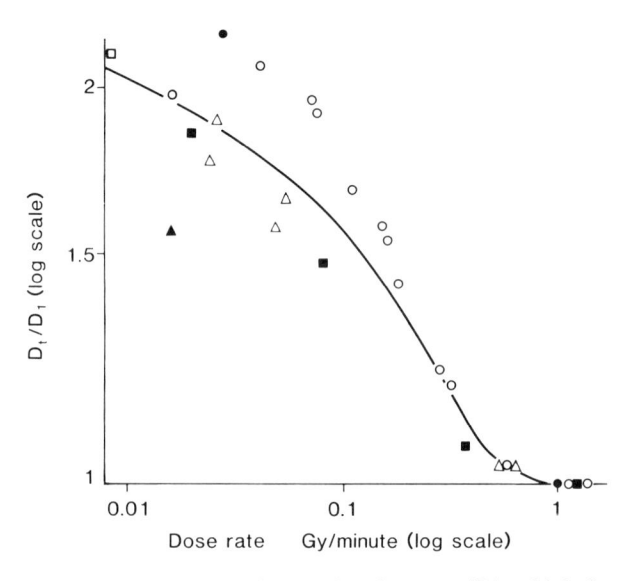

Figure 2.12. Ratios of isoeffect doses given at low dose rate ($D_t$) or high dose rate ($D_1$), for LD50/5-7 (open symbols) or crypt survival at about 50 surviving crypts per circumference (closed symbols). Data from: Krebs & Leong (1970) (open circles); Wambersie et al. (1978) (open triangles); Withers (1972) (closed circles); Lord et al. (1984) (closed triangle); Huczkowski & Trott (1984) (closed squares).

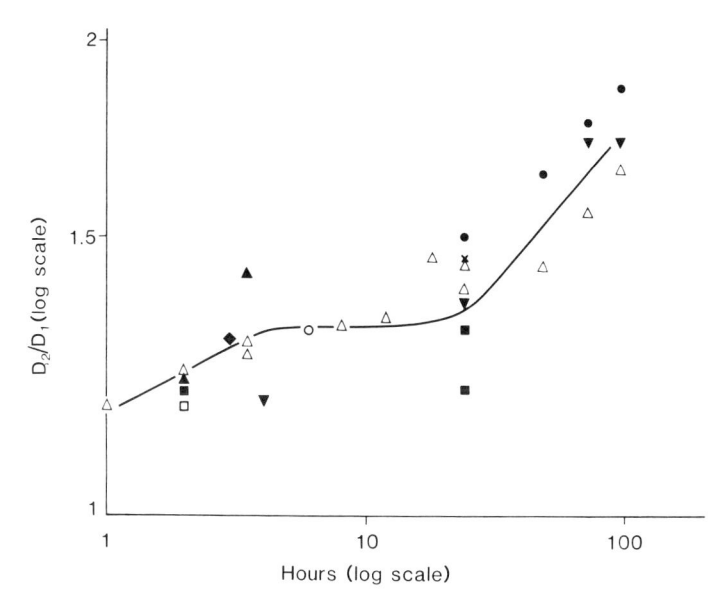

Figure 2.13. Ratios of isoeffect doses given as two doses ($D_2$) separated by various times or as a single dose ($D_1$), for LD50/5−7 (open symbols) or crypt survival at about 50 surviving crypts per circumference (closed symbols). Data from: Hornsey and Vatistas (1963) (open circle); Hornsey (1973a) (open and closed squares); Wambersie et al. (1974) (open triangles); Potten & Hendry (1975) (closed circles); Hornsey et al. (1977) (closed triangles); Potten (1978) (closed inverted triangles); Withers et al. (1975) (closed diamond); Hendry et al. (1975) (cross).

Table 2.4. Dose-modifying factor for 11 different radioprotective chemicals, calculated as the ratio of doses of X-rays with/without each chemical

| Chemical | DMF (X-rays) LD50/6 | 50% crypt survival |
|---|---|---|
| WR−2721 | 1·64 | 1·79 |
| WR−638 | 1·57 | 1·53 |
| WR−77913 | 1·42 | 1·52 |
| WR−2347 | 1·42 | 1·50 |
| AET | 1·42 | 1·50 |
| WR−2823 | 1·32 | 1·23 |
| MEA | 1·26 | 1·43 |
| WR−2822 | 1·23 | 1·44 |
| WR−1607 | 1·18 | 1·16 |
| WR−109342 | 1·17 | 1·06 |
| WR−3689 | 1·12 | 1·32 |
| − | 1·00 | 1·00 |

From Sigdestad (1975)

few hours, when intracellular repair is the dominant effect, to a few days, when cell repopulation becomes important.

Another example of the correspondence between dosage changes measured using LD50/6 and crypt survival may be found in the studies by Sigdestad (1975) concerning the degree of radioprotection achieved using 11 different chemical agents. The dose-modifying factors, listed in Table 2.4 in order of decreasing effectiveness for LD50/6 with X-rays, show close similarities to the values measured using crypt-cell survival with X-rays. With neutrons the ordering was slightly different, and the correspondence was not as clear, partly because of the lower protection achieved with neutrons.

**Epidermis**

Epidermis is another tissue in which measurements of the change in effect or in isoeffective dose with split dose have been made for both clonogens (Withers 1967a; Emery et al. 1970) and tissue reactions (Denekamp et al. 1969). However, there are difficulties in the comparison of dosage changes for the two endpoints, because the measurements for clonogens were made using lower doses (typically $D_1 \simeq 15\,\text{Gy}$, giving 1 colony/mm$^2$) than those used to produce an average skin reaction of 1·5 ($D_1 \simeq 30\,\text{Gy}$, equivalent to $10^{-4}$–$10^{-5}$ colonies/mm$^2$ based on $D_0 = 1\cdot 5\,\text{Gy}$. Because of this, and keeping in mind the general dose dependence of dose-rate or split-dose effects, the split-dose effects would be expected to be less for clonogens than for skin reactions, for example as noted above for the bone marrow, unless the survival curve is exponential over the range of doses used for both endpoints. There is good evidence that this is the case for the epidermis (Withers 1967a; Chen & Hendry 1986), and this supports a comparison in terms of $(D_2 - D_1)$ for the two endpoints at different values of $D_1$. The values of $(D_2 - D_1)$ were 5·25 Gy (1-day interval) and 5·80 Gy (21 days) for skin reactions (Denekamp et al. 1969), and 5·70 Gy (1 day) and 5·80 Gy (21 days) for colony counts (Emery et al. 1970). However, other evidence, including skin reactions in pigs and other species, suggests that $(D_2 - D_1)$ does increase with increasing $D_1$ (Redpath et al. 1984). Nonetheless, it can be concluded, at least for the mouse data where colony techniques have also been applied, that the correspondence between the response of clonogens and the whole tissue using split doses holds reasonably well for the epidermis, as it does for the testis, the bone marrow, and the gut.

## 2.3. Slopes of isoeffect graphs

In the previous section, agreement has been demonstrated between the predictions of target-cell theory and the responses of normal tissues to changing dose rate and fractionation. Additional insight may be gained by an examination of the shapes of the isoeffect graphs (e.g. ED50 versus dose per fraction or dose rate), and in particular their slopes. When proliferation is negligible the slopes of the graphs can be calculated theoretically using the isosurvival-equals-isoeffect assumption and models of the response of cell populations to changes in pattern of dose delivery. Limits are derived on the expected range of values of the slopes and compared with those determined from experimental data.

It will be noted that resort is made to predictions of mathematical models based on the target-cell concept. The justification for this approach is that if the target-cell hypothesis is correct, then survival-model predictions should correlate with observations based on tissue response, particularly if the predictions are independent of values of the parameters. This is the case for the analysis of the number-of-fractions exponent, but not the analysis of the exposure-time coefficient. Again, necessary but not sufficient evidence for the hypothesis is presented.

## Number-of-fractions exponent

Under the assumption that target-cell response is governed by the linear-quadratic model, the number-of-fractions ($n$) exponent is given by (Thames et al. 1982)

$$\mathrm{d}\ln D/\mathrm{d}\ln n = x/(\alpha/\beta + 2x) \tag{2.5}$$

where $x$ is the size of dose per fraction (see Section 3.3 and equation (7.20)). Two predictions of a general nature may be derived from this result. First, the number-of-fractions exponent decreases toward zero as the dose per fraction decreases to zero, whatever the value of $\alpha/\beta$. This is in clear distinction to the Ellis (1967) NSD model, in which the number-of-fractions exponent has the constant value 0.24 and consequently an indefinite increase in isoeffect dose with increasing fraction number is predicted.

The evidence for such a decrease in the number-of-fractions exponent is presented for various tissues in Figure 2.14 and Table 2.5. It is always highest for one to a few fractions, and decreases as the number of fractions increases. That it actually does approach zero is conclusively demonstrated by the studies of Dutreix et al. (1973) and Withers (1975b) on the 'flexure dose'. This is discussed at length in Section 3.5, but for present purposes let it be noted that there seems to be a limit to measurable increases in isoeffect dose when dose per fraction is reduced.

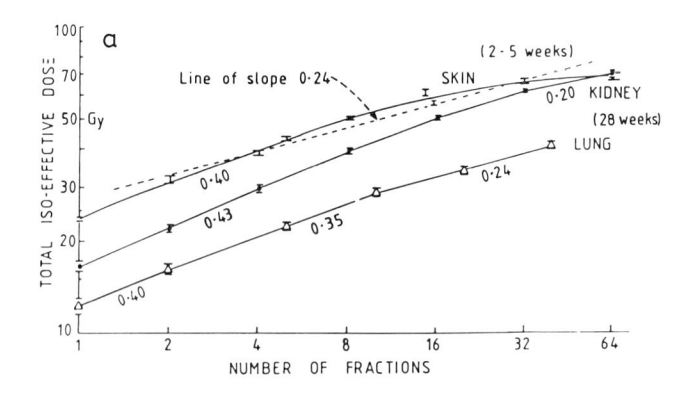

Figure 2.14. Increase of total isoeffect dose with increase in number of fractions for the kidney (Stewart et al. 1984a), for mouse skin desquamation (Douglas & Fowler 1976), and for mouse lung breathing-rate increase (Parkins et al. 1985). The error bars are ±1 SEM. The steeper dependence for kidney and lung than for skin, especially at small doses per fraction, is illustrated. The dotted line corresponds to the NSD formula (From Fowler 1984a with permission of Taylor & Francis Ltd and the author.)

The recovered dose in isoeffective regimens for skin (Dutreix et al. 1973) and gut (Wambersie et al. 1974) was determined when either a single daily dose was given or when this was split into two equal fractions separated by varying time intervals. It was found in both studies that the dependence of total dose on fraction number disappeared as the daily dose to be split decreased below 2 Gy. The same conclusion was reached by Withers (1975b) using colony survival in the gut as the endpoint. Divergence of the single-dose and multifraction responses occurred for fraction sizes larger than about 2 Gy (see Figure 3.19).

The second inference of a general nature that may be drawn from the theoretical equation for the number-of-fractions exponent (equation 2.5) concerns the limit on its value for large dose fractions, namely the prediction that the number-of-fractions exponent observed experimentally will never exceed 0·5 when proliferation is not a factor. This may be appreciated by noting that the number-of-fractions exponent increases with increasing dose per fraction ($x$), until twice the size of the dose per fraction greatly exceeds the $\alpha/\beta$ ratio characteristic of the tissue (cf. Section 3.3). At that time, the exponent approaches the limiting value 0·5. This theoretical upper limit is more likely to be approached for tissues characterized by a small $\alpha/\beta$ ratio, i.e. for late-responding tissues.

The experimental evidence is consistent with these predictions. Generally the exponents range between 0·4 and 0·5 for late reactions and between 0·2 and 0·3 for early responses (Table 2.5). The exceptions to this rule occur in studies in which experiments were designed so that

Table 2.5. Number-of-fractions exponents

| Tissue | Reference | Conditions | Exponent |
|---|---|---|---|
| *Early reacting* | | | |
| Jejunum | Withers et al. (1975) | 1–10 fractions | 0·32 |
| | | 10–20 fractions | 0·30 |
| | Withers (1975b) | 1-h intervals: 1–10 fractions | 0·27 |
| | | 10–20 fractions | 0·08 |
| Skin | Fowler et al. (1974) | 3 fractions/wk ⎫ 2 to 18 days | 0·31 |
| | | 5 fractions/wk ⎭ | 0·35 |
| Lip mucosa | Xu et al. (1984) | 1–4 fractions: 200 cGy/min | 0·5 |
| | | 33 cGy/min | 0·29 |
| Spleen colonies | Withers (1975c) | 1–4 fractions | 0·24 |
| | | 6–12 fractions | 0·08 |
| Colon | Withers & Mason (1974) | 1–10 fractions | 0·32 |
| | | 10–22 fractions | 0·22 |
| Testis | Thames & Withers (1980) | 1–4 fractions | 0·29 |
| | | 10–22 fractions | 0·07 |
| *Late reacting* | | | |
| Cervical cord | van der Kogel (1979) | white-matter necrosis | 0·46 |
| | | vascular damage | 0·42 |
| Kidney | Stewart et al. (1984a) | 1–16 fractions | 0·43 |
| | | 16–64 fractions | 0·24 |
| Lung | Wara et al. (1973) | mice (350 kV X-rays) | 0·38 |
| | | humans ($^{60}$Co, 1 or 4 MV X-rays) | 0·41 |
| | Field et al. (1976) | 1 to 8 fractions | 0·39 |
| | | 8 to 30 fractions | 0·25 |
| | Travis et al. (1987) | 1–4 fractions | 0·36 |
| | | 6–10 fractions | 0·33 |
| Bladder | Stewart et al. (1984b) | 1–2 fractions | 0·50 |
| | | 10–20 fractions | 0·24 |

proliferation *was* a factor. These include measurements of the response of the colonic mucosa (Withers & Mason 1974) using an *in situ* colony assay and studies of the intestinal syndrome (Hagemann & Concannon 1975). The latter workers exposed mice whole-body to a variety of fractionated dose regimens, some of which lasted as long as six weeks. The number-of-fractions exponent, which was undoubtedly influenced by repopulation of survivors, was estimated to be 0·54.

## Exposure-time exponent

The change in isoeffect dose with exposure time may be described by the exposure-time coefficient, that is by the power-law representation, which states that log dose is proportional to log exposure time. For very short and very long exposure times, this coefficient is zero (if proliferation is negligible during irradiation), and therefore is 'constant' and nonzero only over a restricted range of times. This results from the limited range of the dose-rate effect, i. e. most of the change in killing efficiency per unit dose occurs between dose rates of 1 and 100 cGy/min, and it is in this range that such a coefficient is considered to apply. These limits will be variable according to tissue and endpoint, but in general there is a negligible change in killing efficiency per unit dose for changes in dose rate above 1000 cGy/min or below 0·1 cGy/min. Between these limits, clinical observations have led to the approximate value 0·29 for the exposure-time coefficient (Paterson 1963; Ellis 1968a,b; Kirk et al. 1972).

In making these statements we rely on the idealized concept of invariant radiosensitivity during exposure time, an assumption that may be occasionally invalid, e. g. because of localized hypoxia after dose rates as high as 6000 cGy/min (Hornsey & Alper 1966) or accumulation of cells

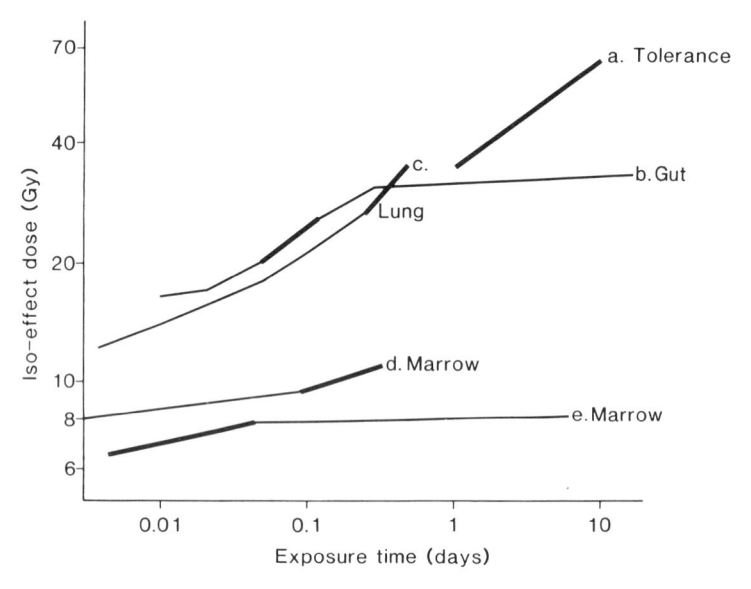

Figure 2.15. Isoeffect doses versus exposure time for continuous irradiation of various tissues in mice and in man. The curves connect data points reported in the literature, and the heavy markings delineate the steepest segments of the curves. The slopes ($m$) of these segments and the authors are as follows:
(a) $m = 0·29$†; Paterson (1963); Ellis (1968). (b) $m = 0·28$; Krebs & Leong (1970). (c) $m = 0·37$; Down et al. (1986). (d) $m = 0·11$; Neal (1960). (e) $m = 0·08$; Puro & Clark (1972).
† The analysis of these data by Orton and Webber (1977) gives $m = 0·26$. Also, the exponent is virtually identical to the value of 0·25 deduced for skin necrosis in 50% of mouse tails, using dose rates between 1 and 3·7 Gy/h and 'daily' exposures with overall times between 5 and 10 days (Wilkinson et al. 1980).

in the radiosensitive $G_2$ and M phases of the cell cycle during protracted low-dose-rate exposures (Kal et al. 1975; Mitchell et al. 1979). If the possibility of such 'reverse dose-rate effects' is ignored, the exposure-time coefficient is given theoretically by equation (7.23). The derivation of the maximum value of this slope is mathematically intractable; it is simpler to derive maximum values numerically from equation (7.23), using values of $\alpha/\beta$ and $T_{1/2}$ typical of the tissues for which studies of the dose-rate effect have been made.

The available experimental data and the Paterson–Ellis clinical rule for 'normal connective-tissue tolerance' are pictured in Figure 2.15. Straight lines have been drawn between the experimental points for clarity, although there is no evidence that they correctly predict isoeffect doses at intermediate times. The maximum slope and the approximate exposure time at which it occurred were estimated from the steepest segment of these lines and compared to that predicted theoretically by equation (7.23). The results are set out in Table 2.6, where the theoretical predictions were calculated from parameter values derived from *fractionation* experiments.

The observed slopes are all less than the predicted maxima, but are close to these values. *The exposure-time coefficient is smaller for the acutely responding tissues* (bone marrow, gut) than for lung. This is in line with the large number-of-fractions exponents (and smaller $\alpha/\beta$ ratios) for late-responding tissue. The predicted maximum slopes are in good agreement with those observed, and furthermore there is rough agreement between predicted and observed values for the exposure time at which maximum steepness will be observed. The isoeffect graph is

Table 2.6. Maximum exposure-time exponents and corresponding exposure time: prediction of target-cell model vs. observed

| Tissue | Predicted Maximum exponent | Time (h) | Observed Maximum exponent | Time (h) | Reference |
| --- | --- | --- | --- | --- | --- |
| Bone marrow | 0·15 | 2·2 | 0·11 0·08 | 2·2–7·2 0·1–1·2 | Neal (1960) Puro & Clark (1972) |
| Gut | 0·28 | 5·5 | 0·28 | 1·2–2·9 | Krebs & Leong (1970) |
| Lung | 0·38 | 12·0 | 0·37 | 9·6–12·0 | Down et al. (1986) |

Assumed parameters:
Bone marrow $(\alpha/\beta = 8\cdot 3\,\text{Gy},\ 100\,\beta/E = 0\cdot 10\,\text{Gy}^{-2};\ \mu = 2\cdot 0\,\text{h}^{-1}$: Thames et al. 1984)
Gut $(\alpha/\beta = 8\cdot 8\,\text{Gy},\ 100\,\beta/E = 0\cdot 15\,\text{Gy}^{-2};\ \mu = 1\cdot 4\,\text{h}^{-1}$: Thames et al. 1984)
Lung $(\alpha/\beta = 3\cdot 2\,\text{Gy},\ 100\,\beta/E = 0\cdot 52\,\text{Gy}^{-2};\ \mu = 0\cdot 8\,\text{h}^{-1}$: Travis et al. 1987)

steepest for lung for exposure times of about 12 hours, whereas maximum dose-rate effects are observed using shorter exposure times for bone marrow and gut.

It is noteworthy that accurate quantitation of tissue response to changing *dose rate* is possible using parameters of the response to changing *fractionation*. These parameters result from simple analyses of target-cell response to alterations in the pattern of dose delivery, coupled with the isoeffect-equals-isosurvival assumption.

In summary, it may be stated that the results of studies of tissue response to fractionated doses are consistent with the predictions of the target-cell model. In particular, the number-of-fractions exponent goes to zero for large numbers of fractions and never reaches the predicted maximum of 0·5 for small numbers of fractions, when proliferation is not a factor. These predictions are independent of any assumptions about parameter values. With responses to low-dose-rate continuous exposures the situation is not as clear-cut, since there are fewer experimental data and the theoretical predictions depend on assumed values of the survival-model parameters. Nevertheless, there were no inconsistencies between the data and the predicted maximum exposure-time exponents derived from target-cell theory. Last, and not least, the target-cell model yields an internally consistent description of fractionation and dose-rate effects with tissues.

The various recovery phenomena that influence tissue responses to fractionated radiation are considered next, always with the target-cell model as working hypothesis.

# Chapter 3
# Response of tissues to fractionated irradiation: effect of repair

The first two chapters present the case for a target-cell concept of tissue injury. This may be summarized roughly as follows. First, cell renewal occurs in a controlled fashion in normal tissues and in a less-controlled fashion in tumours. Renewing populations mature and assume a functional role, which persists until senescence and death after a lifetime that is widely variable among tissues. This state of affairs may be perturbed by cytotoxic injury inflicted by agents that affect either the renewing populations, the functional cells, or both. Radiation is different from other toxic agents in that damage resulting from it may remain latent for days, months, or years. This is so because, with the exceptions of some transient changes that have no known basis in cell killing (e.g. nausea, edema, somnolence) and cells that die during interphase, the killing effect of radiation is expressed only at cell division. Changes at the tissue level may be detected only after depletion of the renewing populations is manifest through a deficit in functional cells, which occurs at least one functional-cell lifetime after this depletion.

The target-cell populations for radiation injury are the precursors of renewing cell populations in a tissue. These have been identified in some tissues (e.g. intestine), but not in others (e.g. lung). Target cells may be studied in terms of clonogenicity and their response to single radiation doses of varying dose rate or LET, under varying oxygenation conditions, different fractionation regimens, etc. The parameters of response can be compared to those derived from the tissues in which they constitute the renewing populations. In a number of cases these parameters show close agreement. In other tissues, when colony survival assays do not exist or when target populations have not been identified, it is possible to demonstrate qualitative agreement between changes in tissue isoeffect doses and the predictions from theory based on the target-cell hypothesis.

This sets the stage for the present chapter, in which the response cf tissues to fractionated radiation is discussed in terms of *cellular* repair processes. Proliferation of survivors is assumed to play a negligible role.

## 3.1. Damage and repair after low-LET radiation

The nature of radiation-induced lesions that reduce the clonogenicity of a cell population is not fully understood, and so lesions have been given operational definitions. These may be derived from the shape of the dose−survival curve or may instead reflect the category of repair processes that modify them. Historically, three types of damage have been recognized: (1) sublethal damage (SLD), (2) potentially lethal damage (PLD), and (3) irreparable or lethal damage (LD). However, proponents of repair models postulate that there is a certain mix of repairable (RD) and irreparable lesions (LD), with relative proportions of these changing with the quality or linear energy transfer (LET) characteristic of the radiation (Section 6.2).

**Sublethal damage and repair**

After a dose of radiation it is supposed that a cell (1) may be completely devoid of ionization lesions and remain undamaged, (2) may suffer an ionizing event within a critical target, resulting in irreparable damage, or (3) may accumulate ionizing events in some, but not all, of its targets (SLD). According to this model SLD can interact with other SLD to produce LD; alternatively, it can be repaired over one to two hours, and a cell can thereby retain its clonogenicity.

This 'multitarget' model of SLD has been complemented by a single-hit exponential component to account for nonzero initial slopes of survival curves. Thus killing at low doses is considered to be primarily of the single-hit type, attributable to a high-LET component of the beam, whereas the killing at higher doses is considered to have an additional component from damage accumulation (Section 6.4).

The time course and extent of the repair of SLD (SLDR) are studied by delivering a test dose at various intervals after an initial dose and measuring the surviving fraction (split-dose recovery). There is an initial sharp increase in survival, which reaches a plateau after a few hours when progression in the cell cycle is negligible. This increase in survival is said to be due to SLDR. When progression in the cell cycle occurs during SLDR, survival does not reach a plateau, but rather a peak that then falls to a valley, which is thought to result from a shift to a more radiosensitive distribution of cells in the division cycle.

When split-dose survival was measured after an interval long enough for SLDR to be practically complete, but under conditions that precluded progression in the cell cycle, it was found that the response to the second dose was the same as that to the first dose (Elkind & Sutton 1959). One would therefore predict that, in the absence of progression in the division cycle and when SLDR is complete, repeated equal doses would each reduce survival by the same proportional amount, and that log survival would be a linear function of total dose. This was the case for up to five fractions *in vitro* (cf. Figure 2.6), while more than this number resulted in a progressive downward bending of the curve (cf. Figure 2.7) that was attributed to saturation of repair (McNally & de Ronde 1976; Zeman & Bedford 1985). However, this bending did not occur when, for example, hepatocytes were irradiated *in vivo* (Fisher & Hendry 1986), as discussed in Section 2.2.

An idealized fractionation experiment is shown in Figure 3.1. The slope of the response to repeated equal fractions depends on the size of the

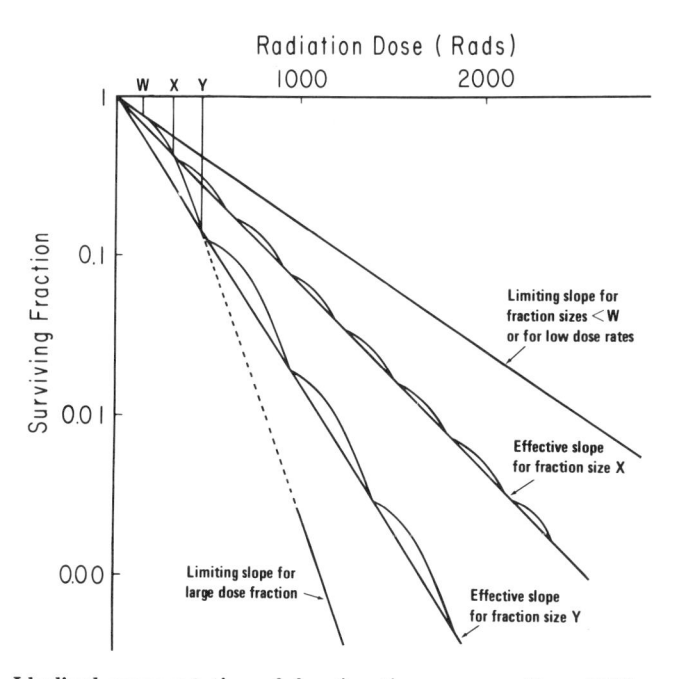

Figure 3.1. Idealized representation of fractionation response (from Withers & Peters 1980). When a radiation dose is equally fractionated and complete repair of sublethal injury occurs between fractions, the net fractionated-dose survival curve becomes a simple exponential function of dose, unless the cell-killing effectiveness of equal dose increments changes during treatment. In the ideal case, the slope of the multifraction curve can be described in terms of an 'effective' $D_0$ for a particular fraction size, and this changes with fraction size such that the response is steeper, the bigger the dose per fraction. The $D_0$ (eff) can never exceed $_1D_0$ (for single-hit killing), nor can it be less than the terminal $D_0$ of the single-dose survival curve. (Reproduced with permission of Lea & Febiger and the authors.)

individual doses and is progressively shallower as these become smaller. If the inter-fraction interval is constant, the effect of reducing fraction size is to reduce the rate of dose delivery, a reduction that results in progressive loss of biological effect per unit dose with decreasing fraction size.

The dose-rate effect consists of a reduction in the biological effect of a given dose as the time over which it is delivered is increased. Obviously, for very long exposure times a dose-rate effect could result from repopulation of survivors. However, it also occurs when conditions are such that repopulation is not possible, as in the experiments with plateau-phase cells shown in Figure 3.2, where repair of some sort must be invoked as a factor. In fact, the qualitative effect on the cell-survival curve of reducing the dose rate is the same as that of reducing the dose

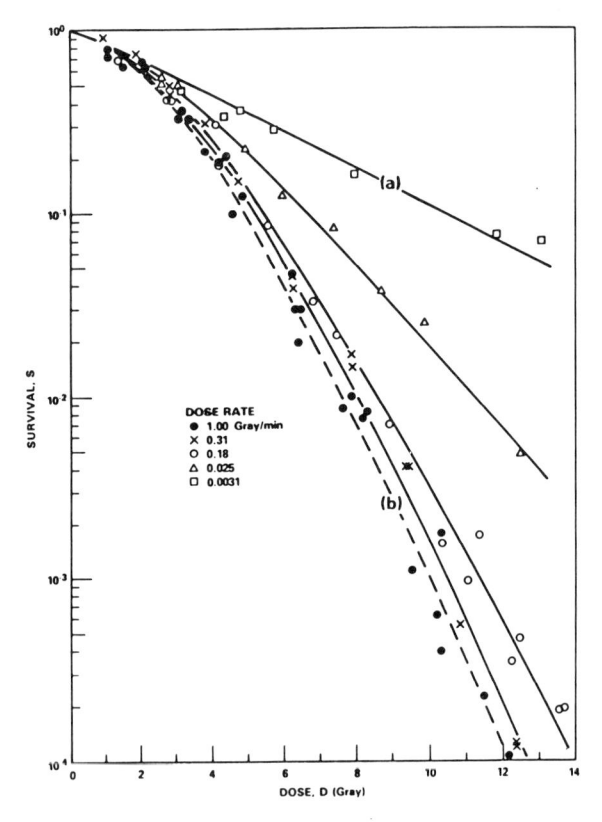

Figure 3.2. Survival curves for plateau-phase CHO cells irradiated with different doses of 250-kVp X-rays given at five different dose rates show substantial reduction in effect with protracted exposure (from Metting et al. 1985). Survival after a 48 hour exposure (a) is 52 times greater than that after the same dose, 9 Gy, delivered in 9 minutes (b). (Reproduced with permission of Academic Press Inc. and the authors.)

per fraction, i.e. a reduction in effect per unit dose. This suggests that when proliferation can be neglected the dose-rate effect is a manifestation of SLDR.

The results in tissues are consistent with this conceptual picture of the relative changes of isoeffective doses with changing fraction size and dose rate. Pertinent comparisons have been set out in Sections 2.2 and 2.3.

## Potentially lethal damage and repair

Potentially lethal damage and its repair (PLDR) were first recognized through a modification of response manifest after varying postirradiation culture conditions (Phillips & Tolmach 1966). It was termed 'potentially lethal' since under ordinary circumstances it resulted in cell death (here ordinary refers to culture conditions that stimulated growth, conditions that might well be considered extraordinary *in vivo*). Generally speaking, PLDR acts to enhance cell survival when postirradiation conditions are suboptimal for growth, achieved, for example, by replacing growth medium with physiologically balanced salt solution or by maintaining the cells in plateau phase by nutrient deprivation or high-density culture.

With increasing postirradiation delay until restitution of optimal growth conditions, survival is progressively enhanced (Figure 3.3). For cells in culture the effect of PLDR is generally dose-modifying, i.e. the ratio of doses required to achieve the same level of killing in the presence and absence of PLDR is independent of dose.

The nature of PLD is as elusive as that of SLD, and so also with the mechanisms of PLDR and SLDR, with current views divided between identical or different lesions and repair mechanisms. On the assumption that entry into the division cycle occurs sooner, the shorter the delay in plating, it may be hypothesized that the effect of PLDR is greater for cells not in cycle because there is more time for repair before some lesions are fixed (e.g. at $G_1/S$ and $G_2/M$ boundaries) or because repair varies in its efficiency with phase of the cell cycle. These ideas are considered in more detail in the next section.

Cells in tissues demonstrate PLDR (reviewed by Hendry 1985c), as shown in Figure 3.4. Measurements have been made with fibroblasts and epithelial cells in kidney and in lung and with marrow fibroblasts, all using *in vitro* assays. Also, transplantation assays (Section 6.3) have been used with mammary, thyroid, and liver parenchymal cells. By contrast, the effect with these tissues is generally *not* dose-modifying, but results in a constant additional dose of about 2 Gy required for equal effect when the assay is delayed, for example, 6 hours after single doses higher than 4 Gy.

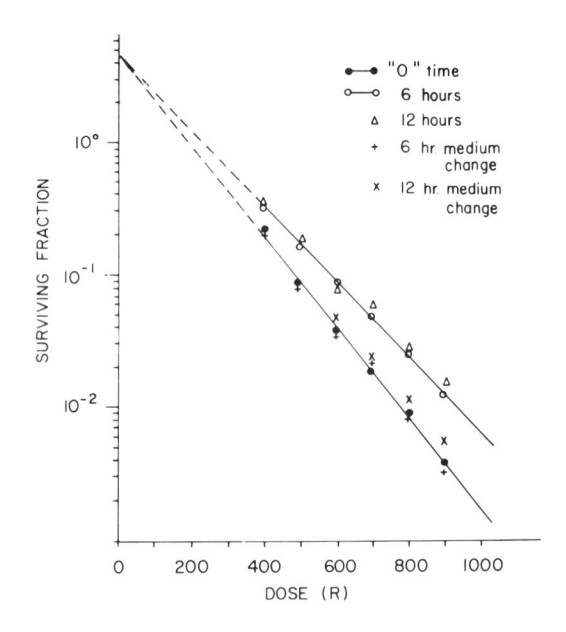

Figure 3.3. Survival curves for stationary-phase Chang liver cells (Little 1971). The lower survival curve was obtained if the cells were plated into fresh medium immediately (closed circles), or if fresh medium was supplied for six hours (+) or 12 hours (X) before plating, whereas the upper curve traces the survival of cells maintained without new medium for 6 hours (open circles) or 12 hours (triangles) after irradiation. The increase in survival, and the consequent decrease in slope of the survival curve for the 'unfed', slowly proliferating cells results from repair of potentially lethal damage. (Reproduced with permission of Taylor & Francis Ltd and the author).

An unusual example is bone marrow, where the opposite effect is seen, namely a reduction in dose by about 1 Gy for equal effect when the assay is delayed after doses greater than 1 Gy. This could result from induced differentiation of the colony-forming cells or a natural rate of differentiation during a period of mitotic delay.

No comparison has been made of PLDR half-times for cells in different types of tissue, in contrast to SLDR where the half-time appears slower in late-responding tissues. When tissues respond naturally *in vivo*, any PLDR will be part of the overall response and hence will not be observed as a separate component. However, PLDR in tissues can be observed when cells are extracted from the tissue and tested for PLDR at different times after irradiation. Late-responding tissues in particular will have ample time for this type of repair, and it has been observed many weeks and months later, not just in the first few hours. Chromosomal injury in the liver and in the thyroid has been observed to decline weeks after irradiation (Curtis 1967; Tates *et al.* 1980; Scott *et al.* 1984). The decline was very much smaller after neutrons, indicating a lesser capability of

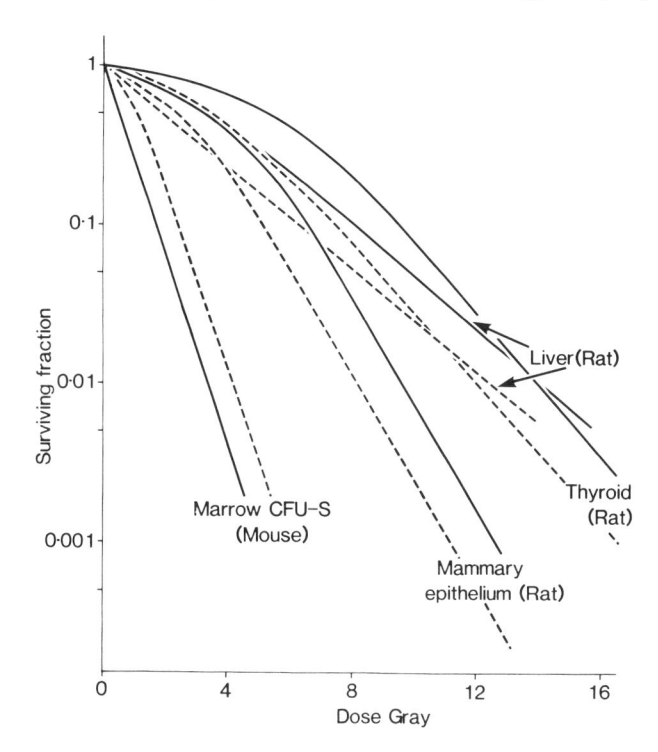

Response of tissues to fractionated irradiation: effect of repair 59

Figure 3.4. Survival curves assessed *in vivo* by transplantation (modified from Hendry 1985c). Broken lines, immediate assay; solid lines, assay at 24 h. Marrow (van Putten *et al.* 1969), mammary epithelium (Gould and Clifton, 1977, 1979), thyroid (Mulcahy *et al.* 1980) and liver (Jirtle *et al.* 1982). Other data for liver show a dose-modifying change in survival (Fisher *et al.* 1987).

repairing high-LET-induced injury and also indicating that naturally infrequent cell division was not the major reason for the loss of damage. The importance of these findings has been shown recently by the observation of a gradual increase in cell survival in the liver when a transplantation assay was used and the delay before assay was increased to many months (Fisher *et al.* 1987).

PLDR *in vivo* has been measured after fractionated treatments only in the case of hepatocytes (Fisher & Hendry 1987). Zeman & Bedford (1986) found that prior exposure of plateau-phase cultures *in vitro* to fractionated radiation reduced the amount of PLDR after a single dose of 9 Gy.

## The survival-curve shoulder as a result of repair

The concept of the shoulder of the survival curve as a consequence of single-hit killing at low doses combined at higher doses with multiple sublethal damage accumulation, as described above, has been challenged by proponents of the *repair models*. On these models the shoulder is attributed to repair of lesions induced by single-hit processes, i.e. to progressive reduction in the biological effect of these lesions on account of repair. The increased effectiveness at higher doses or bending downward of the survival curve is supposed to arise from a reduced effectiveness of the repair process at higher doses (Powers 1962; Orr *et al.* 1966; Calkins 1971; Laurie *et al.* 1972), exhaustion of 'Q factor' (Alper 1979, 1980, 1984), or repair saturation (Goodhead 1980). Alternatively, the downward curvature has been attributed to 'misrepair' (Tobias *et al.* 1980) or damage fixation (Curtis 1982, 1986). The principles of repair models for shouldered survival curves are illustrated in Figure 3.5.

In the absence of repair the survival curve is presumed to be exponential, or nearly so, with the inverse slope equal to the terminal $D_0$. Although this might at first appear surprising, there are known

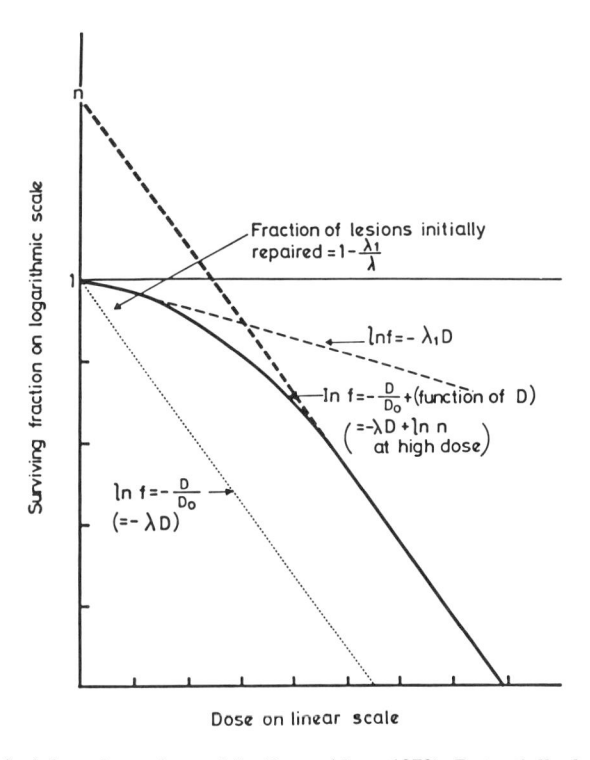

Figure 3.5. Principles of repair models (from Alper 1979). Potentially lethal damage is registered linearly with dose (dotted line). Temporally dependent repair progressively removes this damage, and more efficiently at low (light dashed line) than at high (heavy dashed line) doses. The fraction of unrepaired lesions at long times postirradiation corresponds to a single-hit, irreparable component of damage. (Reproduced with permission of Cambridge University Press and the author.)

Response of tissues to fractionated irradiation: effect of repair 61

instances of exponential survival curves for mammalian cells (e.g. Cox & Masson 1974). Radiation-induced damage is considered to be a combination of lethal, irreparable lesions (LD) and repairable lesions (RD), in proportions dependent on the LET of the radiation. If repair occurred without saturation effects or misrepair, the survival curve would swing upward from that descriptive of both RD and LD (slope $1/D_0$) to that descriptive of LD only (slope $1/_1D_0$, i.e. the initial slope). Because of saturation or misrepair (or other) effects, however, the effectiveness per unit dose increases with dose and the survival curve bends downward.

Thus the shoulder is viewed as resulting from temporally dependent repair processes coupled with saturation or misrepair effects at higher doses. As pointed out by Pohlit & Heyder (1981), no distinction need be drawn between PLDR and SLDR when these recovery phenomena are interpreted using repair models, i.e. the fractionation effect (shoulder) may be considered to result from PLDR. This is illustrated in Figure 3.6, where the effect of plating delay on the survival of human fibroblasts is presented (Deschavannes et al. 1980a). Note that this type of 'holding recovery' or PLDR leads to a considerable decrease in the initial slope

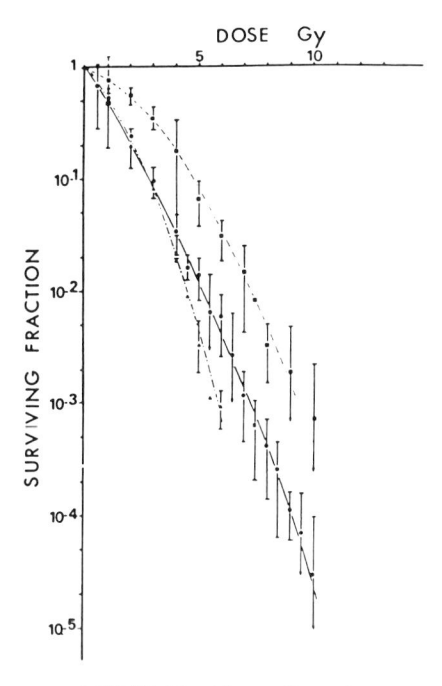

Figure 3.6. Survival curves of HF19 fibroblasts (from Deschavannes et al. 1980a). In exponential growth (circles); in unfed plateau phase plated immediately after irradiation (triangles); in unfed plateau phase plated 24 hours after irradiation (squares). The error bars represent the 95 per cent confidence interval (t test) of the means of five or three experiments. (Reproduced with permission of Taylor & Francis Ltd and the authors.)

of the survival curve, and only a modest decrease in the final slope, with the suggestion that the shoulder is largely a consequence of repair. Although such marked alteration of the initial slope is not observed in all *in vitro* studies, it was found for hepatocytes *in vivo* (Fisher et al., 1987). Repair of damage previously thought to be single-hit and irreparable has been confirmed by other workers (Utsumi et al. 1981). Because of the more pronounced change in initial slope, an increase in the 'curviness' of the survival response of cells would be predicted as more time is available for repair. Therefore, the response to fractionated irradiation, and the amount of SLDR, might be governed by the shoulder arising from PLDR (Thames et al. 1987c), and both types of repair would be considered to be part of a general repair response to damage resulting from single-hit lesions (see Sections 3.3 and 4.2 for applications of this concept).

## 3.2. Damage and repair after high-LET radiation

Whether assayed using cells in culture or *in vivo* using animal tumours,

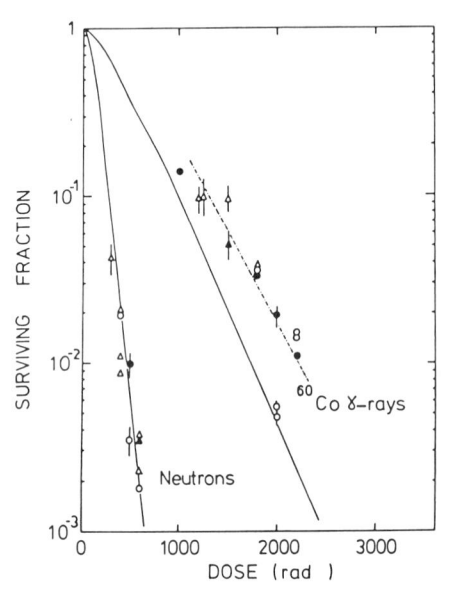

Figure 3.7. Survival data for Lewis lung carcinoma cells irradiated *in situ* with $^{60}$Co γ-rays or neutrons (16-MeV d + Be) (from Shipley et al. 1975). The tumour was removed and the colony-forming ability of the cells was measured. The solid lines are survival curves for cells from tumours removed immediately after irradiation. Closed and open symbols refer respectively to cells from tumours removed 4−8 hours or 18−24 hours after irradiation. There was clear evidence of PLDR in cells exposed to γ-rays, but not in cells exposed to neutrons. (Reproduced with permission of Waverly Press Inc. and the authors.)

Response of tissues to fractionated irradiation: effect of repair 63

PLDR seems to be minimal or nonexistent after high-LET radiation. The data of Shipley et al. (1975) illustrate this point for neutrons (Figure 3.7). Lewis lung carcinomas were irradiated in situ with graded doses of either 16-MeV deuterium-on-beryllium neutrons or cobalt-60 gamma-rays. Tumours were removed either immediately or at various times after exposure, and the surviving fraction of clonogenic cells was assayed. Although survival after gamma-rays was enhanced by delayed removal of the tumours, there was little evidence of such an effect after neutrons.

Split-dose recovery after exposure of cultured human kidney cells to 15-MeV neutrons and X-rays was studied by Broerse & Barendsen (1969). As shown in Figure 3.8, cells exposed to single doses of neutrons (curve 1) were killed much more efficiently than those exposed to single doses of X-rays (curve 4); the neutron survival curve was characterized by a steeper initial slope and very little curvature. In analogy with the split-dose study of Elkind & Sutton (1959), first doses of neutrons or X-rays were followed after 5 hours by various doses of neutrons (curves 2 and 3) or X-rays (curve 5). There was substantial repair of the injury

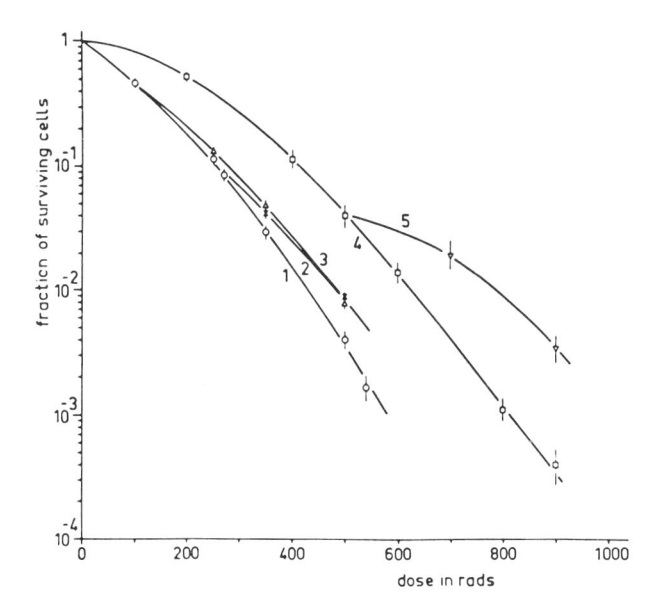

Figure 3.8. Survival of cultured cells of human origin (T − 1g) after single and two-dose exposures of 250 kVp X-rays and 15-MeV neutrons (from Broerse & Barendsen 1969). Curve 1 (circles), single doses of 15-MeV neutrons. Curve 3 (triangles) first dose of 1 Gy of 15-MeV neutrons followed by different doses of 15-MeV neutrons after an interval of 5 hours. Curve 2 (crosses), first dose of 2·5 Gy of 15-MeV neutrons followed by different doses of 15-MeV neutrons after an interval of 5 hours. Curve 4 (squares), single doses of 250-kVp X-rays. Curve 5 (inverted triangles), first dose of 5 Gy of 250-kVp X-rays followed by different doses of 250-kVp X-rays after an interval of 5 hours. (Reproduced with permission of Taylor & Francis Ltd and the authors.)

induced by X-rays, evidenced by repetition of the initial slope shoulder after a first dose of 5 Gy. A similar repetition occurred with the shoulder of the neutron survival curves, but considerably less increase in survival was evident.

There is a small dose-rate effect with neutrons in the energy range of interest for radiotherapy. This has been observed for the 5- and 30-day mortality of whole-body-irradiated mice (Broerse 1969) and for skin reactions in rats and control of a rhabdomyosarcoma (Kal 1974). Griffin & Hornsey (1986) found a small but significant dose-rate effect between 2 and 2250 cGy/min using survival of mouse jejunal crypt cells as the endpoint. This was attributed to repair during irradiation of damage caused by low-LET components (gamma-rays) of the beam.

## 3.3. Tissue response to fractionated irradiation

Almost all cells and tissues are spared some damage when a radiation dose is fractionated. This has been appreciated for a long time (see Chapter 5), although in the early research and clinical practice the components (repair and repopulation) of this 'recovery' were not understood. What was understood was that protracting a treatment led to a decreased biological effect, and thus early attention focused on time as the deciding factor. Later, the importance of fraction size and number was made clear by the experiments of Elkind & Sutton (1960), Fowler *et al.* (1963), and Dutreix *et al.* (1973).

The purpose of the present discussion is to define the concept of *fractionation sensitivity* of tissues, for example the number-of-fractions exponent in isoeffect formulae such as the nominal standard dose (NSD) equation of Ellis (1967). The questions to be answered include: How may fractionation sensitivity be quantified? Are normal tissues different in this respect from each other, and from tumours? How is fractionation sensitivity related to the survival curve of the target cells and to factors such as fraction size and interfraction interval? Throughout, it is assumed that the proliferation of survivors plays a negligible role (see Chapter 4).

**Slopes of isoeffect curves**

After the introduction of survival curves, the shoulder width $D_q$ (Figure 6.4) was often used as a measure of repair capacity in tissues. $D_q$ was obtained by determining the difference between the single and split doses that produced equivalent biological damage, when repair was complete and the doses were big enough to be 'off the shoulder'. $D_q$

values were higher for cells *in vivo* than *in vitro*. However, there was no systematic difference in $D_q$ values between normal tissues and tumours. It is likely that values of $D_q$ and the extrapolation number $N$ have little significance for clinical fractionated-dose radiotherapy, for which the relevant portion of the survival curve is the shoulder region, which is only partially described by these parameters (Withers & Peters 1980). It is the exact shape of the dose−survival curve in the shoulder region that is important, and this can be used to derive a quantitative measure of tissue fractionation sensitivity as follows.

From the idealized picture of fractionation set out in Figure 3.1 it is clear that the slope of the response to multiple equal doses depends on the size of the individual fractional doses. The slopes are given by the ratio of the change in the ordinate (log survival or effect) to the change in the abscissa (dose per fraction). Therefore, the slope of the response to repeated equal doses is the slope of the chord passing through surviving fraction 100% at zero dose and the point on the survival curve corresponding to the given dose per fraction. This slope becomes shallower as the dose per fraction decreases (Figure 3.1).

How are isoeffect doses affected by choice of fraction size, and how does the shape of the survival curve affect this dependency? The situation is illustrated in Figure 3.9 where the influence of changing fraction size on isoeffect dose is shown for two types of target cells, those characterized by a relatively 'flat' survival curve and those characterized by a relatively 'curvy' survival curve. The isoeffect doses are indicated along the constant-survival line at effect 'E', and these are seen to increase as the size of dose per fraction decreases and the fraction of each dose recovered through repair increases (Figure 3.9(c)). However, on account of the difference in shapes, the increase in isoeffect doses is faster for the curvier survival curve of Figure 3.9(b). Therefore, a higher fractionation sensitivity would be ascribed to tissues whose target-cell survival response is curvier, since isoeffect doses for these tissues would change faster with changes in dose per fraction.

If fractionation sensitivity of tissues is related to the curviness of the dose−survival curves of target cells whose depletion results in injury, how might this curviness be quantified? It is shown in the Section 7.7 that the appropriate measure is given by the ratio of slopes of the lines pictured in Figure 3.10. One of these is the chord, whose slope is a measure of the intensity of *response to repeated exposures to fractions of size x* (assuming an equal effect per fraction). The other is the tangent line to the dose−survival curve at the dose $x$, whose slope measures the steepness of *response to single doses of size x*. By comparison of Figures 3.9(a) and 3.9(b) it may be appreciated that this ratio is indeed a measure of the curviness of the dose−survival curves (Thames *et al.* 1982). To be

66 *Fractionation in Radiotherapy*

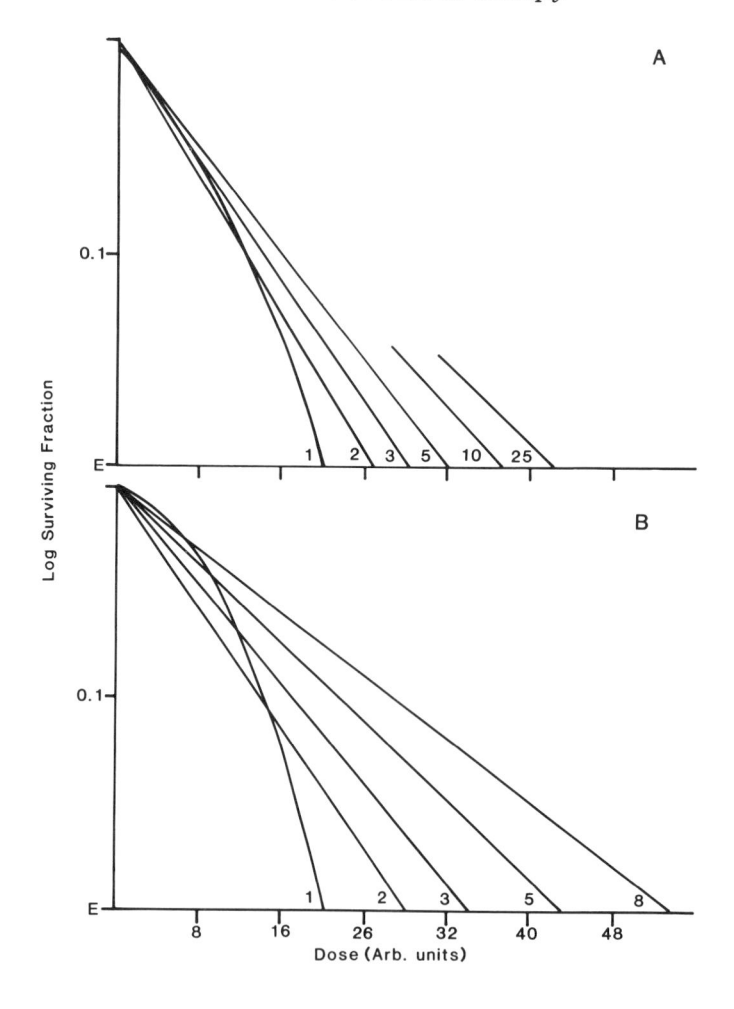

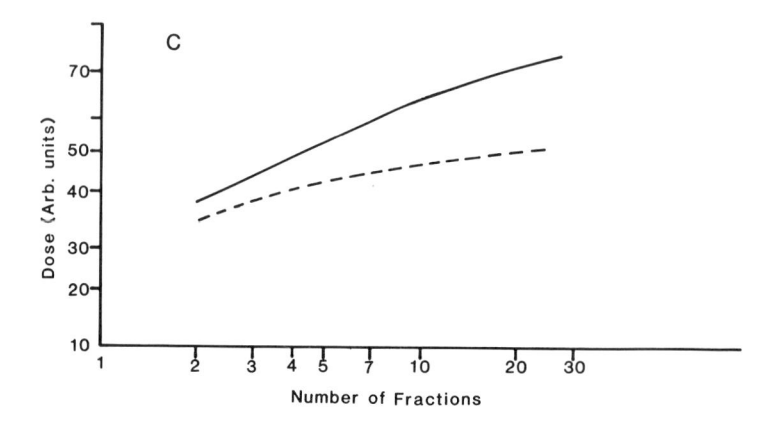

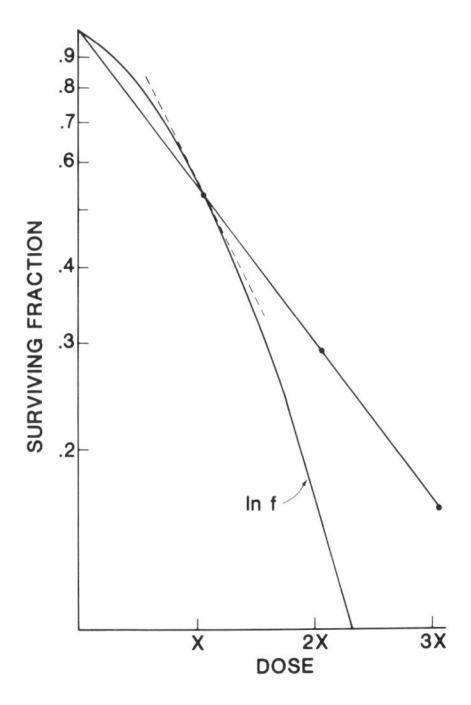

Response of tissues to fractionated irradiation: effect of repair 67

Figure 3.10. The steepness of the response (dashed line) to the single dose x, i.e. the slope of the tangent to the dose—survival curve, d(ln f)/dx, is always greater than the steepness of the multifraction response (solid line) to repeated doses of the same size, i.e. (ln f)/x (from Thames et al. 1982). It is clear that this ratio of slopes will increase with increasing curviness of the survival curve (cf. Figures 3.9(a,b)). (Reproduced with permission of Pergamon Press Inc. and the authors.)

Figure 3.9. Hypothetical responses to repeated equal doses of target-cell populations with different dose—survival curves, illustrating the importance of the low-dose parts of the survival curves. (a) Curve typical of rapidly renewing cell populations, for which the fractionated dose required to reach a given level of cell depletion E (isoeffect) increases with decreasing dose per fraction and increasing fraction number, but not as rapidly as for (b) a curve typical of a slowly regenerating population. This is 'curvier' than in (a), and consequently the fractionated dose for isoeffect increases more rapidly with decreasing fraction size (increasing fraction number). (c) Double-log plot of isoeffect doses read off the horizontal lines at isosurvival level E for increasing fraction number. Dashed curve: isoeffect doses for curve (a); solid curve: isoeffect doses for curve (b). Tissues whose target-cell populations obey a survival response like curve (b) will exhibit greater sensitivity to changes in fraction size than will tissues whose target-cell populations follow a survival response like curve (a). Clearly, the shoulder width $D_q$ is irrelevant for the purpose of distinguishing between tissues on the basis of their fractionation sensitivity. Instead, any measure of fractionation sensitivity must depend on the parameters of the dose—survival curve, but in a combination that serves as a measure of its 'curviness'.

precise (Section 7.7), the slope of the isoeffect curve is given by

$$\text{slope}(\ln D \text{ vs. } \ln x) = (\text{slope of tangent/slope of chord}) - 1 \quad (3.1)$$

when plotted with decreasing dose per fraction $x$.

In the somewhat more familiar isoeffect representation with respect to fraction number as shown in Figure 3.9(c),

$$\text{slope } (\ln D \text{ vs. } \ln n) = 1 - (\text{slope of chord/slope of tangent}). \quad (3.2)$$

These relationships equations (3.1) and (3.2) are *independent of any particular assumptions concerning the survival curve*. They may be summarized by stating that tissue sensitivity to dose fractionation is higher, the greater the difference between sensitivities of the target cells to changes in single doses (single exposure) versus change in dose per fraction (multiple exposures), i.e. between slopes of tangent and chord.

What is the slope of the isoeffect curve when a particular survival model is chosen? For the linear–quadratic model the surviving fraction (s.f.) after $n$ doses of size $x$ is

$$\text{s.f.} = e^{-n(\alpha x + \beta x^2)} \quad (3.3)$$

It is shown in the Appendix (equation (7.20)) that the slope of the $\ln D$ versus $\ln n$ curve is $x/(\alpha/\beta + 2x)$ and thus depends on the size of dose per fraction, $x$. The maximum $n$-exponent should be $0 \cdot 5$ (for large doses per fraction), and the $n$-exponent should decrease with increasing $n$ (decreasing $x$), as observed experimentally for a variety of tissues (cf. Table 2.4).

The ratio $\alpha/\beta$ should be independent of level of effect, if the target-cell hypothesis holds. This assumption was tested for a variety of tissues and endpoints (Thames 1984), and was found to be acceptable for most tissues, especially those for which the target-cells are identifiable. It was not clear whether the assumption of effect-independence held for functional assays in the kidney.

For the two-component model (Section 6.4),

$$\text{s.f.} = e^{-x/_1D_0}[1 - (1 - e^{-x/_ND_0})^N] \quad (3.4)$$

which tends to an exponential response at high doses (as opposed to the linear–quadratic model, equation 3.3, which continues to steepen), fractionation sensitivity may be expressed roughly by the ratio of initial to final $D_0$. It is 1.0 for exponential survival curves, larger for bone marrow progenitor cells, as large as 10 for mouse skin reactions, and infinitely large for some S-phase cells *in vitro* and the alga *Closterium*

Response of tissues to fractionated irradiation: effect of repair 69

*moniliferum* (Elkind 1976, 1977). The ratio can be determined using maximum-likelihood techniques (Taylor & Withers 1985), or graphically from the relative steepness of the single-dose and multifractionated dose—incidence curves.

The ratio $\alpha/\beta$ for a tissue may be derived as follows. Using the logit or probit fits to the typical data shown in the upper panel of Figure 3.11(a) (a redrawing from van der Kogel's (1979) study of hind-leg paralysis following irradiation of the lumbar cord in rats), the doses effective in paralysing 50% of the rats (ED50$_n$) when given in various

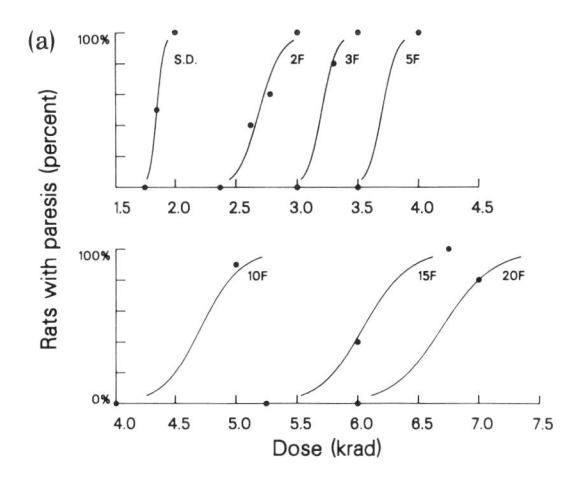

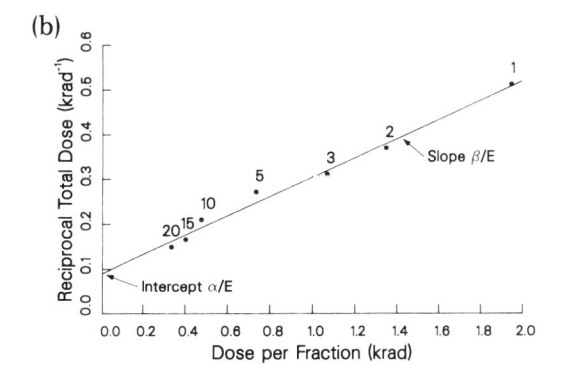

Figure 3.11(a). Proportion of rats with hind-leg paralysis resulting from exposure of the spinal cord to single (S.D.) or multiple doses of radiation (van der Kogel 1979). For each curve, an estimate of ED50 (effective dose for 50% of the animals) is obtained. (b) Reciprocal-dose plot of data of van der Kogel (1979). The line is a least squares fit of the regression model, equation (3.5) (from Tucker & Thames 1983). The intercept-to-slope ratio is an estimate of $\alpha/\beta$. (Reproduced with permission of Pergamon Press Inc. and the authors.)

numbers of fractions are estimated. If this level of injury corresponds to the same level of depletion of target cells ($-$ log of the surviving fraction, designated by $E$), regardless of fractionation scheme, then the reciprocal of the 50% effective dose in $n$ fractions ($ED50_n$) should be related linearly to the dose per fraction, $ED50_n/n$, if the linear−quadratic (LQ) model adequately describes target-cell depletion (Douglas & Fowler 1976):

$$1/ED50_n = (\alpha/E) + (\beta/E)(ED50_n/n) \qquad (3.5)$$

The slope and intercept are respectively, $\alpha/E$ and $\beta/E$. The intercept-to-slope ratio is an estimate of $\alpha/\beta$ (Thames et al. 1982). The fit of equation 3.5 to the data of van der Kogel is illustrated in Fig. 3.11(b).

An alternative method is to fit all the raw data simultaneously using maximum likelihood methods (Thames et al. 1986b). This method, termed the *direct method*, avoids the intermediate step of estimating the ED50s and so may be applied in instances when these cannot be obtained for one or a few fraction numbers. The direct method provides more reliable error estimates than does the reciprocal-dose technique.

A final point concerns the appropriateness of the LQ model for tissue responses. Tucker (1984) has devised a graphical goodness-of-fit test that aims at distinguishing those tissues whose fractionation response is adequately fitted by the LQ model from those for which the model is inappropriate.

## Fractionation sensitivity of normal tissues and tumours

In the foregoing, fractionation sensitivity has been described in terms of the steepness of isoeffect curves: higher fractionation sensitivity indicates a faster change in tissue isoeffect dose with changing dose per fraction (or fraction number). It may be quantified by the ratio $\alpha/\beta$ of LQ survival parameters or the ratio of initial-to-final $D_0$s for the relevant target cells. How does fractionation sensitivity vary for normal tissues in experimental animals?

### *Early and late radiation responses*

The terms early and late, when applied to radiation reactions in normal tissues, refer to the time of development of injury (Chapter 1). Although early reactions can begin as early as a few days after a single dose or the start of a fractionated course of radiation, late responses are delayed in their appearance until several months or more after treatment has been completed. While early reactions have generally been ascribed to the radiation-induced depletion of rapidly renewing populations (e.g. intestinal crypt cells, basal epidermal cells), most late effects have been thought of as tissue damage occurring as a result of and secondarily to

Response of tissues to fractionated irradiation: effect of repair 71

vascular injury (Casarett 1964; Fajardo & Stewart 1971; White 1976; Ullrich & Casarett 1977; Stearner & Christian 1978; Hopewell 1980). An alternative view holds that, since radiation-induced death is the result of damage to the reproductive integrity of the cell and is therefore expressed only if it attempts division, the rate at which radiation injury becomes manifest is a reflection of the rate of turnover of target cells and the lifetime of functional, differentiated cells (Withers et al. 1980; Michalowski 1981). Thus, it is possible to regard early and late radiation effects as analogous in having their pathogenesis in the depletion of parenchymal (or stromal) cells, with late effects differing from early effects only in the rate of turnover of their target cells.

*Experimental data: normal tissues*
The increase in isoeffect dose with decreasing dose per fraction is shown in Figure 3.12 for various early (dashed curves) and late (solid curves) effects. The data used for the acute-effects curves were restricted to experiments in which the overall treatment time was kept short by using 3- or 4-hour fractionation intervals, or in which an effect of regeneration of target cells was shown to be unlikely. For one 'late' endpoint,

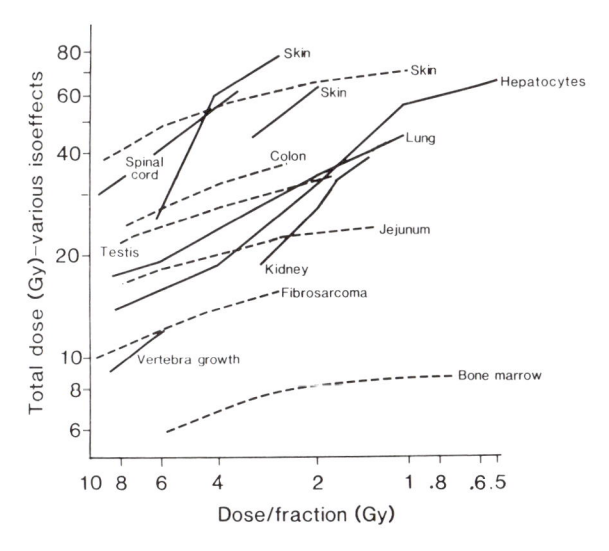

Figure 3.12. Increase in isoeffect dose with decreasing dose per fraction for various early-responding tissues and a tumour (dashed curves), and late-responding tissues (solid curves). Slopes are steeper for the late-responding tissues, which are more sensitive to change in fraction size and whose target-cell populations were correspondingly characterized by lower $\alpha/\beta$ ratios. Regeneration was minimal in the early-responding tissues surveyed but to the extent that this may have occurred the dashed isoeffect curves would be artificially steep; therefore when corrected for this effect the dashed curves would flatten and the disparity between slopes of dashed and solid lines would be even greater (Adapted from Thames et al. 1982 and Fisher and Hendry 1987).

Table 3.1. Estimates of $\alpha/\beta$ for normal tissues

|  | Reference | $\alpha/\beta$ (Gy) |
|---|---|---|
| *Early reactions* | | |
| Skin (desquamation) | Fowler et al. (1974) | 9·4 (6·1−14·3) |
|  | Douglas & Fowler (1976) | 11·7 (9·1−15·4) |
|  | Moulder & Fischer (1976) | 21·0 (16·2−27·8) |
|  | Joiner et al. (1986) | 10·5 (8·5−12·5) |
| Hair follicles (epilation) | Withers et al. (1987) | |
| (anagen) |  | 7·7 (7·4−8·0)* |
| (telogen) |  | 5·5 (5·2−5·8)* |
| Lip Mucosa (desquamation) | Ang et al. (1985c) | 7·9 (1·8−25·8) |
| Jejunum (clones) | Withers et al. (1975) | 7·1 (6·8−7·5)* |
| Colon (clones) | Tucker et al. (1983) | 8·4 (8·3−8·5)* |
| Testis (clones) | Thames & Withers (1980) | 13·9 (13·4−14·3)* |
| Spleen (clones) | Withers (1975c) | 8·9 (7·5−10·9) |
| *Late reactions* | | |
| Spinal cord (paralysis) | | |
| (cervical) | van der Kogel (1979) | 2·5 (−0·7−7·7) |
| (cervical) | Ang et al. (1987b) | 3·4 (2·7−4·3) |
| (lumbar) | van der Kogel (1979) | 4·1 (2·2−6·5) |
| (lumbar) | Hornsey et al. (1981b) | 5·2 (2·0−10·2) |
| Brain (LD50/10 months) | Hornsey et al. (1981b) | 2·1 (−1·1−14·4) |
| Eye (cataracts) | Schenken and Hagemann (1975) | 1·2 (0·6−2·1)† |
| Kidney | | |
| Rabbit | Caldwell (1975) | 0·4 (−0·8−3·4) |
| Mouse | Williams & Denekamp (1984) | |
| (urination frequency) |  | 1·6 (0·7−2·4) |
| (weight) |  | 1·6 (1·0−2·7) |
| ($^{51}$Cr-EDTA clearance) |  | 4·1 (3·1−5·2) |
| Bladder | Stewart et al. (1984a) | |
| (urination frequency) |  | 7·2 (1·3−18·1) |
| (contraction) |  | 7·8 (2·6−17·0) |
| Lung (LD50/pneumonitis) | Wara et al. (1973) | 2·1 (0·2−5·2) |
|  | Hornsey et al. (1975) | 2·5 (2·0−3·2) |
|  | Field et al. (1976) | 4·3 (3·8−4·9) |
|  | Parkins and Fowler (1985) | 3·0 (2·4−3·6) |
|  | Vegesna et al. (1985) | 3·7 (3·2−4·3) |
|  | Travis et al. (1987) | 3·7 (2·8−4·5) |
| Bowel (stricture/perforation) | Terry and Denekamp (1984) | 3·0−5·0(−1·6−22·0) |
| Dermis/subcutis (skin contraction) Pig | Withers et al. (1978) | 0·3 < $\alpha/\beta$ < 2·4 |
| Total-body irradiation (LD50/1 year) | Travis et al. (1985) | 5·1 (−1·5−15·0) |

*Calculated according to Tucker et al. (1987). 95% confidence range in parentheses.
†Direct analysis of published data by present authors.

pneumonitis, the effect of regeneration was unknown; a correction based on the author's best estimates was applied.

The slopes of the isoeffect curves are steeper for late effects, indicating a greater fractionation sensitivity (and susceptibility to sparing from dose fractionation) in slowly responding tissues. Proliferation, if it occurred, would probably have increased the isoeffect doses for acutely responding tissues, and preferentially at the smaller fraction sizes. Therefore, the steepness of the dashed lines in Figure 3.12 might be slightly exaggerated, and the difference between the slopes for acute and late isoeffects attributable to repair could be even greater than that shown. Estimates of $\alpha/\beta$ are set out in Table 3.1: *$\alpha/\beta$ is smaller in the late-responding normal tissues.*

These conclusions, although presented in terms of the LQ model, are independent of the survival model that describes target-cell killing. The reader may recall from Figure 3.10 that the fractionation sensitivity increases with increasing difference between the sensitivity of the target cells to changes in single doses (slope of tangent of survival curve) vs. changes in dose per fraction (slope of chord). Therefore, fractionation sensitivity can always be related to the dose—survival curves of the relevant target cells, even when measures as simple as the ratio $\alpha/\beta$ cannot be derived (c.f. Section 7.7).

A further point of consideration is the steepness of the dose—response curve bracketing the isoeffect level under consideration. As the initial slope of the target-cell survival curve is the major contribution to the slope for fractionated exposures, it might be expected that dose—incidence curves would be less steep for late-responding than for early-responding tissues. This is based on the idea that the $\alpha/\beta$ ratios of late-responding tissue are smaller mainly because of smaller $\alpha$'s, a conclusion that would follow from the repair-model arguments of the next section ('Why do tissues differ in their fractionation sensitivity?'). However, in general the dose-response curves are *steeper for late than for early effects*, a feature remarked upon by several investigators but quantified only recently (Thames *et al.*, 1987a). This can be deduced from the direct analysis of fractionation data to give *absolute values of $\alpha$ and $\beta$* (Table 3.2). The effective $D_0$ is $1/(\alpha+2\beta x)$ for a dose—response curve generated by increasing the size $x$ of each of a constant number of fractions, and $1/(\alpha+\beta x)$ by increasing the number of fractions of constant size $x$. The greater steepness for late effects applies for both high single doses and for low fractional doses ($\alpha$ dominant) e.g. by comparing examples 1 (typical values for early-responding tissues, Tucker *et al.*, 1987) and 7 (Table 3.2). In the kidney, the deduced $D_0$ for high single doses is $0 \cdot 6 - 0 \cdot 7$ Gy, in contrast to $1 \cdot 5$ Gy for clonogen survival (Withers *et al.*, 1986). One explanation for this discrepancy (not observed for early-responding tissues (Section 2.1)), is that two or three

Table 3.2. Fractionation parameters for various tissues (from Thames et al. 1987a)

| | $K$ | $10\alpha(Gy^{-1})$ | $100\ \beta(Gy^{-2})$ | $\alpha/\beta(Gy)$ |
|---|---|---|---|---|
| 1. Epidermal healing | $2 \times 10^4$ <br> $(3 \times 10^3 - 2 \times 10^5)$† | 1·3 <br> (1·0−1·5) | 0·78 <br> (0·61−0·95) | 16 <br> (15−18) |
| 2. Skin atrophy | 4 <br> (3-5) | 0·33 <br> (0·25−0·41) | 0·12 <br> (0·04−0·12) | 29 <br> (15−130) |
| 3. Spinal cord | $4 \times 10^6$ <br> $(2 \times 10^5 - 9 \times 10^7)$ | 0·93 <br> (0·67−1·19) | 2·7 <br> (2·2−3·2) | 3·4 <br> (2·7−4·3) |
| 4. Lung | 100 <br> (50−180) | 0·56 <br> (0·45−0·68) | 2·2 <br> (1·9−2·5) | 2·5 <br> (2·0−3·2) |
| 5. Lung | $8 \times 10^6$ <br> $(2 \times 10^4 - 3 \times 10^9)$ | 1·9 <br> (1·5−2·3) | 5·2 <br> (4·5−5·9) | 3·7 <br> (2·8−4·5) |
| 6. Lung | $1 \times 10^5$ <br> $(2 \times 10^4 - 4 \times 10^5)$ | 1·9 <br> (1·6−2·2) | 5·2 <br> (4·5−5·8) | 3·7 <br> (3·2−4·3) |
| 7. Kidney | | | | |
| Urination frequency | $6 \times 10^3$ <br> $(3 \times 10^2 - 1 \times 10^5)$ | 0·75 <br> (0·34−1·2) | 4·8 <br> (3·3−6·2) | 1·6 <br> (0·7−2·4) |
| Kidney weight | $3 \times 10^5$ <br> $(2 \times 10^3 - 5 \times 10^7)$ | 0·92 <br> (0·53−1·3) | 5·9 <br> (3·2−8·6) | 1·6 <br> (1·0−2·7) |
| $^{51}$Cr-EDTA clearance | $5 \times 10^5$ <br> $(6 \times 10^3 - 5 \times 10^7)$ | 1·9 <br> (1·2−2·6) | 4·7 <br> (3·1−6·4) | 4·1 <br> (3·1−5·2) |

Data sources:
1. Hendry et al. (1980)
2. Hendry (1987)
3. Ang et al. (1987b)
4. Hornsey et al. (1975)
5. Travis et al. (1987)
6. Vegesna et al. (1985)
7. Williams and Denekamp (1984)
†95% confidence intervals

clonogens are required to regenerate a nephron. This would also give unexpectedly high values for the number of TRU, i.e. $K$, and it could relate to different epithelial cell types constituting a nephron.

This feature of greater steepness is in addition to the lower $\alpha/\beta$ ratio. The clinical implication is that the *accuracy of dose prescription* is more important for late than for early effects.

*Experimental data: tumours*

Williams et al. (1985) have reviewed the available fractionation data for experimental tumours assayed *in situ* after irradiation either clamped or unclamped. These are characterized by heterogeneous populations of oxic and hypoxic cells, the proportions of which may change during a course of fractionated irradiation because of reoxygenation and regeneration. To minimize the influence of these factors, Williams et al.

included data where an attempt had been made to render all tumour cells uniformly radiosensitive (with misonidazole or hyperbaric oxygen) or uniformly resistant (by clamping). It was then assumed that the overall sensitivity of misonidazole-treated tumours was close to that of well oxygenated cells, whereas all dose values for clamped tumours had to be divided by an assumed OER.

The results of the analyses of Williams et al. (1985) are summarized in Table 3.3. The 95% confidence levels for the individual values are wide, and are in reality wider because of technical reasons. However, there is a clear tendency for $\alpha/\beta$ values obtained for tumours to exceed those for late-responding normal tissues, and in some cases also those for early-reacting tissues. Notably, only 4 of 48 tumours studied had an $\alpha/\beta$ ratio of less than 5 Gy.

The influence of reoxygenation and regeneration on $\alpha/\beta$ ratios for tumours is difficult to predict, although some broad generalizations may be made. It can be shown that reoxygenation should decrease the $\alpha/\beta$ ratio (Thames et al. 1985). However, there may be variations in the value of the oxygen enhancement ratio (OER) with dose, and this would preclude any easy statements of the effect of reoxygenation on the $\alpha/\beta$ ratio. Regeneration tends to increase the isoeffect dose as treatment time is protracted and would therefore steepen the isoeffect curve relative to the slope reflecting repair only. Therefore, lower $\alpha/\beta$ values would be expected. There may be exceptions to this, however, since synchrony effects can reverse the increase in isoeffect dose expected with regeneration.

In conclusion, the results of experimental studies indicate that the late-responding normal tissues are more sensitive to changes in size of dose per fraction than are those that respond acutely, with the implication that the dose-survival curve of late-effects target cells is 'curvier' than that of acute-effects target cells. The same relationship holds between late-effects tissues and tumours. Although these survival-curve characteristics are independent of the survival curve chosen to represent them, they may be expressed as a lower $\alpha/\beta$ ratio of LQ survival-model parameters for late-responding tissues.

*Clinical data*
When conventional radiotherapy treatment schedules have been changed to fewer fractions and larger doses per fraction, an increase in late complications has resulted with little or no difference in the severity of the acute responses (Montague 1968; Arcangeli et al. 1974; Bates & Peters 1975; Fletcher et al. 1974; Fletcher & Shukovsky 1975; Kim et al. 1975). Examples of the dissociation between acute and late effects with changes in dose per fraction are shown in Tables 3.4 and 3.5. Similarly, experimental studies of early and late radiation response in pigskin

Table 3.3. (a) $\alpha/\beta$ ratios for tumours irradiated and assayed in situ

| Tumour | Assay | Conditions | Numbers of fractions | Interfraction interval (hours) | Maximum overall time (days) | Dose per fraction (Gy) | $\alpha/\beta$ ratio (Gy) | 95% C.L. (regression of reciprocal-dose plot) | Ref. no. |
|---|---|---|---|---|---|---|---|---|---|
| 1. Mam.Ca N.T. | G.D. | MISO 0·67 mg/g | 1,2,5 | 48 | 9 | 6–19 | 17·9 | 17·3–18·5 | 9 |
| 2. Mam.Ca..N.T. | G.D. | MISO 0·67 mg/g | 1,2,5 | 48 | 9 | 6–14 | 16·2 | 13·4–19·1 | 7 |
| 3. Fibrosarcoma A | G.D. | MISO 0·67 mg/g | 1,2,5 | 24 | 4 | 7–22 | 19·5 | 7·1–31·9 | 9 |
| 4. C3H Mam.Ca | TCD50 | MISO 0·67 mg/g | 1,3,5 | 24 | 4 | 9–15 | 12·2 | 9·4–15·1 | 21 |
| 5. Fibrosarcoma FSA | in situ growth | 'oxic' microscopic lung colonies | 1,2,5 | 3 | 0·5 | 3–10 | 9·2 | 8·6–9·8 | 34 |
| 6. Mam.Ca. N.T. | G.D. | MISO 1·0 mg/g | 1,2,5 | 24 | 4 | 5–15 | 5·1 | 4·4–5·9 | a |
| 7. Slow Sarcoma S | G.D. | MISO 0·67 mg/g | 1,2,5 | 24 | 4 | 5–18 | 36·0 | 25·5–47·5 | b |
| 8. Ca M.T. anaplastic | TCD50 | MISO 0·2 mg/g | 5,20 | 12–24 | 9 | 5–14 | 25·7 | — | 42 |
| 9. Fibrosarcoma Sa FAa | G.D. | MISO 0·67 mg/g | 1,5 | 24 | 4 | 8–24 | 20·3 | — | 8 |
| 10. Fibrosarcoma SA FAb | G.D. | MISO 0·67 mg/g | 1,5 | 24 | 4 | 7–24 | 31·8 | — | 8 |
| 11. Slow sarcoma S | G.D. | MISO 0·67 mg/g | 1,5 | 24 | 4 | 5–19 | 30·1 | — | b |

Note: The cells were either 'naturally oxic' or sensitized by misonidazole
[a] Joiner & Denekamp (unpublished)
[b] Terry & Denekamp (unpublished)
Median $\alpha/\beta = 19\cdot 5$; Mean $\alpha/\beta = 20\cdot 4$; S.D. $= \pm 9\cdot 7$.

(b) $\alpha/\beta$ ratios for clamped tumours irradiated and assayed in situ

| Tumour | Assay | Numbers of fractions | Interfraction interval (hours) | Maximum overall time (days) | Dose per fraction (Gy) | $\alpha/\beta$ ratio (Gy) | 95% C.L. (regression of reciprocal-dose plot) | Ref. no. |
|---|---|---|---|---|---|---|---|---|
| 12. Mam.Ca.N.T. | G.D. | 1,3,6,9, | 12 | 4 | 8–36 | 7·3 | 6·1–8·4 | c |
| 13. Mam.Ca.A.T. 17 | G.D. | 1,2,4,6 | | | 10–36 | 10·8 | 8·5–13·0 | d |
| 14. C3H Mam Ca. | TCD50 | 1,2,10 | 24 | 9 | 8–46 | 15·3 | 1·4–29·3 | 49 |
| 15. C3H Mam.Ca | TCD50 | 1,2,5,10,20 | 12–24 | 10 | 8–70 | 18·8 | 13·2–24·5 | 45 |
| 16. Slow sarcoma S | G.D. | 1,2,5 | 24 | 4 | 9–31 | 19·3 | 3·0–35·7 | e |
| 17. Mam.Ca.N.T. | G.D. | 1,2,5 | 24 | 4 | 12–35 | 9·1 | 7·9–10·3 | c |
| 18. Mam.Ca.N.T. | G.D. | 1,3,6,9 | 3 | 1 | 8–40 | 15·5 | 10·6–20·5 | c |
| 19. DBA Mam.Ca. | TCD50 | 1,10 | 24 | 9 | 11–51 | 9·0 | — | 46 |
| 20. C3H Mam.Ca | TCD50 | 1,10 | 24 | 9 | 12–58 | 9·9 | — | 47 |
| 21. Squamous Ca. | TCD50 | 1,10 | 24 | 9 | 10–50 | 12·1 | — | 48 |
| 22. Fibrosarcoma | TCD50 | 1,10 | 24 | 9 | 10–35 | 0·9 | — | 48 |

[c] Rojas & Denekamp unpublished
[d] Kummermehr personal communication
[e] Terry & Denekamp unpublished
Values divided by an assumed OER of 2·7.
Median $\alpha/\beta = 10·8$; Mean $\alpha/\beta = 11·6$; S.D. = ± 5·3.
From Williams et al. (1985), where the references can be found.

(Berry et al. 1974; Withers et al. 1978) and epilation and spinal-cord paralysis (Masuda et al. 1977) indicate that the severity of late responses after larger doses per fraction cannot be adequately judged from early skin reactions. For example, to achieve the same effect in 13 fractions over 6½ weeks as resulted from 64 Gy given in 32 fractions in the same time period, required about 60 Gy for desquamation but less than 47 Gy for late contraction (Withers et al. 1978). These results can be interpreted

Table 3.4. Incidence of late complications for regimens yielding acute responses of approximately equal severity

| Complication | Treatment schedule (rad) | Dose/fract (rad) | % Incidence | Reference |
|---|---|---|---|---|
| Necrosis of laryngeal cartilage | 5500/3 weeks | 366 | 7 | 25 |
| | 6000/5 1/2 weeks | 200−225 | 1 | 13 |
| | 7000/6 1/2 weeks | | | |
| Severe oedema of vocal cords | 5500/4 weeks | 260−275 | 9 | |
| | 6500/5 weeks | | | 14 |
| | 6000/5 1/2 weeks | 200 | 1 | |
| | 7000/6 1/2 weeks | | | |
| Subcutaneous fibrosis of chest wall | 4900/32 days | 490 | 33 | |
| | 4410/30 days | 490 | 2·1 | 22 |
| | 5000/18 days | 385 | 17 | |
| | 4600/28 days | 230 | 4·4 | |

From Thames et al. (1982), where the references can be found.

Table 3.5. Late complications after irradiation of the breast[a]

| Complication | 3500−4000 rad/4 weeks 5 × weekly (88 pts) % (dose in rad per fraction) | 3500−4000 rad/4 weeks 3 × weekly (30 pts) % (dose in rad per fraction) |
|---|---|---|
| Severe chest wall fibrosis | 2 (200) | 20 (>500) |
| Rib fracture | 7 (200) | 10 (>500) |
| Severe pneumonitis | 2 (200) | 13 (>500) |
| Severe axillary fibrosis and frozen shoulder | 2 (200) | 20 (333) |
| Posterior scapular fibrosis | 0 (200) | 7 (333) |
| Arm oedema | 1 (200) | 10 (>500) |
| Severe supraclavicular fibrosis | 0 (200) | 17 (333) |
| Brachialplexopathy | 0 (200) | 3 (333) |

[a] From Montague (1968): acute responses were similar in all groups.
Based on assessment of damage resulting primarily from either anterior−posterior supraclavicular fields (333 rad per fraction) or alternating tangential breast beams (500 to 600 rad per fraction).

From Thames et al. (1982)

# Response of tissues to fractionated irradiation: effect of repair

to indicate that the dose–survival characteristics of target cells for late injuries are different from those for acutely responding tissues.

This difference, namely, that the target-cell survival curve for late-responding tissues is 'curvier' than that for acutely responding tissues, as deduced in the previous section, may be applied to explain the dissociation between acute and late effects observed clinically with variations in fractionation pattern; this is illustrated in Figure 3.13. Survival curve parameters were chosen to yield equal reduction in survival to $10^{-6}$ for target cells for early response in two fractionation patterns: 30 fractions of 2 Gy and 12 fractions of 4 Gy. Thus, based on the assumptions, 2 Gy given five times weekly is equivalent for acutely responding tissues to 4 Gy given twice weekly. By virtue of the smaller

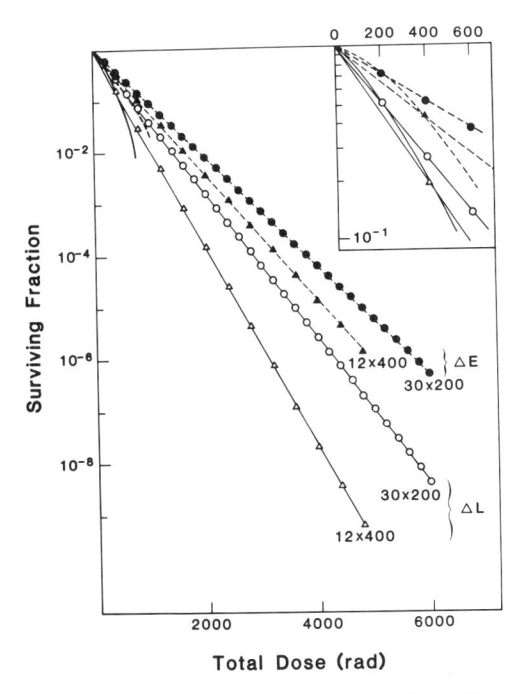

Figure 3.13. Interpretation of the dissociation between acute and late reactions when the dose per fraction is increased (from Thames et al. 1982). Equivalent early reactions ($\Delta E \simeq 0$) are obtained after 200 rad given 5 times weekly and 4 Gy given twice weekly in 6 weeks' overall time (fractionation responses are indicated by solid circles and triangles connected by dashed lines). There is a significant increase ($\Delta L$) in late response, however, equivalent in cell killing to approximately 8 Gy. This results from the smaller $\alpha/\beta$ ratio of the dose-survival curve for late effects target cells (solid curve, upper left and inset), which makes it 'curvier', so that the slope of the response to doses of 4 Gy (open triangles) is sharply steeper than that of the response to multiple doses of 2 Gy (open circles). On a sigmoid dose-response curve for late complications, a noticeable increase in frequency would result from the 100-fold reduction in survival of late-effects target cells. (Reproduced with permission of Pergamon Journals Ltd.)

$\alpha/\beta$ ratio for late responses, however, a two-decade reduction in survival of late-effects target cells results from replacing 2 Gy five times weekly with 4 Gy given twice weekly. That this reduction might result in a significant increase in late complications can be appreciated by noting that equivalence for late response occurs at about 10 times 4 Gy rather than 12 times 4 Gy. On a sigmoid dose–response curve for frequency of late complications, the extra 8 Gy would cause a noticeable increase from the 'acceptable' frequency resulting from 30 times 2 Gy by virtue of the steep slope of the multifraction response for late effects (Thames et al. 1987a) at this relatively high dose per fraction (see Section 6.10). At this point it is worth noting that tumour-related injuries may modify the steepness of the dose–response curves for late-responding normal tissues (see Section 6.9). Also, there are few dose–response curves for human tissues in the literature where fractionated doses are not presented in transformed units, e.g. values of NSD (Moore et al. 1983).

There are very few results on the fractionation sensitivity of human tumours. Douglas (1982a) analysed published data from human tumours and obtained values for $\alpha/\beta$ of 3·9 Gy for breast cancer and 10 Gy for squamous carcinoma. These values may have reflected the influences of reoxygenation and regeneration. However, analyses of the results of treatment of larynx (Maciejewski et al. 1983) and skin (Hliniak et al. 1983) tumours with widely varying overall treatment times and fraction sizes indicated that the latter were not a significant factor, and this is consistent with a high value of $\alpha/\beta$ for these tumours (see Section 4.3).

The results of treatment of liposarcomas were surveyed by Reitan & Kaalhus (1980), who derived a large number-of-fractions exponent (0·5) indicative of the high fractionation sensitivity of this tumour. The data were also analysed by Thames & Suit (1986), who estimated $\alpha/\beta$ at 0·4 Gy, which correlates with the large number-of-fractions exponent. However, the 95% confidence interval (−1·4, 5·4) Gy was wide, and the result should be accepted as a qualitative indication, rather than quantitative measure, of high fractionation sensitivity.

A comparison of $\alpha/\beta$ ratios for normal tissues derived from clinical and experimental data is presented in Section 3.5 (see Table 3.7).

## Why do tissues differ in their fractionation sensitivity?

Two explanations of the higher fractionation sensitivity of the late-responding tissues have been put forward, one having to do with the postirradiation proliferative response of tissues and the other with differences in shapes of target-cell survival curves, i.e. repair capacity, as outlined in the preceding section. The interpretation in terms of differences in postirradiation kinetic behaviour of early and late-responding tissues (Wheldon et al. 1982) is based on the observation of dose-dependent differences in division potential of radiation-sterilized cells (Puck & Marcus 1956; Elkind et al. 1963). Because of this, cells sterilized by low doses may complete several divisions, whereas those sterilized by high doses are more likely to fail at the first attempted division. Therefore, a dose–response curve for functional capacity of a tissue might display an enhanced shoulder at low doses, on account of residual functional activity of cells radiation-sterilized but still capable of a few divisions, and more so in the late-responding than in the early-responding tissues. In this way the dose–response curve for functional changes (the usual endpoint in assays of radiation effects in late-responding tissues) would be 'curvier' than that for clonogenic survival. If this effect can be extrapolated to high total-dose multifractionated treatments, then it in itself would explain the increased fractionation sensitivity in late-effect tissues.

This hypothesis was tested by Thames et al. (1986a) by determining the colony-size distributions of radiation-sterilized, plateau-phase cells exposed to isoeffective gamma-ray doses in different fractionation regimens. Although the division potential of radiation-sterilized cells decreased with increasing single doses in accord with the results of Elkind et al. (1963), there was no trend with size of dose per fraction in isosurvival fractionation regimens (Figure 3.14). Therefore, when

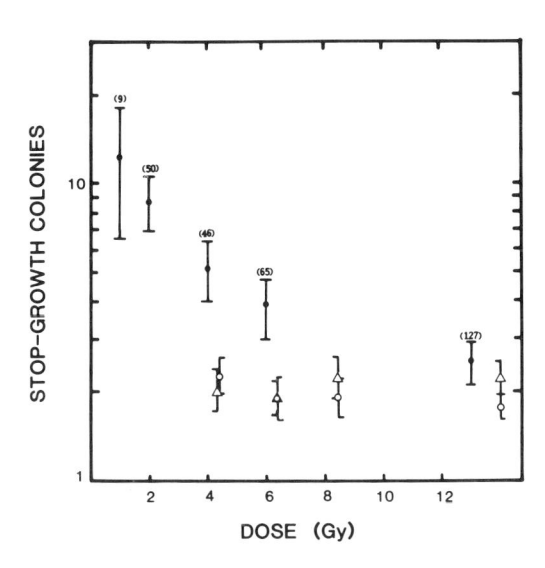

Figure 3.14. Maximum colony size as a function of dose per fraction after isoeffective fractionated doses (from Thames et al. 1986a). Experiment 1 (open circles), Experiment 2 (open triangles). Data from single-dose exposures are included for comparison (closed circles). Error bars show 95% confidence limits. (Reproduced with permission of Macmillan Press Ltd.)

survival was reduced to about 0·5%, sterilized cells seemed capable of about one division on average, regardless of dose per fraction. If applicable to target cells *in vivo*, these results were not consistent with differences in postirradiation kinetic behaviour as an explanation of differences in fractionation sensitivity.

Concerning repair, two possibly related explanations have been advanced: differences in redistribution (Zeman & Bedford 1984) and differences in the time available for repair prior to fixation of repairable damage consequent upon movement in the division cycle (Thames 1985: equation 43), or equivalently, variable repair capacity in the division cycle. The latter explanation is closely related to the repair models described in Section 3.1 and to the view that the survival-curve shoulder is a consequence of PLDR. To illustrate, consider the presentation of plating-delay results in Figure 3.6. The basis for our argument is the assumption that immediate or very slightly delayed plating causes cells to enter the cycle quickly, and that as a result their response resembles that of target cells in 'acutely responding' tissues, whereas long-delayed plating prevents entry of cells into the division cycle, and thus permits the response of 'late responding' tissues to irradiation to be simulated.

From the results of Deschavannes *et al.* (1980a) set out in Figure 3.6, it can be seen that as plating delay increased, there was a progressive decrease in the initial slope of the survival curve and a smaller change in the final slope, with the result of a smaller $\alpha/\beta$ ratio with long plating delays. On this speculative interpretation, then, the initial slope is altered to a greater extent by postirradiation repair than is the final slope. Therefore, the consequence is a smaller $\alpha/\beta$ ratio in those tissues in which more repair occurs, i.e. the slowly turning-over tissues that manifest late effects. However, in the studies by Fisher & Hendry (1987) with hepatocytes *in vivo*, the final slope decreased markedly with long delays (up to 1 year) before cell transplantation. With fractionation, the $\alpha$ component decreased slightly with time and the $\beta$ component decreased more. However, the $(\alpha/\beta)$ ratio remained very low ($1-2$ Gy) at all times of assay. These interpretations will be considered further in Section 4.2, in connection with the possibility that $\alpha/\beta$ ratios of acutely responding tissues change when these undergo a proliferative response to radiation injury.

## 3.4. Repair kinetics

The kinetics of split-dose recovery has been studied in terms of the effect of the time between two doses on cell survival. Survival increases steeply for intervals of up to 1 or 2 hours, on account of repair. Longer intervals may produce a dip, which is attributed to progression of survivors to more sensitive phases of the cell cycle. This dip can be avoided *in vitro* by special techniques (Elkind *et al.* 1965), such as maintenance of cells at room temperature, which minimize progression in the division cycle. The recovery curve, after its steep initial increase, gradually reaches a plateau of maximum recovery, e.g. Figure 6.6. The shapes of such curves are readily fitted by exponential functions, resulting in the notion of exponential repair kinetics (e.g. Lea 1938; Lajtha & Oliver 1961).

Exponential, or first-order, repair kinetics might at first glance seem an oversimplification, since it is likely that a myriad of enzymatic reactions contributes to the increase in survival that is measured. However, it is possible that the slowest of these, which limits the rate of recovery, may on average obey simple first-order enzyme kinetics, according to which the rate of repair is proportional to the number of lesions to be repaired:

$$dL/dt = -\mu L \qquad (3.6)$$

and the relative number of lesions decreases according to the function

$$\exp(-\mu t)$$

The repair constant $\mu$ is assumed to be independent of dose, or equivalently the initial number of repairable lesions, when first-order kinetics is used. This assumption was tested for a variety of tissues (Thames 1984) and found acceptable. There is, however, evidence from DNA repair studies *in vitro* that repair saturates after higher doses, and is slower than after low doses (Wheeler and Nelson 1987).

## Incomplete-repair models

Incomplete-repair (IR) models, whose derivation is presented in Section 7.2, are based on generalizations of the concept of 'dose-equivalent of incomplete repair' (Oliver 1964). This is illustrated in Figure 3.15. Two acute doses of size $x$ are given, with interfraction interval $\Delta t$, to a homogeneous population with the hypothetical survival curve as shown. If $\Delta t = 0$, i.e. the two doses are given as one, then the survival response will be described by the unbroken continuation of the first segment of the curve, indicated by the lower of the three curves in the inset. On the other hand, if $\Delta t$ is long and repair is complete, the response to the second dose will be the same as to the first dose (upper curve in the inset), i.e. a repetition of all of the first segment. Oliver envisaged that, in intermediate cases, a variable portion of the initial segment would be repeated, depending on $\Delta t$ (heavy part of first segment and middle curve in inset), with the exclusion of an initial segment equivalent to an

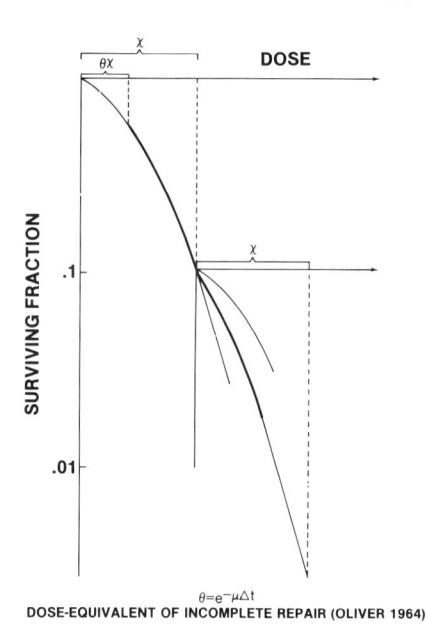

Figure 3.15. Dose-equivalent of incomplete repair (from Thames et al. 1984). The heavy portion of the dose-survival curve is repeated after a second dose of size $x$; the initial segment $\theta x = x \exp(-\mu \Delta t)$ is not repeated. As $\Delta t$ increases, an increasingly larger part of the initial segment is repeated, until for large $\Delta t$ the entire segment is recovered. (Reproduced with permission of Macmillan Press Ltd.)

'unrepaired part of the dose'. This was taken to be a fraction $\theta$ of the first dose $x$. Hence for $\Delta t = 0$ we must have $\theta = 1$ (none of the shoulder repeated) and $\theta$ should decrease toward zero as $\Delta t$ increases. Because of the shape of split-dose recovery curves, an exponential decrease with $\Delta t$ was postulated (Lajtha & Oliver 1961; Oliver 1964):

$$\theta = e^{-\mu \Delta t} \qquad (3.7)$$

which is equivalent to the rate law of equation 3.6.

The calculations may be generalized to arrive at a representation of survival after $n$ doses, with variable fractionation interval (Section 7.2). It is necessary to assume a form for the survival curve if data are to be analysed; the formulae presented in Section 7.2 are based on the LQ model (equation 3.3).

A model of survival response to continuous exposure is derived (Section 7.3) by allowing the number of fractions ($n$) in the IR model to approach infinity, with ever-smaller dose per fraction and interfraction interval ($\Delta t$), but in such a way that total dose and overall time are held constant.

Other exponential-repair models have been derived. In each case exponential recovery is the result of assumptions equivalent to that described by equation 3.6. First, there are formulations based on interactions between two or more sublethal events, where the probability of these interactions is assumed to decay exponentially (Swann & del Rosario 1931; Hoffman & Reinhard 1934; Lea 1938; Kellerer & Rossi 1972; Payne & Garrett 1975a,b; Roesch 1978). Second, there are models with explicit first-order repair (equation 3.6) combined with quadratic (dose-squared) misrepair or sublesion-interaction processes (Tobias et al. 1980; Curtis 1982, 1986), which lead to the same exponential decay over time of the probability of interaction between sublesions. Third, there is a pool model (Laurie et al. 1972), in which first-order repair and a downward-bending survival curve result from exhaustion of the limited pool of substances required for repair.

### Exponential-repair accumulation models

Roesch (1978) and Braby & Roesch (1978) have classified some of the exponential-repair models as accumulation models, on the basis that accumulation models lead to a better description of the dose-rate effect. These include the models of Lajtha & Oliver (1961), Kellerer & Rossi (1972), Payne & Garrett (1975a,b), Roesch (1978), Tobias et al. (1980), Curtis (1982, 1986), and Thames (1985). What distinguishes an accumu-

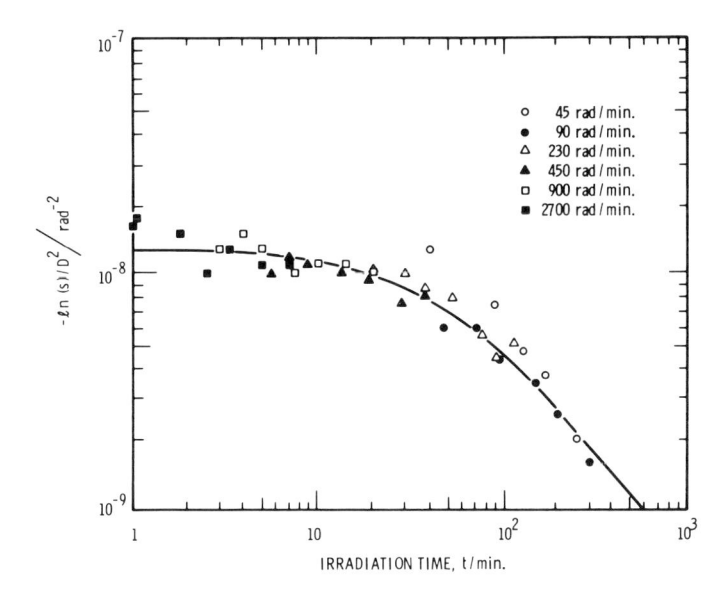

Figure 3.16. The survival data for *C. reinhardi* plotted as $-\ln(S)/D^2$. (From Braby & Roesch 1978; reproduced with permission of Academic Press Inc. and the authors.)

lation model from other exponential-repair models, is that the probability of killing per energy deposition event increases with each event because of the accumulation of products with which a lethal interaction can occur. In nonaccumulation models this probability is constant. In the Swann–del Rosario model, for example, once a cell has been damaged its chance of being killed is not enhanced by any further damage.

Braby & Roesch (1978) measured the survival of *Chlamydomonas reinhardi* after exposure to 1·5-MeV electrons at dose rates ranging from 45 to 2700 cGy/min, with exposure times ranging from 1 to 300 min. When the data were plotted as the quotient of the negative log surviving fraction by the square of the dose versus irradiation time, they fell essentially on a single curve (Figure 3.16), regardless of dose rate, in accord with the prediction of accumulation models. The other models (Swann–del Rosario 1931; Rajewski & Danzer 1934; Kappos & Pohlit 1972; Laurie *et al.* 1972) predicted families of curves, one for each dose rate.

Exponential repair accumulation models may be similar across restricted dose ranges. Thus, for low doses per fraction and for low dose rates the IR model is equivalent to the LPL (lethal, potentially lethal) model of Curtis (1982, 1986) although they arise from what seem to be quite different assumptions (Thames 1985).

**Repair kinetics in tissues**

Repair kinetics have been studied in tissues using both short fractionation intervals (e.g. Thames *et al.* 1984) and changes in dose rate (e.g. Steel *et al.* 1986). In tissues where colony assays have been developed, the models may be used to fit survival responses in fractionation regimens in which repair is incomplete, or very nearly complete. The data of Withers (1975b and unpublished) shown in Figure 3.17 illustrate the effect of repair on the survival of jejunal crypt cells after fractionated doses with 3-hour versus 1-hour intervals.

When survival cannot be measured, repair kinetics in tissues is determined from functional assays of response. The data of Ang *et al.* (1987) for paralysis of rat spinal cord are shown in Figure 3.18. With quantal (all-or-nothing) responses like this, the data are fitted using direct (maximum-likelihood) analysis (Thames *et al.* 1986b). On the other hand, with graded reaction scores of response, e.g. as measured with skin and lip mucosa, isoeffect doses must be estimated for each individual fractionation regimen or dose rate and the reciprocal-dose technique employed (see Section 3.3). (Alternatively, the proportions of individuals in a group with reactions greater than a specified level can be used as quantal data). The plot of reciprocal isoeffect doses versus dose per

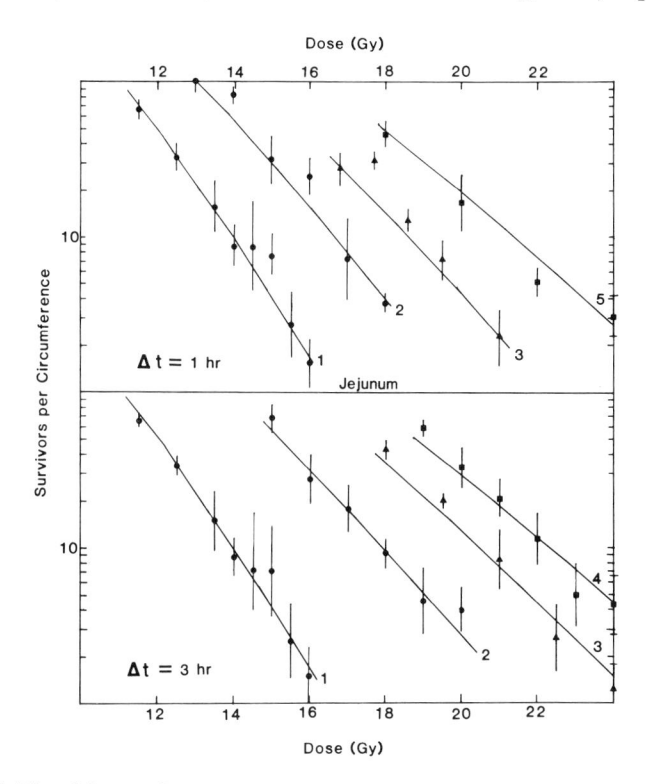

Figure 3.17. Fit of incomplete-repair model; data of Withers (1975b and unpublished). Goodness of fit to observed response of jejunal mucosa to fractionated regimens with intervals of 1 (upper) and 3 (lower) hours. (From Thames et al. 1984; reproduced with permission of Macmillan Press Ltd and the authors.)

fraction—linear when repair is complete—is curved when repair is incomplete (Thames 1985).

The results of analyses of published data are set out in Table 3.6, for both fractionation and low-dose-rate studies. Repair half-times are longer in the skin and spinal cord, shortest in jejunum, and intermediate in lung and colon. The longer time (1·5 h) derived from the results of Vegesna et al. (1985) does not agree with the results of two other studies. This may be so because incomplete repair was not the only cause of curvature in the reciprocal-dose plot. The assumption of an exponential tail to the dose−survival curve (Taylor & Withers 1985) explained the data as well as did the assumption of incomplete repair (Thames et al. 1984).

The *effect of fraction size* on repair kinetics has attracted considerable attention recently, because of the clinical importance of determining the minimum interfraction interval for treatment two or more times daily. Catastrophic late complications occurred in patients who received 8

88  *Fractionation in Radiotherapy*

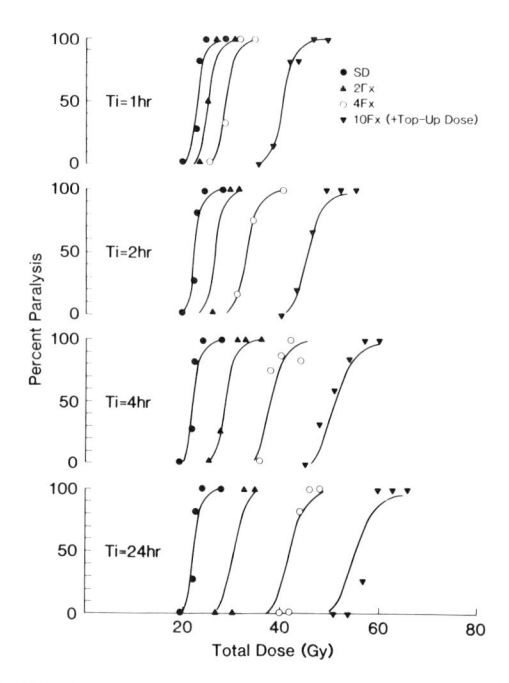

Figure 3.18. Repair kinetics in the spinal cord (from Ang *et al.* 1987b). The effect of repair is evidenced by increasing displacement of the curves to the right with increasing fractionation interval. Significant repair occurred between 4 and 24 hours. (Reproduced with permission of Pergamon Journals Ltd. and the authors.)

Table 3.6. Tissue repair half-times

| Tissue (ref.) | Dose delivery[a] | $T_{1/2}$ (hours) |
|---|---|---|
| Jejunum (Thames *et al.* 1984) | Fx | 0·45(0·43,0·47) |
| (Huczkowski & Trott 1986; Dale *et al.* 1987) | LDR | 0·2−0·7 |
| Colon (Thames *et al.* 1984) | Fx | 0·79(0·76,0·83) |
| Skin (Henkleman *et al.* 1980) | LDR | 1·3(1·0,1·6) |
| Lip mucosa (Ang *et al.* 1985c, 1987a) | Fx | 0·8(0·6,1·3) |
| Hair follicles (Withers *et al.* 1987) | Fx | 1·5(1·4,1·6) (telogen) |
|  |  | 0·63(0·58,0·7) (anagen) |
| Lung (Vegesna *et al.* 1985) | Fx | 1·5(1·2,1·9) |
| (Down *et al.* 1986) | LDR | 0·68(0·55,0·89) |
| (Travis *et al.* 1987) | Fx | 0·74(0·68,0·81) |
| Spinal cord (Ang *et al.* 1987b) | Fx | 1·55(1·40,1·73) |

95% confidence intervals enclosed in parentheses.
[a] Fx = fractionated with short intervals: LDR = low dose rate.

fractions/day separated by 2 hours (Nguyen et al. 1985). Although Ang et al. (1984) reported faster repair in the *spinal cord* after small fraction sizes, in a subsequent publication (Ang et al. 1987b) with more extensive data it was shown that the half-time was about 1·6 h regardless of fraction size, with an (insignificant) trend in the 2-fraction data toward a longer repair half-time (1·9 h). For the *lung*, Travis et al. (1987) found a half-time (0·76 h) close to that reported by Down et al. (1986) from low-dose-rate exposures (0·68 h). There was however, a trend toward shorter half times (0·6 h) with the large fraction sizes than with the small fraction sizes (0·8 h) in the data of Travis et al. (1987).

Rojas et al. (1987) have investigated the influence of fraction size on repair kinetics in *skin* and *kidney*. For the skin the half-time was shorter (about 1 h) for fraction sizes in the range 2 to 4 Gy, and longer (about 3 h) for doses per fraction of 10·5 Gy. This trend was the opposite of that seen in the lung by Travis et al. (1987), and of the results of Rojas and colleagues for kidney, namely shorter (about 1 h) repair half-times for 7 Gy fractions than for 2 Gy fractions (about 2 h).

The effect of *dose rate* on repair kinetics has also shed light on the question of dose-dependent kinetics. with survival *in vitro* using cell lines derived from human tumour xenografts, repair was faster after low dose-rate irradiation than deduced from split-dose studies (Steel et al., 1987). For crypt-cell colonies repair was faster, the lower the dose rate (Dale et al., 1987; range of $T_{1/2}$ in Table 3.6).

## 3.5. Response of normal tissues to low doses

The increase in tissue isoeffect dose with decreasing dose per fraction is steeper for late-responding tissues than for those that respond acutely. A clinically important question then arises: is there any limit to this increase, and if so, at what dose per fraction? The isoeffect models can give little information on this point, since such low doses represent an extrapolation well beyond the range of experimental data in which the models were fitted. The NSD formula predicts an unlimited increase in isoeffect dose with decreasing dose per fraction, as does any model employing a power of the number of fractions. The survival-curve models, such as those of Barendsen (1982) or Withers et al. (1983), predict a bounded isoeffect dose as dose per-fraction goes to zero, but the limiting isoeffect dose is usually so much larger than those used in clinical practice that radiotherapists could reasonably ask whether such predictions are meaningful.

By reference to Figure 2.14 it may be seen that isoeffect doses tend to an upper limit when the fraction size is so small as to be in the approximately linear initial region of the survival curve. Therefore we are led to the idea of a limiting fraction size for effective fractionation. This concept was introduced by Dutreix et al. (1973) and subsequently elaborated by Withers (1977), who labelled this dose per fraction the *flexure dose*. More recently, various definitions of the flexure dose have been introduced (Tucker & Thames, 1983; Fowler et al. 1983) and used to calculate a range of such doses for a number of therapeutically relevant tissues.

**Incremental dose per fraction for isoeffect**

The method introduced by Dutreix et al. (1973) for the investigation of the flexure dose was to measure the increase in isoeffect dose when the size of dose per fraction was reduced by half. One definition of the flexure dose would be a dose per fraction that when halved led to no further increase in isoeffect dose. This approach was applied in studies of response to multifraction radiation of human skin (Dutreix et al. 1973) and mouse jejunum (Wambersie et al. 1974). No detectable increases in isoeffect dose occurred when doses per fraction of approximately 2 Gy were halved, and thus 2 Gy was taken as the flexure dose for skin and gut.

Withers (1975b) generalized this approach by calculating the incremental dose per fraction ($\Delta D_r$) required for an effect when the fraction number was increased but not necessarily doubled. With increasing fractionation the survival curves for jejunal crypt cells were displaced to the right, until the dose was divided into more than 15 fractions: the 15- and 20-fraction data were fitted by approximately the same survival curve. Thus, when doses per fraction of 110 to 165 cGy were given 20 times, the response was the same as that obtained with 15 doses of 150 to 230 cGy. In other words, Withers found no significant additional recovery when doses per fraction were less than about 230 cGy. This implies that the dose-survival curve was indistinguishable from an exponential between its origin and 230 cGy.

Estimates of the flexure dose may be derived by selecting isoeffect levels. Depending on the survival level chosen, however, the value of $D_s$ at which $D_r = 0$ will appear to be different. For example, if the isoeffect were 100 survivors per circumference, we would obtain $D_r = 0$ for 140 cGy per fraction, whereas at 1 survivor per circumference $D_r = 0$ for 230 cGy per fraction. Thus, there are some uncertainties in the estimate of the dose at which $D_r = 0$.

**Divergence of multifraction and single-dose survival curves**

If the survival curve is exponential in the initial region and then bends downward, the single dose and multifraction curves should begin

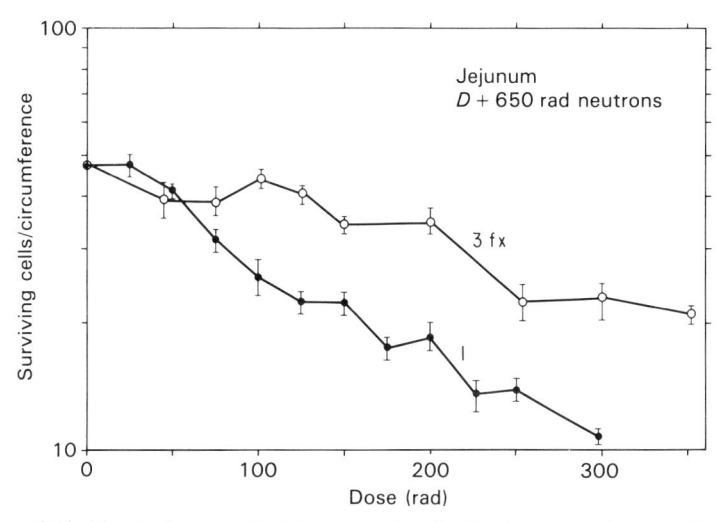

*Response of tissues to fractionated irradiation: effect of repair* 91

Figure 3.19. Survival curves for jejunal crypt cells of mice exposed to γ-radiation given as a single exposure or in three fractions separated by 3 hours (from Withers 1975b). The curves were obtained from cellular survival measurements when the γ-ray doses plotted on the abscissa were supplemented by a single dose of 6·5 Gy neutrons to reduce cellular survival to levels that could be assayed. The curves diverge after about 1 Gy. (Reproduced with permission of John Wiley, the Institute of Physics and the author.)

diverging when doses per fraction are greater than the dose at which the single-dose curve begins diverging from the exponential, i.e. the flexure dose. Survival curves for jejunal crypt cells exposed to low doses of gamma-rays given as single doses or as three fractions separated by 3 hours were obtained by delivering test doses and subsequently, after an interval of 4 hours, a dose of 6·5 Gy neutrons to reduce cellular survival to levels readily counted using a microcolony technique (Withers 1975b). In Figure 3.19 the points are not fitted by straight lines, but have been joined by lines to simplify visual resolution. The single-dose and 3-fraction data diverged from one another at total doses of about 1 Gy. If artefacts, due for example to synchrony from division cycle delays during the 3-fraction experiments, did not cause the divergence, the curves in Figure 3.19 suggest that repair of sublethal injury affected the jejunal response at doses above 0·75−1·0 Gy. Therefore, the flexure dose for jejunum could be lower than that expected from the dose (2 Gy) derived by the incremental-dose-for-isoeffect method.

### Estimates of the flexure dose

The above discrepancy, and the difficulties associated with level of effect in the estimation of $D_r$ as set out above, may be circumvented by various methods of estimating the flexure dose (Tucker & Thames 1983). A number of possible definitions for the flexure dose were considered:

*1. Limited resolution between fractional doses*: If the dose-survival curve for some target-cell population had an initial linear region, the response would be independent of fraction number for fractional doses less than the flexure dose, provided that the fraction number $n$ is large enough. When the level of resolution is taken as some value such as 5%, the flexure dose is found to be a multiple of the ratio $\alpha/\beta : 0\cdot053\ \alpha/\beta$.

*2. Sacrifice of total dose*: As the dose per fraction decreases, the total dose required to reach a given biological effect approaches a limiting value. The flexure dose could be defined by specifying what percentage the isoeffect total dose should be of this limiting value. Again it follows that the flexure dose is a multiple of the ratio $\alpha/\beta$. When the specified resolution is 5%, the flexure dose is given by $0\cdot05\ \alpha/\beta$.

*3. Statistical formulation*: If the isoeffect assay is repeated, the resulting data would differ from those obtained previously, and consequently the estimates of the isoeffect dose would differ by some amount. Suppose that $D$ and $D'$ are theoretical values of the isoeffect dose and that $D'$ corresponds to a smaller dose per fraction than does $D$. Then it would be expected that $D'$ is greater than $D$. Because of statistical variation in the data, however, there is some probability of obtaining estimates of $D$ and $D'$ such that $D'$ is less than or equal to $D$. The isoeffect doses $D$ and $D'$ could be considered essentially equal if the probability of observing $D'$ less than or equal to $D$ is sufficiently high. This leads to the following definition of the flexure dose: let $d_f$ be the largest fractional dose for which the probability of obtaining estimates $D$ and $D'$ with $D'$ less than or equal to $D$ exceed some prescribed value $p$, where $D$ is the value of isoeffect dose corresponding to the dose per fraction $d_f$, and where $D'$ is any value of the isoeffect dose corresponding to a dose per fraction smaller than $d_f$. The resulting expression for the flexure dose is consistent with each of the previously derived expressions for the flexure dose in that it is a multiple of the ratio $\alpha/\beta$.

Other definitions of the flexure dose are possible, and each of them leads to a definition of flexure dose as some constant multiple of the ratio $\alpha/\beta$, lying in the range $0\cdot05\alpha/\beta$ to $0\cdot15\alpha/\beta$ in agreement with Fowler *et al.* (1983). The simplest summary of the results would therefore be: 'the flexure dose is smallest for late-reacting normal tissues, and largest for tumours and acutely responding normal tissues'.

The LQ model was used to derive each of the expressions for the flexure dose. It is possible that the dose–response characteristics of a cell population are better described by some other model, such as the two-component model, which may be more nearly exponential in the low-dose region. In this case, the LQ model can be viewed as an approximation to the true curve over some dose range. One pitfall, however, is that the flexure dose may well be larger than approximated by the LQ model if the true dose—survival curve of the target cells is exponential over some appreciable initial region. That this may well be the case is suggested by Ang et al. (1985b), who found that isoeffective doses for spinal cord paralysis predicted by the LQ model were higher than those measured experimentally for fraction sizes in the range 1 to 2 Gy. Similarly, Stewart et al. (1987) found that the fit of the LQ model was poor for isoeffect doses for kidney damage when doses per fraction were lower than 2 Gy. These discrepancies might be explained, however, by incomplete repair during the relatively short intervals (4 hours—cord; 5 hours—kidney) used in some of the experiments (Thames 1987b).

## Correlation between clinical and experimental $\alpha/\beta$ values for late effects

Suppose that the level of late complications may be assessed clinically in two fractionation schemes. In the first of these the total dose $D_1$ is given in fractions of size $d_1$, while on average in the second regimen the total dose $D_2$ is given in fractions of size $d_2$. By algebraic manipulation it can be shown that if reactions are more severe in the first fractionation scheme, then

$$\alpha/\beta < \frac{d_2 D_2 - d_1 D_1}{D_1 - D_2} \tag{3.8}$$

while the opposite inequality holds if reactions are more severe in the second fractionation scheme. To illustrate how equation (3.8) can be used, it may be recalled that late reactions are more severe after the use of large dose fractions. If the larger dose per fraction is denoted by $d_1$, the equation above shows that an upper bound for the $\alpha/\beta$ ratio may be derived, if the differences in responses are statistically significant. For example, Atkins (1964) found that muscular atrophy was more severe after treatment with 2 fractions of 1250 cGy than it was after treatment with 20 fractions of 250 cGy. Therefore, we may deduce that the $\alpha/\beta$ ratio that describes muscular atrophy in humans is less than $7\cdot 5$ Gy as shown by the following calculation:

$$\alpha/\beta < \frac{2\cdot 5(50) - 12\cdot 5(25)}{25 - 50} = 7\cdot 5.$$

The results of similar comparisons are presented for a variety of normal tissues in Table 3.7. Values of $\alpha/\beta$ for a variety of late effects are presented, as are the experimental animals in which they were studied, the authors, and the results of clinical comparisons calculated as described in the foregoing. The experimental data do not conflict with the

Table 3.7. Late effects $\alpha/\beta$ (Gy): experimental and clinical

| Tissue (endpoints) | Experimental | Clinical |
|---|---|---|
| Dermis/subcutis (fibrosis contraction telangiectasia) | Mouse: 4·6 (Masuda et al. 1980)<br><br>Pig: $0·3 < \alpha/\beta < 2·4$ (Withers et al. 1978) | < 7·5 (Atkins 1964)<br>< 10 (Sause et al. 1981)<br>< 6 (Overgaard 1984b)<br>3—5 (Turesson and Notter 1984a) |
| Cartilage or bone (necrosis) | | < 4·4 (Horiot et al. 1972)<br>< 4·2 (Stell & Morrison 1973; Fletcher et al. 1974)<br>< 10·6 (Kok 1973)<br>3·4 (Henk & James 1977)<br>4·5 (Horiot et al. 1985) |
| Lung (pneumonitis) | Mouse: 3—6 (Field et al. 1976<br>Wara et al. 1973<br>Travis et al. 1987<br>Vegesna et al. 1985<br>Parkins et al. 1985) | 4·2 (Katz and Alberts 1983)<br><br>4·7 (Overgard 1984) |
| Spinal cord (myelopathy) | Rat: 1·7—4 (Masuda et al. 1977<br>White & Hornsey 1978<br>van der Kogel 1979<br>Ang et al. 1987) | < 3·3 (Dische et al. 1981)<br><br>< 7·0 (Abbatucci et al. 1978) |
| Bowel (stricture perforation) | Rat: 9·6 (Breiter & Trott 1986)<br>Mouse: 3—5 (Terry & Denekamp 1984) | < 6 (Bennett 1978)<br>< 8 (Singh 1978)<br>$\geqslant$ 2·2 (Edsmyr et al. 1984) |

clinical data for any of the late endpoints, with the possible exception of bowel.

By and large, the lowest dose per fraction used in the experimental studies is higher than the dose per fraction used in the clinical comparison. This is a matter of some concern, since extrapolation of the isoeffect curve outside the range of the experimental data for which it is valid could result in serious error. As mentioned above, there has been some indication of a discrepancy in the experimental studies employing doses per fraction in the range 1 Gy to 2 Gy. Even if this was due to incomplete repair, it is important that the $\alpha/\beta$ model be validated over the entire range (in terms of dose per fraction and fractionation interval) in which it might conceivably be used, for example in hyperfractionated radiotherapy.

In summary, there would seem to be no contradiction between experimental and clinical results, with the possible exception of late complications in the bowel. A great deal of caution is called for, however, in employing the LQ model at doses per fraction outside the range in which estimates of $\alpha/\beta$ have been determined.

Practical examples of dosage calculations when changing schedules are given in Section 6.10, for changes in dose per fraction, fractionation interval in twice-a-day schedules, and dose rate.

## 3.6. Hyperfractionation

Suppose that a conventional radiotherapy treatment of 35 fractions of 2 Gy per fraction in 7 weeks was modified so that the dose per fraction was significantly reduced, but the overall time remained the same. The total dose is increased to exploit increased late normal-tissue tolerance, so that two or three fractions per day would have to be given, with account taken of the time necessary for complete repair. There are reasons for believing that a therapeutic gain would result from this strategy, called hyperfractionation, in treatment situations where late normal-tissue reactions are dose-limiting (Thames *et al.* 1982, 1983; Douglas 1982a, b; Barendsen 1982; Withers *et al.* 1982a, b; Peters *et al.* 1982; Fowler 1984a,b).

**Rationales for hyperfractionation**

*Redistribution*
Cells surviving a dose of radiation will be grouped predominantly in the more resistant phases of the cell cycle. Allowing these to redistribute themselves through the cycle will improve the efficiency of killing by the next dose. Since redistribution occurs in all cycling cells, normal and neoplastic, no therapeutic gain will occur relative to normal epithelial cells, which determine acute reactions. However, the cells generally considered responsible for late reactions are very slowly cycling. They will be less sensitized by redistribution, resulting in less severe late reactions for a given level of tumour control, or conversely better tumour control for a given level of late reactions (Withers 1975a). Redistribution would be expected to cause some self-sensitization in proliferative normal tissues, increasing the severity of acute normal-tissue reactions.

*Higher fractionation sensitivity of late-effects tissues*
It is reasonable to postulate that tumours with an actively dividing clonogenic population would respond like acutely reacting normal tissues, while those with slowly dividing clonogens may mimic slowly reacting normal tissues in their response to multifractionated radiotherapy. Therefore, relative to both acutely responding normal tissues and most tumours, late-responding normal tissues (and slowly

proliferating tumours) would be spared by hyperfractionation of dose. This rationale for a therapeutic gain is illustrated in Figure 3.20. By *decreasing* the size of dose per fraction below 2 Gy, it should be possible to increase the total dose for equivalent late effects (Figure 3.20(a)). Because of the less curvy survival curve for acute effects, this increase in total dose will significantly increase the kill of acute-effects target cells (Figure 3.20(b)). Inasmuch as the response of many tumours to radiation is more like that of acute- than of late-responding normal tissues (since it is determined by depopulation of actively proliferating cells), it can be predicted that the tumour-cell kill would be increased, for the same level of late reactions, so that the therapeutic ratio with respect to late normal-tissue injury would be improved by hyperfractionation. A corollary of this is that acute normal-tissue reactions would be exacerbated by hyperfractionation (Withers *et al.* 1982a), and that no therapeutic gain would be realized between these and the tumour.

Other rationales for hyperfractionation have been proposed. Littbrand *et al.* (1975) pointed out that the OER may be reduced at low doses per fraction and an opportunity to circumvent the protection afforded by hypoxia might be gained by significant reduction of the fraction size. Later, a reduction in OER after low doses was confirmed (Palcic and Skarsgard 1984).

### Clinical experience with hyperfractionation

Reported clinical experience with predominantly hyperfractionated regimens (Table 3.8) has been limited. Edsmyr *et al.* (1985) treated carcinoma of the bladder with three small (1 Gy) doses per day to a total dose of 84 Gy, with a two-week rest interval after 42 Gy. Their original rationale was that, in view of the likely decrease of the OER with decreasing dose per fraction, there would be reduced protection of hypoxic tumour cells at doses per fraction of 1 Gy (Littbrand *et al.* 1975). There was a clear indication of an improvement in results (e.g. improved survival in T3 patients: $p < 0.01$), with complications similar to, but significantly worse than, those encountered in conventional treatment. In the hyperfractionation group, 10/83 patients had complications requiring surgery, as opposed to 4/85 in the conventionally treated group. However, a split course was used for the conventional arm and the total dose was only 64 Gy, so that it is likely these patients were relatively underdosed and consequently did not constitute a valid control group.

Parsons *et al.* (1984) reported the results of twice-a-day irradiation for moderately advanced and advanced squamous cell carcinomas of the head and neck in 50 patients; similar to the technique used by Meoz *et al.* (1984), the time was somewhat shorter (6 − 6·5 weeks) than with

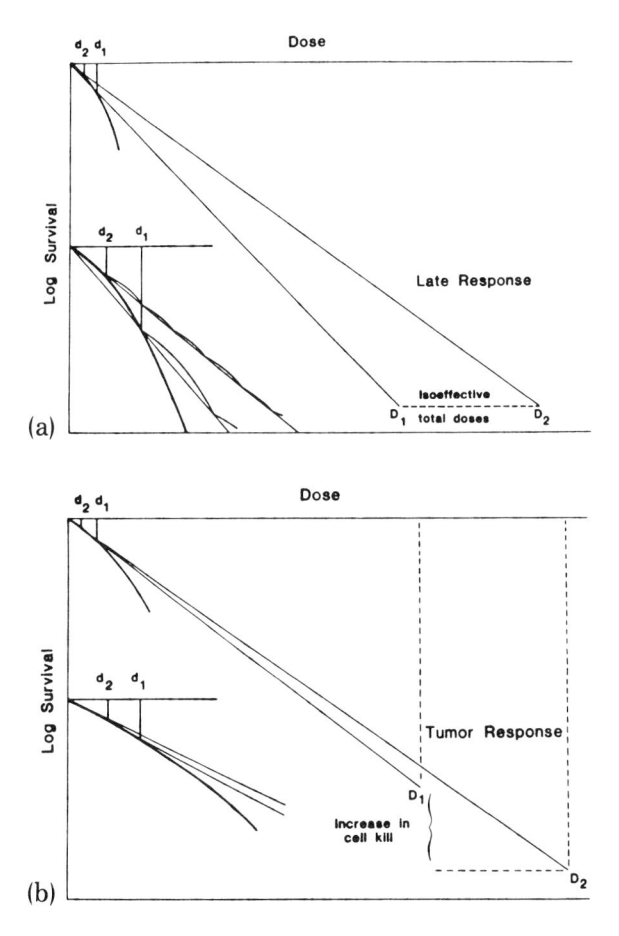

Figure 3.20. Therapeutic gain from hyperfractionation based on late reactions (from Thames et al. 1983). The single-dose survival curve for late effects is 'curvier' in the dose range of clinical interest than is that for acute effects (b). The inserts in (a) and (b) show the reduction in survival after single doses $d_2$ to $d_1$ in more detail. (a) A given level of late injury results when the total dose $D_1$ is fractionated into multiple doses of size $d_1$. Reduction in size of dose per fraction from $d_1$ to $d_2$ decreases the slope of the fractionated response (insert) allowing the total dose for a given level of late injury to be increased from $D_1$ to $D_2$. (b) Kinetically, tumour response is analogous to an acute normal-tissue reaction since both are determined by depopulation of actively proliferating cells. Therefore, the same changes in dose per fraction and total dose would result in a greater degree of depopulation in tumour cells having a less curvy dose—survival curve. If the daily dose were increased from $d_1$ to $(D_2/D_1)d_1$ by giving multiple fractions daily of size $d_2$, the total dose $D_2$ would be delivered in the same overall time as the smaller dose $D_1$, with the same level of late responses and an increased rate of tumour control. (Reproduced with permission of Pergamon Journals Ltd.)

Table 3.8. Clinical studies of predominantly hyperfractionated regimens

| Site | No. of pts | T(wks) | Fx/day | Dose/Fx (Gy) | Total dose (Gy) | Reference |
|---|---|---|---|---|---|---|
| Bladder ($T_2-T_4$) | 83 | 8[a] | 3 | 1 | 84 | Edsmyr et al. (1985) |
| Head and neck | 17 | 9[a] | 3 | 1 | 84 | Bäckstrom et al. (1973) |
| Head and neck | 21 | 7−8 | 2 | 1·1 | 75 | Medini et al. (1985) |
| Head and neck | 65 | 5−6½ | 2 | 1·1−1·2 | 60−75 | Meoz et al. (1984) |
| Head and neck | 126 | 7−8 | 2 | 1·15 | 80·5 | Horiot et al. (1985) |
| Head and neck | 450 | 6−6·5 | 2 | 1·2 | 74·4−76·8 | Parsons et al. (1984) |

[a] Split course: 2-week rest after 42 Gy.

conventional treatment (7 weeks), so that these series may be better described as combined rationales—a mixture of hyperfractionation and accelerated fractionation (Section 4.3). Local control was achieved in 11/13 T3 lesions that received ⩾ 74·4 Gy; although 74·4 Gy controlled only 1/10 T4 tumours, doses higher than this controlled 3/8 of these lesions. There was one severe complication of irradiation and two of salvage surgery. The authors considered these results at least as good as those obtained with conventional once-a-day fractionation.

Horiot et al. (1985) reported the results of a randomized trial of hyperfractionation given to 254 patients with advanced head and neck cancer using 2×1·15 Gy daily, with a total of 80·5 Gy given in seven weeks. At 36 months local control was 72% in the hyperfractionation arm and 56% in the control (70 Gy in 35 fractions in seven weeks) arm ($p=0·15$). However, in patients with Karnovsky status 90−100, the results were 72% and 42%, respectively ($p=0·09$). In April 1987, the difference in favour of hyperfractionation was significant for all patients ($p=0·05$), but even more so ($p=0·001$) for Karnovsky status 90−100 (Horiot, private communication). There were no significant differences in complications, although maximum acute tolerance was approached in the hyperfractionation arm.

Medini et al. (1985) reported that a better response was obtained by treating patients who had massive advanced squamous cell carcinoma of the head and neck with 2 × 1·1 Gy daily to a total dose of 75 Gy than with 70 Gy given in 2 Gy fractions; 53% (8/15) of the patients showed no evidence of primary tumour at the end of therapy, and 60% showed complete regression of cervical lymphadenopathy. Meoz et al. (1984) reported on the treatment of 65 patients with advanced squamous cell carcinoma of the head and neck (primary or advanced neck disease) with hyperfractionation, defined as 11 to 12 Gy per week, given in 10 fractions of 1·1−1·2 Gy to a total dose of 60−75 Gy in 5 to 6½ weeks. The time interval between fractions was 3 to 6 hours (some intervals were possibly too short for complete repair in late-effects tissues). Of 38 evaluated patients with advanced primary disease, 13 (38%) were controlled, and of 20 patients with advanced neck disease, 54% were controlled for at least 1 year. The incidence of late complications was 17% (11/65), of which three were fatal. These results were considered encouraging, given the advanced state of the disease.

Bäckstrom et al. (1973) gave hyperfractionated therapy (Table 3.8) to 17 patients with advanced squamous cell carcinomas of the upper respiratory and digestive tracts; of these, 8 were initially considered operable and 9 inoperable. Response to radiation rendered 5 of these 9 suitable for surgery. Of the remaining 4, 2 had local control. Hyperfractionation was employed in the treatment of 12 patients with noninflammatory breast disease (T3 + T4) who did not respond to chemotherapy and whose tumours were clinically unresectable (Montague, private communication). Of 12 patients treated between 1974 and 1977, tumours in 11 were controlled locally.

The importance of sufficient intervals between fractions, probably 6 hours or more, is emphasized by the results of Nguyen et al. (1985). A practical case is considered in example 6 of section 6.10.

To summarize, a therapeutic gain is expected from hyperfractionation because of differences in *repair* between tumours and normal tissues. The experience with it has been somewhat limited, but implies that a benefit may be realized when late-responding normal tissues are dose limiting, because of the possibility of giving larger doses with equivalent late sequelae. This emphasizes the point that the potential advantages of hyperfractionation might be lost if significant increases in the total dose do not accompany the use of markedly reduced fraction sizes.

# Chapter 4
# Proliferative response to radiation injury

In the previous chapter the role of cellular repair processes in tissue recovery from radiation injury has been considered. The sensitivity of target-cell populations was assumed constant throughout fractionated and low-dose-rate exposures in this discussion. This assumption is valid in many late-responding normal tissues; however, the target cells of tumours and acutely responding normal tissues cycle sufficiently rapidly when treatment is protracted for their response to be determined to a substantial degree by fluctuating sensitivity and the outright repopulation of survivors.

After large single doses of radiation, the ensuing proliferative response may be studied in the absence of considerations involving altered radiosensitivity, since the latter does not occur during the acute dose delivery. The same is approximately true of closely spaced fractionated exposures given in overall times short enough for progression and proliferation of slowly cycling stem cells in normal tissues to be negligible during treatment; in addition the radiation may 'freeze' the cells at one or more blocks in the division cycle. However, when treatment is spread over a long enough time for (stimulated) progression and repopulation to begin to occur, the situation is different, since the cycling status of cell populations may affect their radiosensitivity, the number of cells at risk changes, reoxygenation may occur in tumours, etc. These considerations suggest that a distinction should be drawn between a proliferative response *following* radiation injury, and proliferation that occurs *during* a fractionated or low-dose-rate exposure.

In this chapter proliferative responses in various tissues and tumours following single or fractionated doses are described. Attention then turns to a consideration of the response of tissues and tumours in which the target cells are in, or are induced into, active proliferation during fractionated or continuous radiation exposures, and to changes in fractionation sensitivity that might ensue. The clinical application of these ideas is discussed, as well as their implications for retreatment.

## 4.1. Proliferative response following single and fractionated doses

Following a single dose, the response of cell populations follows a consistent sequence of events. First, there is a delay in progression through the division cycle (mitotic delay) that is linearly related to the dose of radiation and to the cycle time (Denekamp 1975, Chwalinski and Potten 1986). Cells accumulate at the $G_2/M$ boundary and, in the more slowly renewing populations, probably also at the $G_1/S$ boundary (Nagasawa *et al.* 1984). Some of the cells die of the radiation-induced damage at a subsequent mitosis. For example, cells *in vitro* will be delayed approximately one cycle time after 10 Gy, and will then progress through $G_2$ into mitosis, where they will lyse and die. At lower radiation doses cells that have been lethally damaged may undergo successful divisions only to die at a subsequent mitosis. Similar events occur *in vivo*, and when the cell cycle time is longer than it is *in vitro* the time of cell death is delayed correspondingly (here we ignore the exceptions to the rule of death at mitosis, e.g. lymphocytes, which can die during interphase). Second, following the death of appreciable numbers of cells in tissues, there is a homeostatic response in most normal tissues and perhaps in some tumours as well. Whether it is triggered by the death of proliferative cells or by an ensuing deficit of cells in the nonproliferative functional compartment is unknown, but it seems likely that the earliest time of setting off faster cycling and repopulation of stem cells would be after actively proliferating cells had died. Accordingly, the latest possible time would be related to the lifetime of cells in the functional compartment. The last step is the expression of tissue injury, which occurs at a time related to the transit times of cells through any resistant last divisions of proliferative cells and through the functional compartment. A more detailed treatment of these topics can be found in Chapter 1.

### Early-responding normal tissues

*Skin*
The timing of the radiation response following single or fractionated doses is correlated with the turnover kinetics of skin (reviewed by Denekamp & Fowler 1977; Potten 1985a). The basal cells in mouse skin (cf. Figure 1.2) have an average cell-cycle time of 4 to 5 days, and a transit time through the superficial layers of 10 to 15 days (Hegazy &

Fowler 1973). Desquamation occurs after doses of 20 to 30 Gy at 15 to 20 days following exposure, and this is equal approximately to the transit time from the least-differentiated resistant transit cell to the surface (Potten 1981). By contrast, skin that has been stimulated prior to irradiation by plucking of hairs develops a reaction earlier, and this may be considered a system in which active proliferation can occur during protracted irradiation. Considerable mitotic delay occurs after large doses, followed by cell death in the basal layer; however, the rate of progression of cells into the superficial layers remains unchanged for several days (Etoh et al. 1975; Potten 1981). Ultimately, the failure of cell production in the basal layer results in a deficit of cell supply to the superficial layers, and desquamation results. The deficit of basal cells may be a signal for rapid compensatory proliferation in transit and in stem cells, a response that is delayed about one to two weeks after large single doses or after multiple small doses of radiation. After surgical or mechanical wounding, however, the loss of basal cells is more rapid and enhanced proliferation occurs within 24 hours. This also occurs after UV irradiation, possibly because of the prompt sterilization of both stem and transit basal cells (Potten 1981).

As a result of cell depletion the average cycle time of the basal cells is reduced from the 4 to 5 days characteristic of unirradiated cells to 2 days after moderate damage, or to 1 day after severe depletion (Denekamp 1973; Denekamp et al. 1976). Denekamp (1973) gave 4, 9, or 14 daily doses of 3 Gy to the feet of mice and measured the degree of recovery by determining the dose increment required subsequently to induce a specified level of injury. After 4 fractions there was no measurable repopulation for two weeks. After 9 fractions about 0·5 Gy/day was required to counteract repopulation. After 14 fractions, 1·3 Gy/day was needed during the first week after treatment, and this fell to about 0·2 Gy/day in the second week. This was interpreted to mean that no repopulation had occurred after the first week of treatment (at the rate of 3 Gy/day). After two weeks the epithelial cells had increased their proliferation rate by a factor of 2, and after three weeks the average cell cycle time had been reduced by a factor of 4 or 5 (Denekamp et al. 1976).

*GI tract*

The mucosal lining of the gastrointestinal (GI) tract is the most rapidly renewing system in the body. In the mouse, average cell-cycle times of 10 to 12 hours have been measured in the proliferative zone in the crypts (Lesher et al. 1966). The crypts rapidly recognize radiation injury by accelerated proliferation (Hageman et al. 1971, 1972). During compensatory proliferation, the average cell-cycle time of the transit cells is as short as 6 hours (Lesher & Bauman 1969).

The shortening of the cell cycle time measured by Lesher & Bauman (1969) occurred very rapidly. One day after an acute dose of 3 Gy, they noticed a reduction in cycle time to 10·4 hours (relative to the control value of 13·1 hours). This returned to normal by 4 to 8 days. After 10 Gy they observed a remarkable shortening of the cycle time to less than 7 hours. The cycle time of the stem cells is normally about 24 hours (Potten & Hendry 1983a), but during compensatory proliferation it decreases markedly and probably approaches that of the transit cells. However, the doubling time is longer than the cycle time because of the continued differentiation of stem cells into the transit compartment. The doubling time of clonogenic cells following severe depletion is probably about 24 hours (Potten & Hendry 1975; Hendry 1979b), although there are much lower estimates (Withers & Elkind 1969). The timing of the proliferative response varies with the turnover time in the unperturbed state: it is fastest in the jejunum and stomach and slower in the colon. Using colony assays, postirradiation delays before repopulation of colony-forming cells have been reported to be 2·5 days in jejunum (Withers & Elkind 1969), 1 day in the stomach (Chen & Withers 1972), and 4 days in the colon (Withers 1971). In the stomach, where the proliferative cells have an average cell-cycle time of 28 hours (Frankfurt 1967), repopulation occurred more gradually than in the jejunum and colon, after a lag of 1 day and with a doubling time of 43 hours (Chen & Withers 1972).

*Bone marrow*
The haematopoietic system may be divided into three major classifications of cells: the pluripotent stem cells, the committed precursor cells, and the morphologically recognizable maturing cells that lead directly to functional end cells. Proliferation may occur in any of the immature cell populations, and control over cell proliferation is possible at any point in their sequence of development (reviewed by Lord 1986).

The pluripotent stem cell is normally defined by the spleen-colony assay (Till & McCulloch 1961) as a colony-forming unit (CFU-S). The precursor cell committed to granulocyte/macrophage production is defined by an *in vitro* colony test as a GM−CFC, and pre-GM−CFC can be assayed using diffusion chambers implanted *in vivo*. *In vitro* tests of erythrocyte precursor cells involve the production of colonies (CFU-E) or clusters (BFU-E) of erythroid cells, and *in vivo* the erythropoietin responsive (ERC) cell is defined by its ability to produce erythrocytes in the polycythemic mouse. CFU-S are mostly nonproliferating or have very slow turnover times (Becker *et al.* 1965), and the other precursor cells are cycling more rapidly. Following the initial depletion of CFU-S by radiation, there is a post-irradiation 'dip' in CFU-S numbers which has not been satisfactorily explained. Between 0·5 and 4·5 Gy there is a dose-independent decrease in CFU-S of about 50% over a period of 4–6 hours (Hendry & Lord 1983). Possible reasons invoked have been radiation-induced CFU-S differentiation (Lahiri & van Putten 1972) or continued natural differentiation during a period of mitotic delay (Wu & Lajtha 1975).

Following 3- or 4·5-Gy X-rays and this delay, the CFU-S population in mice regrows with a doubling time of about 24 hours in the femur, with approximately one half of them in S phase (reviewed by Hendry & Lord 1983). It has been deduced that this is compatible with a cycle time as short as 6 hours, and a 40% rate of differentiation in each cycle (Lajtha *et al.* 1971). Subsequently, the proportion of cells in S phase decreases, with a slowing growth rate as recovery nears completion. An interesting feature of this recovery was that it occurred over a long time. It is a common finding that when CFU-S in the bone marrow reach 30% of normal, subsequent recovery is extremely slow (Valeriote *et al.* 1968; Guzman & Lajtha 1970; Hendry & Lajtha 1972).

Following depopulation, red-cell production and the ERC population recover faster from damage than the CFU-S or GM-CFC (Blackett *et al.* 1964; Chervenick & Boggs 1971; Testa *et al.* 1974). Thus, when the ERC recover completely, differentiation pressure on the CFU-S is released and CFU-S turnover declines. This seems to occur at a time well before the CFU-S population has fully recovered.

It has been demonstrated that during a continuous daily X-ray exposure of 0·5 to 0·84 Gy, the erythroid and granulocytic cells in rat bone marrow compensate for the depletion in stem cell levels by increasing their net proliferation rates. This is achieved by increasing the number of cell cycles during maturation and by shortening their average time, leading to an enhanced level of cell production (Lord 1964, 1965, 1968).

*Lip mucosa*

Lip mucosa in mice has been used recently as another example of the response of mucosal tissue to fractionated irradiation, although there is little knowledge of its proliferative characteristics after injury.

The overall reaction period for the mouse lip mucosa after radiation injury is shorter than for skin (Parkins *et al.* 1983; Xu *et al.* 1984). Comparing the pattern of the reaction of lip mucosa to that of foot skin of mice of the same strain allows several conclusions. First, the peak of the mucosal reaction is reached earlier (day 11 to 12 versus 17 to 18), and recovery takes place in a correspondingly shorter interval (about 7 versus 12 days). This suggests that the cycle time of the renewing populations in the lip mucosa is shorter than that of the basal cells of the epidermis. Second, lip mucosa is much more sensitive to radiation than skin. A single dose of 16·5 Gy induces confluent desquamation of the mucosa, while a similar epidermal reaction requires 31 Gy. Split-dose experiments showed that repopulation started within 3 days after the first irradiation (Ang et al. 1985a). One would conclude, therefore, that in the mouse the proliferative response in lip mucosa is faster than that of skin, but slower than that of the jejunal epithelium. There are, however, no data to show a definite acceleration of growth following radiation injury.

## Tumours

Denekamp & Fowler (1977) reviewed studies performed to determine whether cells in irradiated tumours can show a compensatory proliferative response after large single doses. In these studies changes were measured in the average cell-cycle time after irradiation, as well as changes in cell survival, cell density, and growth fraction. In other studies, the average rate of tumour-cell repopulation was derived from the connection between cell survival shortly after treatment and the ensuing growth delay (Stephens & Steel 1980). The sequential measurement of cell survival at various times after treatment allowed changes in repopulation during tumour regeneration to be detected.

In studies reviewed by Denekamp (1975), only two of the ten solid tumours showed a shortened cell-cycle time after irradiation (Hermens & Barendsen 1969; van Peperzeel 1970, 1972). Six others showed no change in cycle time (Denekamp & Thomlinson 1971; Tubiana et al. 1968; Nelson et al. 1976), whereas two showed elongated cell-cycle times (Brown 1970; Szczepanski & Trott 1975). In the rhabdomyosarcoma studied by Hermens and Barendsen, the response was associated with changes in density of cells. Thus, the cell cycle shortened to a value similar to that of an earlier phase of tumour growth, when the cell density decreased as a consequence of loss of dead cells. This change in cycle time was also shown by ascites tumours of different ages and cell densities.

Another way cell production increases is by increasing the fraction of cells in growth (the growth fraction). This results from an active triggering stimulus in normal tissues, but in tumours it seems more likely to result from an improvement in nutritional or oxygenation status on account of, for example, death of neighbouring cells or changes in vasculature. The death of some of the well oxygenated, radiosensitive cells lying close to the vasculature will reduce the rate of utilization of nutrients. Previously hypoxic or nutritionally deprived cells then gain access to an improved nutritional oxygen supply, which may enable them to re-enter the cell cycle. An increase in the growth fraction was observed in five of eight of the tumours reviewed by Denekamp (1975). Barendsen et al. (1973) found that labelled colonies of tumour cells originated from both proliferating (P) and quiescent (Q) cells. Thus, Q cells could be the main source of cells that repopulate a tumour after radiation, especially after single doses so large that only hypoxic Q cells would be expected to survive.

An increased rate of tumour growth might also result from a reduction in the rate of cell loss after radiation. Although some studies reported faster volume doubling rates in lung tumours after radiation (van Peperzeel 1970; Malaise et al. 1972), Denekamp (1975) concluded that most studies showed a slower growth rate and increased rate of cell loss after radiation injury.

Stephens & Steel (1980) described the use of tumour cell survival and growth delay after treatment to study cell repopulation patterns in two experimental mouse tumours. When the median time for Lewis lung tumours to grow to four times their treatment volume was plotted against surviving fraction after radiation, a nonlinear relationship was obtained, regardless of whether the tumours were hypoxic and treated with misonidazole or oxic in mice breathing air. Growth delay was not linearly related to log survival as would be expected if repopulation occurred at a constant rate independent of the cell kill. The observed growth delay became longer as the extent of cell killing increased. Although this might indicate a gradual decrease in the repopulation rate with increasing radiation dose, the interpretation of the data at levels where there is little cell killing would be difficult. Thus, when the median time to grow to four times treatment volume was small, the tumour volume might have been influenced by factors other than tumour cell repopulation, such as the rate of resorption of killed cells.

Cell-survival assays were performed sequentially on the tumours of mice irradiated with several doses of gamma rays while the mice were breathing air, and these showed that the repopulation doubling time of clonogenic cells ranged from about 1 to 1½ days, with an apparent decrease as the extent of tumour killing increased (Figure 4.1). There was also a gradual increase in the lag period before the rate of clonogenic tumour-cell repopulation reached its maximum (Stephens et al. 1978). These results agreed with those reported by Barendsen & Broerse (1970), who used the rat R1 rhabdomyosarcoma and sequential survival assays to study repopulation after fractionated X-rays and neutrons. There was a lag phase before clonogenic tumour cells began repopulation, but the maximum repopulation rates did not depend on dose.

Steel (1968, 1977) emphasized the role of the cell-loss factor in the change in tumour volume after radiation injury. After severe radiation injury and the resulting interruption of cell production, tumours with high cell-loss factors generally show a rapid volume reduction and those with low cell-loss factors shrink slowly (Denekamp 1972; Denekamp & Fowler 1977). Therefore, as in normal tissues, the time at which cell depletion is recognized is determined by the normal rate of turnover of these cells in tumours. It is interesting to note that in general the

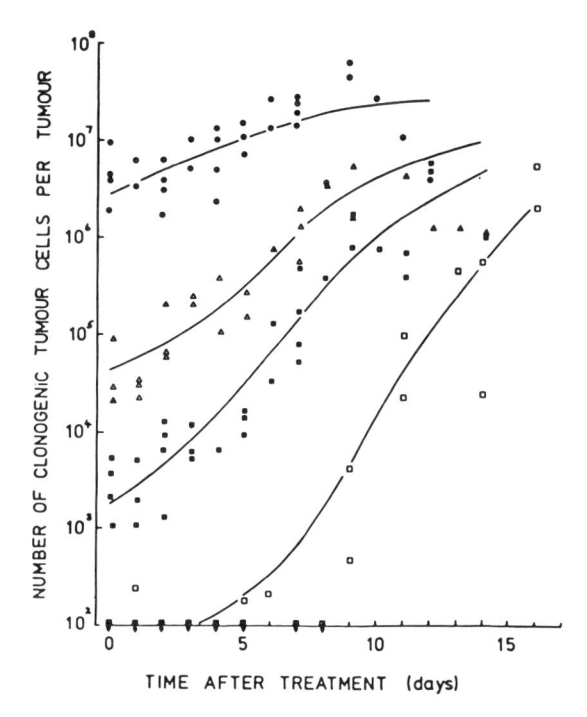

Figure 4.1. Tumour-cell repopulation in the Lewis lung carcinoma following irradiation (from Stephens & Steel 1980). Intramuscular tumours of approximately 0.15 g were irradiated locally with various doses of $^{60}$Co γ-rays in air-breathing mice. Treatments are (triangles) 15 Gy, (closed squares) 25 Gy, (open squares) 35 Gy, and (circles) untreated control. At approximately daily intervals after treatment, pairs of mice were killed and cell survival measured by an *in vitro* clonogenic cell assay. (Reproduced with permission of Raven Press Inc. and the authors.)

tumours with high cell-loss factors (and rapid volume reduction) are carcinomas, which arise from epithelial tissues that are typically in a state of cell production from a minority of precursor cells, with balanced cell loss (MacKillop *et al.* 1983). The sarcomas, on the other hand, exhibit low-cell loss factors and delayed volume reduction after radiation injury. These derive from mesodermal structures, in which the cells are more slowly dividing and more homogeneous in proliferative ability, and where proliferation is marked only following depletion. These differences in proliferative organization emphasize the potential difficulties in correlating the average kinetics of cell populations in tumours with the response of the tumour as a whole (Moore 1983; Steel & Stephens 1983).

To summarize, the rapidly renewing normal tissues and some tumours recover *after* radiation injury by means of a regenerative response. This is preceded by a dose-dependent time lag, and in most tissues and some tumours is characterized by acceleration of growth. This is usually accomplished by means of a shortened cycle time and an increase in the growth fraction. The proliferative response occurs after a time that correlates with the turnover kinetics in the unperturbed state, and in particular is delayed for weeks or months following radiation injury to late-responding tissues.

**Late-responding normal tissues**

In lung, spinal cord, bladder, brain, and kidney, there is very little recovery when the overall irradiation time is prolonged from 1 day to periods as long as 3 months. Although there may be a relatively minor 'slow repair' process manifest over a period of several weeks (Reinhold & Buisman 1973; Field et al. 1976), a proliferative response probably does not occur for many weeks or months after the beginning of radiation treatment. This is in accord with the slow rate of turnover of renewing populations in these tissues. Indeed, the very structural organization of these tissues, which differs from that of the hierarchical, rapidly responding tissues, may dictate a different pattern of proliferative response (Michalowski 1981; Wheldon et al. 1982). In this picture, late-responding normal tissues are 'flexible' in that after radiation injury functional cells can enter the division cycle. Therefore, the loss of any cell might induce a neighbouring cell to attempt division to replace it; this is in contrast to the hierarchical tissues discussed above, where natural cell loss occurs only from the differentiated compartment. Therefore, in addition to the influence of cell kinetic parameters, it is necessary to consider how the tissues will recognize cell depletion and trigger a compensatory response.

## 4.2. Proliferation during fractionated or low-dose-rate exposures

Fractionated or continuous radiation may be considered to have at least three possible effects on the rate of increase in cell number when administered to a dividing population: it may completely stop growth, accelerate growth, or result in behaviour intermediate between these. This will depend on the rate of dose delivery, the radiosensitivity and cell-cycle characteristics of the irradiated population, and homeostatic feedback mechanisms active after recognition of injury by tissues. Concomitantly with altered growth rate, changes in radiosensitivity may occur.

## Dose rate to stop growth

The dose rate necessary to stop growth was different among different cell lines (Szechter et al. 1978; Mitchell et al. 1979). For example, V79 and pig kidney cells required dose rates in excess of 2·7 Gy/h, whereas growth of HeLa cells was stopped by radiation administered at 0·37 Gy/h. For V79 cells, 0·37 Gy/h had little or no effect on growth over three population doublings. Interestingly, the daily dose to stop growth seemed the same, whether given continuously or as fractionated, acute exposures in the studies of Mitchell & Bedford (1977), whereas Szechter et al. (1978) found that continuous irradiation was generally less efficient in slowing growth and cell inactivation than fractionated regimens with similar average dose rates.

Different properties of various cell lines were studied to determine whether any were correlated with the critical dose rate necessary to stop population growth. There was for example no correlation between the dose rate to stop growth and the population doubling time of the controls, even though cell lines had been selected with considerable variation in doubling time. Szechter et al. (1978) observed that, in two cell lines of similar radiosensitivity but different growth rates, the effects of continuous and fractionated irradiation were more pronounced in the line with slower growth rate.

There was, however, an inverse correlation between division delay,

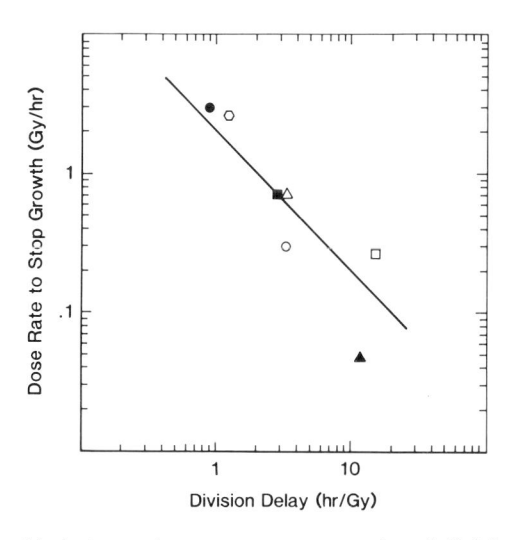

Figure 4.2. Relationship between dose rate to stop growth and division delay, from data of Mitchell et al. (1979). Division delay was the only parameter that showed consistent variation with the dose rate to stop growth; the product of these is dimensionless and approximately equal to 2 for the cell lines studied.

which differed widely between the lines, and the dose rate to stop growth. The data of Mitchell et al. (1979) have been replotted in Figure 4.2, which illustrates that the two are related approximately as (division delay) × (dose rate to stop growth) = constant ≃ 2. The division delay was the only cell-line characteristic that correlated with the dose rate to slow or stop population growth. Interestingly, Szechter et al. (1978) found that the largest effect of changing the dose rate occurred at dose rates of between one and two times the critical dose rate to stop growth.

Changes in sensitivity were observed in the studies of Mitchell et al. (1979), and these were attributed to redistribution and the G2 block. When no division occurred during the radiation exposures, there was a reverse dose-rate effect, i.e. the lower dose rates were more effective in cell killing per unit dose than the higher dose rates (Figure 4.3(b)). This increase in the average radiosensitivity of the population for longer exposure times was attributed to a build up in the radiosensitive $G_2$ phase, when there was negligible cell division. Figure 4.3(a) illustrates that when some division did occur, the reverse dose-rate was lost, possibly because of redistribution into more radioresistant phases of the division cycle.

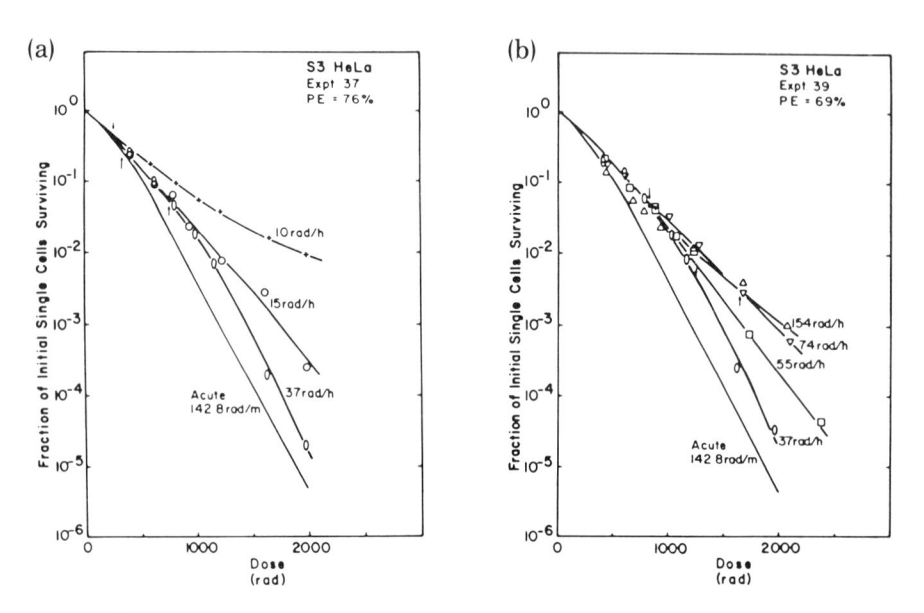

Figure 4.3. Survival curves for log-phase S3 HeLa cells irradiated at different dose rates (caesium-137 gamma-rays) (from Mitchell et al. 1979). (b) illustrates the survival curves in which cell division was not appreciable during exposures. (a) illustrates survival curves for which, in some cases (10 cGy/h and 15 cGy/h), appreciable cell division did occur during exposures. Vertical arrows on the curves indicate the accumulated dose for each dose rate after a time equivalent to one generation time for unirradiated cultures. (Reproduced with permission of Academic Press Inc. and the authors.)

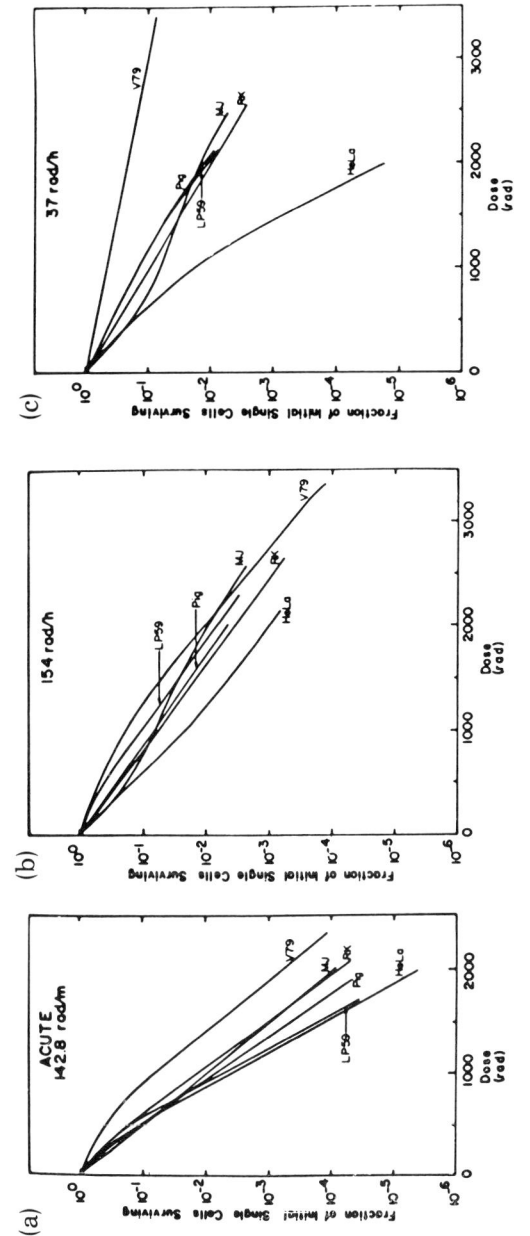

Figure 4.4. A comparison of dose–survival curves for log-phase cultures of six different cell lines irradiated at different dose rates (from Bedford et al. 1980). (a) acute, 142·8 cGy per minute. (b) 154 cGy per hour. (c) 37 cGy per hour. The cell lines were Chinese hamster (V79), Indian muntjac (MJ), rat kangaroo (RK), PK15 pig kidney (Pig), mouse L-P59 (LP59), and human S3 HeLa (HeLa). (Reproduced with permission of Raven Press Inc. and the authors.)

Differences in survival measured after acute doses for the various cell lines were much smaller than those measured at lower dose rates. Figure 4.4 shows a comparison of dose−survival curves for log-phase cultures of six different cell lines and illustrates how differences are accentuated as the dose rate is lowered (Mitchell et al. 1979). These changes cannot be attributed in any significant sense to differences in repair capacity among the cell lines, a point illustrated in Figure 4.5 for two lines that exhibit the widest divergence of behaviour in Figure 4.4, V79 and HeLa. Plateau-phase cultures were irradiated at different dose rates; the reduction in dose rate reduced the effect per unit dose about the same extent for both cell lines. Since cell-cycle effects were eliminated for these $G_0$-like cells, we may conclude that significant sparing from repair occurred in both lines. Therefore the difference between log-phase cultures of V79 and HeLa cells (Figure 4.4), and also among other cell lines, must be attributed to different radiation-induced cell-cycle perturbations in the different lines (Bedford et al. 1980).

## Accelerated growth

In the previous section, data have been presented that indicate a proliferative response in irradiated normal tissues and some tumours after a dose-dependent time lag. In this section the question is whether this can occur *during* fractionated or protracted exposures.

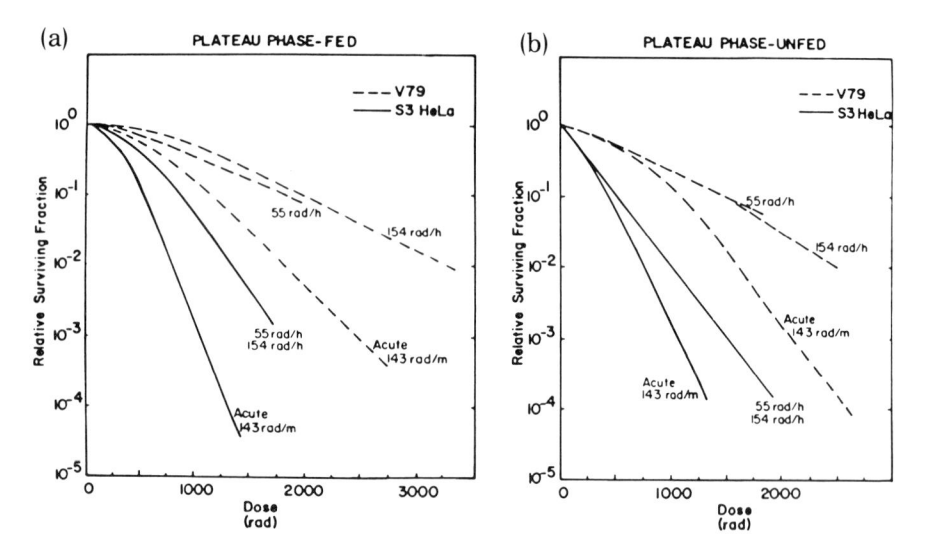

Figure 4.5. A summary of survival curves at different dose rates for fed (a) and unfed (b) plateau-phase cultures (from Mitchell et al. 1979). The dashed lines refer to results for V79 Chinese hamster cells and the solid lines for HeLa cells. (Reproduced with permission of Academic Press Inc. and the authors.)

## Colonic mucosa

Withers & Mason (1974) studied the survival of mouse colonic clonogens after 1 to 20 fractions of gamma rays separated by intervals of 3, 12, and 24 hours. As shown in Figure 4.6, after five fractions the 3-hour interval curve is displaced from the single-dose (0-hour) curve by about 9·4 Gy at a survival of 50 clonogens per circumference. This displacement results almost exclusively from intracellular repair. When the five fractions were separated by 12 hours, a slight displacement (1·5 Gy) to the right occurred, and a bigger displacement (5·5 Gy) resulted with 24-hour intervals. These additional displacements of the survival curves were attributed to regeneration of survivors. The relative roles of repair and regeneration when the dose was divided into ten fractions can be appreciated from Figure 4.7 and Table 4.1. The separation of the 10-fraction, 3-hour curve and the single-dose curve is a measure of repair: at the 50-clonogen survival level it is roughly 15·3 Gy. The separation of the 10-fraction, 24-hour curve from the 10-fraction, 3-hour curve is a measure of additional recovery due to regeneration during the increased overall treatment time (27 hours to 9 days). At the 50-clonogen survival level this is roughly 18·4 Gy. Comparing the 5- and 10-fraction results, it can be seen that recovery results predominantly from repair during the first few (4) days, with regeneration becoming more important as

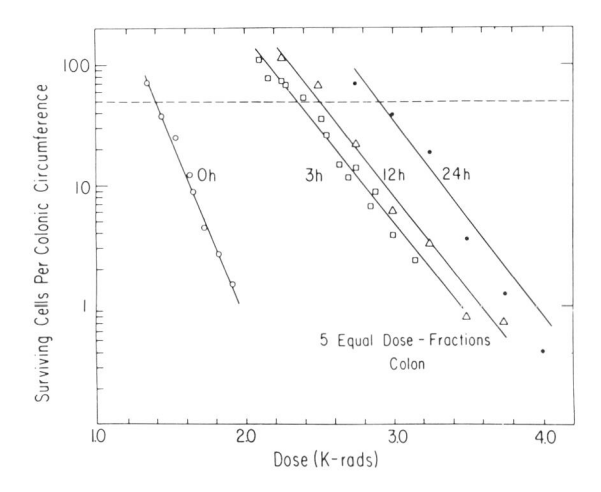

Figure 4.6. Dose−survival curves for colonic crypt cells exposed to single doses or to five fractions separated by 3, 12, or 24 hours (from Withers & Mason 1974). The displacement of the 3-hour curve from the single-dose curve (9·4 Gy at a survival level of 50 cells/circumference) is attributable to repair of sublethal injury during the four fractionation intervals. The additional displacement of the 12-hour and 24-hour curves from the 3-hour curve may be attributed to regeneration of surviving cells between doses. The 24-hour curve is displaced from the 3-hour curve by 5·5 Gy at 50 survivors per circumference. (Reproduced with permission of J.B. Lippincott Inc. and the authors.)

114                  *Fractionation in Radiotherapy*

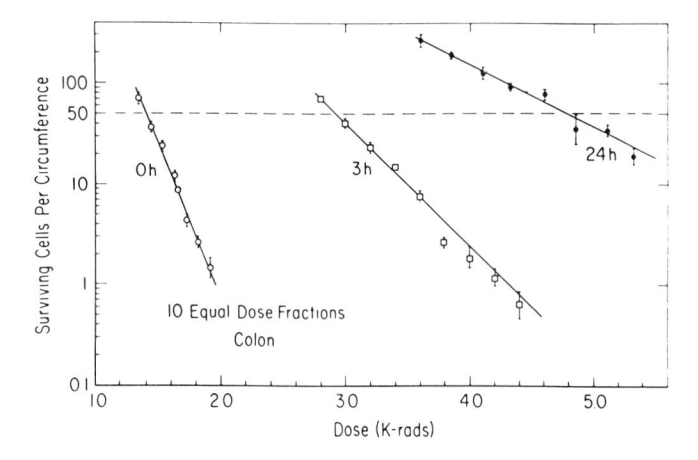

Figure 4.7. Dose—survival curves for colonic crypt cells exposed to single doses or to ten fractions separated by 3 or 24 hours (from Withers & Mason 1974). Displacement of the 3-hour curve (15·3 Gy at 50 survivors per circumference) is attributable to repair of sublethal injury during nine fractionation intervals. The additional displacement of the 24-hour curve (18·4 Gy at 50 survivors per circumference) is attributable to regeneration of surviving cells during the nine days over-all treatment time. (Reproduced with permission of J.B. Lippincott Inc. and the authors.)

treatment time is increased to 9 days. Does this reflect accelerated regeneration of survivors, or simply an increased overall time together with a gradual slowdown in the increase of isoeffect dose with increasing fraction number (cf. Figure 3.9(c))?

Regeneration is reflected in the divergence of the 12- and 24-hour isoeffect doses (repair plus regeneration) from the 3-hour curve (repair only), as illustrated in Table 4.1. Regeneration is slow initially ($t < 2$ days), as illustrated by the slight divergence between isoeffect doses up to three

Table 4.1. Doses (Gy) for an isoeffect of 50 surviving cells per colonic circumference

| Number of fractions | Fractionation intervals (hours) | | |
|---|---|---|---|
| | 3 | 12 | 24 |
| 1 | 11·10 | 11·10 | 11·10 |
| 2 | 18·50 | 17·80 | 19·25 |
| 3 | 20·40 | | 21·85 |
| 4 | | | 25·60 |
| 5 | 23·50 | 25·00 | 29·00 |
| 6 | | | 34·80 |
| 8 | | | 41·00 |
| 10 | 29·40 | 35·10 | 47·80 |
| 15 | 31·00 | | |
| 20 | 34·00 | | |

(Withers & Mason 1974)

fractions (21·9 − 20·4 = 1·5 Gy). After five fractions, the dose attributable to regeneration is 29 − 23·5 = 5·5 Gy. Thus, between the second and fourth days after the beginning of treatment, regeneration accounted for about 4 Gy, or 2 Gy per day, as opposed to 1·5 Gy, or about 0·75 Gy per day, during the first two days. When the total treatment time was extended to nine days (10 fractions), the dose recovered because of regeneration was 18·4 Gy. Therefore, in the five days between four and nine days after the beginning of treatment, regeneration accounted for 18·4 − 5·5 = 12·9 Gy, an average of nearly 2·6 Gy per day.

There is the possibility that repair was incomplete during the 3-hour intervals in those experiments, given the repair half-time of about 0·8 hours (Table 3.6). This would not change the conclusions, but rather would underestimate somewhat the total recovery achievable from repair and regeneration.

From calculations such as these, Withers & Mason (1974) concluded that the doubling time of surviving clonogens shortened as treatment progressed: 48 hours during the first two days, 24 hours between days two and four, and 21·5 hours between four and nine days. Thus, even when division delays were accounted for, there was clear evidence of accelerated growth in colonic mucosa.

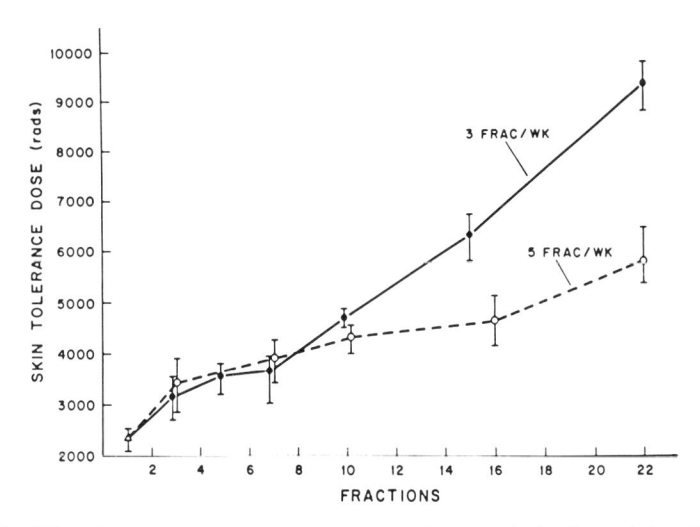

Figure 4.8. Skin-tolerance dose versus fraction number for single doses (triangles), three fractions per week treatments (closed circles), and five fractions per week treatments (open circles) (from Moulder & Fischer 1976). The skin tolerance doses are the doses required to produce acute partial moist desquamation in 50% of animals treated. 95% confidence limits are shown. (Reproduced with permission of J.B. Lippincott Inc. and the authors.)

## Skin

Moulder & Fischer (1976) studied acute skin reactions in the hind legs of rats after X-ray treatment with a wide variety of fraction numbers and treatment times. Their results are presented in Figure 4.8. No significant time-dependent recovery was observed for total times less than 17 days. For longer periods the amount of recovery increased, from about 7·5 Gy/day between 21 and 31 days and 1·25 Gy/day between 31 and 63 days. These daily averages were based on the assumption of constant radiosensitivity (see below, Section 4.3).

There have been reports of a shortening of the average cell-cycle time of basal cells of the epidermis (Devik 1962; Brown & Berry 1969; Hegazy & Fowler 1973; Denekamp et al. 1976). This shortening was moderate (about 25%) in some studies (Brown & Berry 1969) and more pronounced in others (Devik 1962; Denekamp et al. 1976). However, instances of pronounced reduction in cycle time, such as the reduction from 4−5 days in controls to less than 1 day three weeks after fractionated radiation observed by Denekamp et al. (1976), have always occurred after completion of irradiation. It seems reasonable to conclude that *acceleration of regeneration in the skin during fractionated irradiation is not as pronounced as that in the intestinal mucosa.*

## Lip mucosa

Ang et al. (1985a) studied repopulation effects in irradiated mouse lip mucosa during different fractionation regimens. One group received 3 fractions per day, separated by 4 hours (assumed sufficient for complete repair) to a total of 10 fractions. The second group received one exposure per day five times a week, to 10 fractions in 11 days. The third group received a split-course, 3-fractions-per-day schedule in which 5 fractions were given in the first 1·5 days and again after a rest period of 8 days. There was also a split-dose study in which 2 fractions were separated by 1, 3, 5, 7, or 10 days.

Some repopulation was evident in the split-dose study after 3 days. The authors concluded that repopulation accelerated as the time between doses increased, although the differences were small (i.e. 0·4 Gy/day for days 1–3, 0·5 Gy/day between days 3 and 5, 0·6 Gy/day between days 5 and 7, and 1 Gy/day between days 7 and 10). Nevertheless, a trend was evident.

When 10 fractions were given in a split course, an additional recovery of about 5 Gy was observed in excess of the recovery resulting from protraction of treatment to 11 days with 10 daily irradiations. A plausible explanation for this is that repopulation was faster during the rest period between the two courses than during continuous daily irradiations. This interpretation is consistent with the observation of greatly accelerated proliferation in mouse skin *after* irradiation

(Denekamp et al. 1976), but to a smaller degree in rat skin *during* irradiation (Moulder & Fischer 1976). As a corollary, continuous daily irradiation suppressed repopulation for the lip mucosa relative to that potentially achievable in its absence, i.e. with the 8-day rest period.

*Tumours*
Although faster growth after irradiation has been documented for some experimental tumours (reviewed by Denekamp & Fowler 1977) and human lung metastases (van Peperzeel 1970; van Peperzeel 1972; Malaise et al. 1972), there have been few attempts to document this phenomenon during a fractionated or continuous low-dose-rate treatment. Certainly, regeneration of tumour clonogens can occur during treatment. Clinical results with T3 and T4 carcinomas of the larynx were worse when overall times were prolonged (Maciejewski et al. 1983) and the same was true for the treatment of skin tumours (Hliniak et al. 1983). A more difficult issue is whether the *rate* of regeneration increases during treatment, in analogy with normal tissues such as the colonic mucosa. If the volume doubling time (VDT) of tumours reflects the doubling time of their clonogens (growth fraction and cell loss factor assumed constant), then the long VDT of two months for many human tumours suggests that there should be little effect of changing overall treatment times by a few weeks. This is in contrast to the above observations, suggesting that there is accelerated regeneration during treatment.

The data for experimental tumours (Kummermehr & Trott 1982; Kummermehr et al. 1986; and Kummermehr, personal communication) show that repopulation in some types of murine tumours may be accelerated during treatment. Kummermehr's experimental design is illustrated schematically in Figure 4.9. The aim was to determine the degree of repopulation during each week of a three-week treatment. All doses were given under clamp hypoxia to exclude the effects of re-oxygenation. Tumours in the conventional arm were given 6 × 7 Gy per week for 1, 2, or 3 weeks (Figure 4.9(a), middle curves), followed by a test dose (TD). In the comparison arm tumours were given the same doses, except that in the comparison week (1, 2, or 3) the weekly dose was concentrated and given as 6 × 7 Gy/1·5 days, and this was again followed by a test dose to complete treatment (Figure 4.9(b), left curves). This dose per fraction corresponds roughly to 2·5 Gy/fraction in air-breathing animals. The endpoint depicted in Figure 4.9(a) is regrowth delay, and (b) shows the use of local tumour control to address the same question. The curves in (b) correspond to the two left-most curves in (a).

The increment in test dose increased progressively from the first to the third week for the squamous cell carcinoma AT 478, indicating an acceleration of repopulation during treatment (Kummermehr et al. 1986).

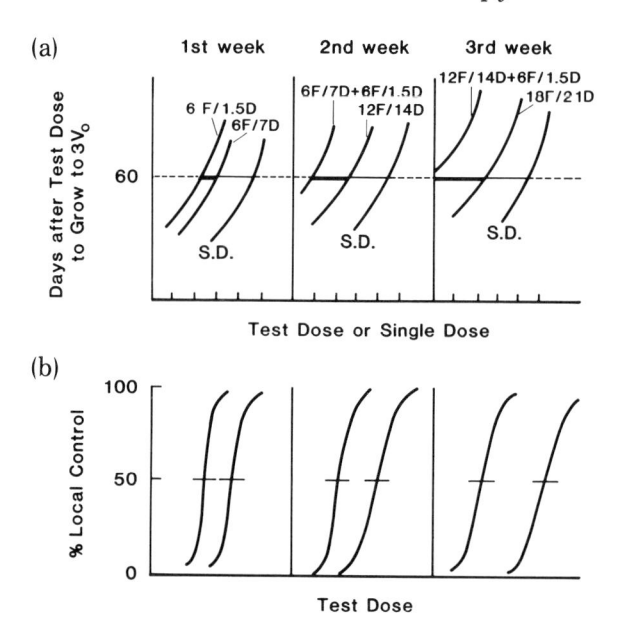

Figure 4.9. Illustration of design of study to assess accelerated growth in tumours during either the first, second or third week of fractionated radiotherapy, using regrowth delay (a) or tumour control (b) (Kummermehr et al. 1986 and Kummermehr, personal communication). The control treatment was $6 \times 7$ Gy per week, and this was continued for one, two, or three weeks after which a range of test doses (TD) was given and regrowth delay (middle curves in (a)) was measured. The same treatment was given in the comparison arm, except that during the week of interest (1, 2, or 3) treatment was compressed to $6 \times 7 \, \text{Gy}/1 \cdot 5$ days + TD, and regrowth delay and tumour control were measured (left curves in (a) and (b)). The displacement of the two leftmost curves is a measure of 'repopulated dose'; in the figure the results suggest a progressive acceleration of growth during the three weeks of treatment.

This was true for both endpoints used, and is similar to the acceleration of growth during treatment seen for the epithelium of normal tissues such as gut. The results in four other mouse tumours were variable during two weeks of treatment. Acceleration of growth occurred for a mammary carcinoma, but the growth rate decreased during the second week for a sarcoma and repopulation appeared to stop completely in the second week for two adenocarcinomas. These results suggest that degree of proliferation varies with histology. Moreover, it was not predictable from any of the cell-kinetic parameters that were determined in conjunction with these studies. However, it generally bore a closer relationship to the potential doubling time than to the overall volume doubling time.

In contrast to the findings of Ang et al. (1985a) that repopulation in the lip mucosa was faster during a rest period between two courses of treatment than during continuous daily irradiations, Kummermehr et al.

(1986) found that the repopulation rate in the squamous cell carcinoma AT 478 stayed constant and then slowed when treatment (6 × 7 Gy/per week) was suspended after two weeks. This indicates a somewhat slower regeneration rate than was measured during the third week when treatment was continued. Clinical results (Parsons et al. 1980a, b), however, indicate no therapeutic benefit from split-course treatment.

To summarize, the data indicate that proliferation does occur in normal tissues and tumours during treatment. Acceleration of growth during treatment has been demonstrated in colonic mucosa and skin, and in some tumours. Repopulation may be faster during a rest interval between two courses of treatment for normal tissues. Therefore fractionated treatment without rest periods seems to suppress repopulation (even though this might be ongoing or even accelerated) relative to what might occur when treatment is discontinued. The opposite behaviour has been observed in one tumour, but in general clinical results do not indicate any therapeutic gain from split-course treatment.

## Change in fractionation sensitivity with accelerated growth

In Section 3.3 it was argued that tissues may differ in their fractionation sensitivity by virtue of differences in cell-cycle time, with longer repair times available to the more slowly turning-over target cell populations in late-effects tissues. The survival curve interpretation was formulated in terms of repair models, in which the shoulder of the survival curve is considered to result from a combination of repair processes and the downward bending caused by an increased killing efficiency per unit dose at higher doses. When viewed in terms of postirradiation repair phenomena, e.g. PLDR (Phillips & Tolmach 1966) or in situ repair (Gould & Clifton 1979), the initial slope would be diminished faster than the final slope with increasing times available for repair; lower $\alpha/\beta$ ratios for slowly cycling target-cell populations would result.

If this hypothesis is correct, the $\alpha/\beta$ ratios for acutely responding tissues could be expected to depend on their proliferative status, increasing when these tissues are stimulated to regenerate after radiation injury. If this occurred, acutely responding tissues would become relatively more sensitive to fractionation regimens with multiple small doses or low dose rate than to those with fewer, larger doses per fraction or higher dose rates. The same would be true of tumours, but to a greater or lesser extent depending on the relative degree to which these are capable of a proliferative response to cell depletion during a course of fractionated irradiation.

The evidence that may be adduced for such changes in $\alpha/\beta$ ratios with changing proliferative status includes both clinical and experimental findings. Although somewhat sparse, it does present a consistent picture.

*Clinical evidence*
Turesson & Notter (1984a) used reflectance spectrophotometry to quantify the acute skin response of patients. They found that early skin reaction (erythema) was more pronounced with three times daily than with once daily fractionation. This relationship was made more precise in another study by the same authors (Turesson & Notter 1984b), where degree of erythema was followed twice weekly in patients receiving 5 × 2 Gy versus 2 × 4 Gy per week. For up to 4 weeks overall time, the acute responses were the same; at 5 and 6 weeks, however, they were worse in the patients receiving 5 × 2 Gy weekly; with 10 weeks split-course therapy with a rest period during the fifth to seventh week, the acute responses were again the same. This timing (4 weeks) is characteristic of the change from steady-state slow turnover of basal cells in humans to a compensatory proliferative response to the radiation injury for a limited time period. Further, contrary to the acute response, the isoeffect relationship for the late response was independent of the overall treatment time (Turesson & Notter 1986).

The idea that tumours might respond better to more highly fractionated treatment is old—see, for example, Coutard's report (1932) on the first successful treatments of deep-seated tumours. His technique involved using once- or twice-a-day treatments given at low dose rates and overall times of 2 or more weeks, aiming for brisk skin and mucosal reactions on the rationale that the radiosensitivity of the cancer cells was the same as that of the regenerative cells of the tissue of origin (see Chapter 5). Cox *et al.* (1980) reported on the treatment of patients with fewer than five fractions per week using megavoltage photons. Fraction size and total doses were varied according to the NSD formula (Ellis 1967). The most frequently used regimen was three fractions per week. The results were compared with those obtained with patients treated in the prior years with five fractions per week. There were 262 patients with inoperable or unresectable carcinoma of the lung of all cell types, including 55% squamous carcinoma, 17% small cell carcinoma, 12% adenocarcinoma, 9% large cell carcinoma, and others. A second group consisted of 94 patients with squamous carcinoma of the oral cavity and oral pharynx. For the lung patients treated with one or two fractions per week, there was a decrease in local control relative to that experienced by patients treated with five fractions per week. In the head and neck patients there was a clear-cut difference, with higher local control in patients treated five times a week compared with those treated three times a week.

In the British Institute of Radiology Study (Wiernik *et al.* 1978) of three versus five fractions per week, there was a tendency toward a higher recurrence rate in patients with glottic tumours who received three fractions per week (hypofractionation). This difference, although significant at first, later became statistically insignificant. Similarly, results of the Medical Research Council trials of hyperbaric oxygen used with radiotherapy for advanced carcinoma of the cervix showed an advantage in local control and survival for patients with stage III disease treated with oxygen (Watson et al. 1978). Two of the four institutions used hypofractionation and two treated patients five times weekly. The difference among institutions is striking in recurrence-free rates in the *control* patients (i.e. those treated without hyperbaric oxygen): there was a significant difference in favour of five fractions per week.

A similar indication of higher tumour responsiveness to more highly fractionated treatment is evident from a comparison between low-dose-rate and high-dose-rate fractionated radiation in moderately advanced cancer of the oropharynx (Pierquin et al. 1985). At 3 years' follow-up, the number of local recurrences in the patients treated with low-dose-rate fractionated radiotherapy (21%) was less than half that for patients treated with conventional fractionation at high dose rates (54%), even though roughly the same total doses were delivered in approximately the same overall time (7−8 weeks).

Clearly no firm conclusions can be drawn from such disparate material. However, there are few exceptions to the rule of higher tumour responsiveness to more, as opposed to fewer, treatments with smaller dose fractions (versus large dose fractions). Melanomas (Overgaard 1986) and liposarcomas (Reitan & Kaalhus 1980; Thames & Suit 1986) are possible examples.

*Experimental evidence*
The study of Moulder & Fisher (1976) of acute skin reaction in the hind leg of rats, as summarized in Table 4.2, resulted in some unusual combinations of isoeffect doses when different numbers of fractions were given in the same overall time in schedules of either three or five fractions per week. If the same amount of regeneration took place after the 17-day lag and radiosensitivity was not changed by the proliferative response, one would expect higher isoeffect doses in the schedule with a higher number of fractions. However, by comparing 10 and 16 fractions given in 21 days, it may be seen that this was not the case (isoeffect doses of 46·85 and 46·7 Gy, respectively). One interpretation of this anomaly is that the $\alpha/\beta$ ratio increased when the proliferative response set in, making the skin more sensitive to the regimen with smaller, more numerous fractions. Similarly, if $\alpha/\beta$ had had the constant value 10 Gy, repair alone would have resulted in an increase from 54·45 Gy (10F/31D)

Table 4.2. Response of rat skin to fractionated irradiation

| Fractionation (frac/days) regimen | Number of animals analysed | Dose range (Gy) tested | Skin tolerance dose (Gy) | |
|---|---|---|---|---|
| Single dose | 135 | 12·05– 67·95 | 23·30 | (21·05–25·25) |
| 3F/ 2D | 36 | 23·60– 59·00 | 34·30 | (28·60–38·95) |
| 3F/ 4D | 60 | 17·70– 67·95 | 31·70 | (27·15–35·28) |
| 5F/ 9D | 57 | 23·60– 64·90 | 35·60 | (32·05–38·20) |
| 7F/ 8D | 44 | 19·75– 67·95 | 39·25 | (34·30–42·80) |
| 7F/14D | 67 | 23·60– 82·60 | 36·45 | (30·30–39·65) |
| 10F/ 9D | 44 | 29·60– 61·50 | 41·15 | (38·25–44·90) |
| 10F/11D | 81 | 23·60– 70·80 | 42·95 | (39·80–45·40) |
| 10F/15D | 46 | 33·05– 61·50 | 43·00 | (40·25–45·70) |
| 10F/21D | 111 | 23·60– 82·60 | 46·85 | (45·05–48·60) |
| 10F/31D | 76 | 35·40– 88·50 | 54·45 | (49·10–57·40) |
| 10F/63D | 46 | 47·20–112·10 | 94·55 | (88·70–99·45) |
| 15F/32D | 65 | 41·30– 88·50 | 63·05 | (58·30–67·30) |
| 16F/21D | 36 | 43·00– 82·60 | 46·70 | (41·50–51·20) |
| 22F/29D | 41 | 43·30–106·20 | 57·95 | (53·45–64·55) |
| 22F/49D | 51 | 62·50–123·90 | 93·00 | (87·45–97·35) |

Dose producing acute partial moist desquamation in 50% of animals treated shown with 95% confidence limits (from Moulder & Fischer 1976).

to 64·9 Gy in isoeffect dose for 22F/29D (as opposed to 57·95 Gy observed). The expected increase in isoeffect dose from repair, assuming the same amount of regeneration, occurred only when 10 fractions in 31 days (54·45 Gy) was increased to 15 fractions in 31 days (63 Gy).

The response of colony-forming cells in the hair follicle of the mouse to fractionated X-rays was assayed by counting regenerating hairs in an irradiated area surrounded by a radiation-sterilized 'moat' (Withers et al. 1987). The hairs in this area were plucked either one day following completion of treatment in the resting telogen state or two days before beginning the treatment (i.e. treatments were given to hairs in the growing anagen phase). The results were analysed using a technique that allowed determination of the clonogens per follicle, survival parameters, and the half-time for Elkind-type repair, and they showed that the number of clonogenic cells per follicle had roughly doubled in the perturbed, anagen state. As shown in Table 4.3, there was an increase in $\alpha/\beta$ from 5·5 to 7·7 Gy.

Deschavannes et al. (1980a), in a study of the survival response of human fibroblasts, determined the effect of plating delay on survival of plateau-phase cultures. Their results are shown in Figure 3.6. One possible interpretation of these results is to assume that cells resuspended and plated immediately after irradiation entered the cycle more quickly than those whose resuspension and plating were delayed. It can be seen that as plating delay increased, there was a progressive decrease in the

Table 4.3. Effect of proliferative status of hair-follicle clonogens on fractionation sensitivity and repair kinetics

|  | Telogen (resting) | Anagen (proliferating) |
|---|---|---|
| $K$ | 67 (61, 73) | 131 (107, 161) |
| $T_{1/2}$ (min) | 90 (85, 95) | 38 (35, 42) |
| $10\alpha$ (Gy$^{-1}$) | 1·48 (1·42, 1·54) | 1·61 (1·55, 1·66) |
| $100\beta$ (Gy$^{-2}$) | 2·69 (2·63, 2·74) | 2·09 (2·00, 2·19) |
| $\alpha/\beta$ (Gy) | 5·5 (5·2, 5·8) | 7·7 (7·4, 8·0) |

$K$ = estimated number of clonogens per hair follicle; parentheses enclose 95% confidence limits (from Withers et al. 1987)

initial slope of the survival curve and a much smaller change in the final slope, resulting in progressively smaller $\alpha/\beta$ ratios. Although such marked alteration of the initial slope is not observed in all *in vitro* studies, it was found for hepatocytes *in vivo* (Fisher et al. 1987).

Zeman & Bedford (1985a) studied gamma-ray dose-fractionation effects in plateau-phase cultures of C3H 10T1/2 cells and in their transformed

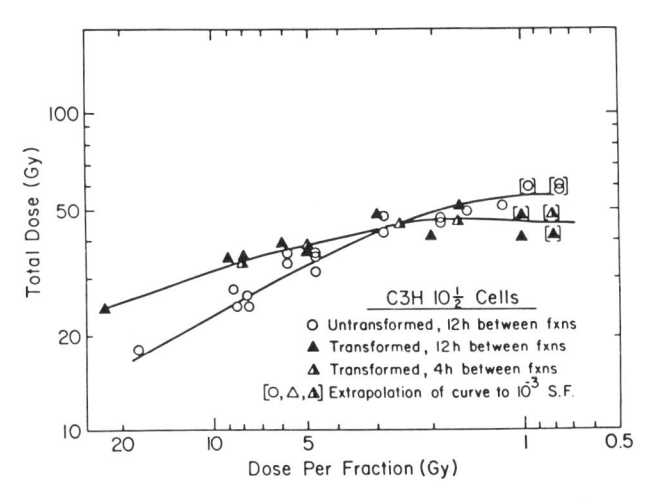

Figure 4.10. Total isoeffect dose as a function of dose per fraction, using a survival level of $10^{-3}$ as an isoeffect (from Zeman & Bedford 1985a). Open symbols refer to data obtained from several dose-fractionation experiments using untransformed 10T½ cells and closed symbols refer to data similarly derived for the transformed cells. Points shown in brackets were taken from multifraction survival curves that required extrapolation to reach the $10^{-3}$ survival level. The isoeffect curve for the more rapidly cycling transformed cells is shallower than that for the more slowly cycling untransformed cells, a finding consistent with the shapes of isoeffect curves for various early and late effects *in vivo*. These curves appear to flatten out at the lower doses per fraction owing to the presumed dose-rate or dose-fractionation independent component of radiation damage. (Reproduced with permission of Academic Press Inc. and the authors.)

counterparts to test the hypothesis that the status of cell populations with respect to their turnover rates might be an important factor influencing dose-fractionation effects. The rate of turnover was three times higher in the plateau-phase transformed cultures, whereas the untransformed cells had a greater capacity to repair potentially lethal damage in plateau phase. The isoeffect curve for the slowly cycling, untransformed cells was found to be appreciably steeper (lower $\alpha/\beta$ ratio) than that of the more rapidly cycling, transformed cells (Figure 4.10).

Thus, there are data to indicate that the $\alpha/\beta$ ratios (fractionation sensitivity) of tissues change with changes in proliferative state and are lower in the relatively slowly cycling, unperturbed state than in the more rapidly cycling state characteristic of the proliferative response to radiation injury. This would have the clinical implication that acutely responding tissues would be relatively more sensitive to more highly fractionated treatments after initiation of a proliferative response, which is to say after about 10–14 days for the oral mucosa and 3–4 weeks for skin.

## 4.3. Clinical implications of regeneration during fractionated radiotherapy

### Effect of tumour clonogen proliferation

The influence of tumour clonogen regeneration on the outcome of radiotherapy can be inferred from both clinical and experimental data.

*Clonogen-doubling versus volume-doubling time*
Time-to-recurrence data suggest that tumour clonogens proliferate more rapidly than indicated by pretreatment volume-doubling times. Cumulative times to recurrence for some squamous cell carcinomas of the upper respiratory and digestive tracts are shown in Table 4.4. It is possible to derive a value for tumour clonogen-doubling times from these data. For example, after a treatment regimen that reduces clonogen survival by the factor $10^8$, it is to be expected that, in a large clinical population where the number of clonogens per tumour is distributed in an unknown way (Figure 4.11($a$)) between about $10^6$ and $10^9$, tumours controlled locally (Figure 4.11($b$)) would have contained approximately $2 \times 10^7$ to $2 \times 10^8$ clonogenic cells, with tumour control probability between 15 and 85%. At the lower end of this range, i.e. $2 \times 10^7$ clonogens, where a tumour-control probability of 85% means that 85% of the tumours contain zero surviving clonogens, there must be

Table 4.4. Cumulative rate of appearance of recurrences of squamous cell carcinomas

| Site | Treatment | % Recurrences by month | | | | |
|---|---|---|---|---|---|---|
| | | 6 | 12 | 18 | 24 | 36 |
| Oropharynx and oral cavity[a] | Surgery + Postop XRT | 53% (20/38) | 74% (28/38) | 76% (29/38) | 92% (35/38) | 100% (38/38) |
| Supraglottic larynx (T1 + T2) | XRT | | 66·5% (10/15) | | 93% (14/15) | 100% (15/15) |

[a] Disease recurring above the clavicles.
From Thames et al. (1983).

recurrences that result from regrowth of a very few surviving clonogens among the 15% that fail locally (Figure 4.11(c)).

Assuming a fairly constant doubling rate, recurrences from few surviving clonogens would be the last to appear, and would be preceded by regrowths from very large primaries or residua of geographical misses. These last-appearing recurrences in several head and neck tumour sites appear after two to three years (Table 4.4). Assuming that these regrow from a single cell and that about $5 \times 10^8$ cells are required for a clinically detectable recurrence, about 30 doublings must have occurred. From the time for occurrences to manifest themselves, the potential doubling time of the tumour can be computed (Thames et al. 1983) for different values of the cell loss factor (CLF), e.g. 6 days for CLF = 75%, 13 days for CLF = 50%, 19 days for CLF = 25%, and 25 days for CLF = 0%. There is no way of determining the appropriate CLF for recurrent tumour growth. However, studies of the responses of human pulmonary metastases to radiation (van Peperzeel 1972) indicate that the CLF is reduced in irradiated tumours, i.e. a regenerative response is triggered. Although a regenerative response can be inferred from these data, its effect on the outcome of fractionated radiotherapy depends also on its time of onset after initiation of treatment. The data of van Peperzeel (1972) suggest that regeneration began well within the 6- to 7-week period typical of conventional courses of radiotherapy (albeit after a single dose or only a few dose fractions).

*Potential doubling times of tumours*

It has been noted above that acceleration of the growth rate can occur during treatment, and this would reduce the potential doubling time (Section 6.8). It is not known whether such acceleration occurs in human tumours where, with the exception of rapidly growing tumours such as Burkitt's lymphoma, the data indicate that potential doubling times range upward from 4 days (Iversen et al. 1976; Sasaki et al. 1980). If cell

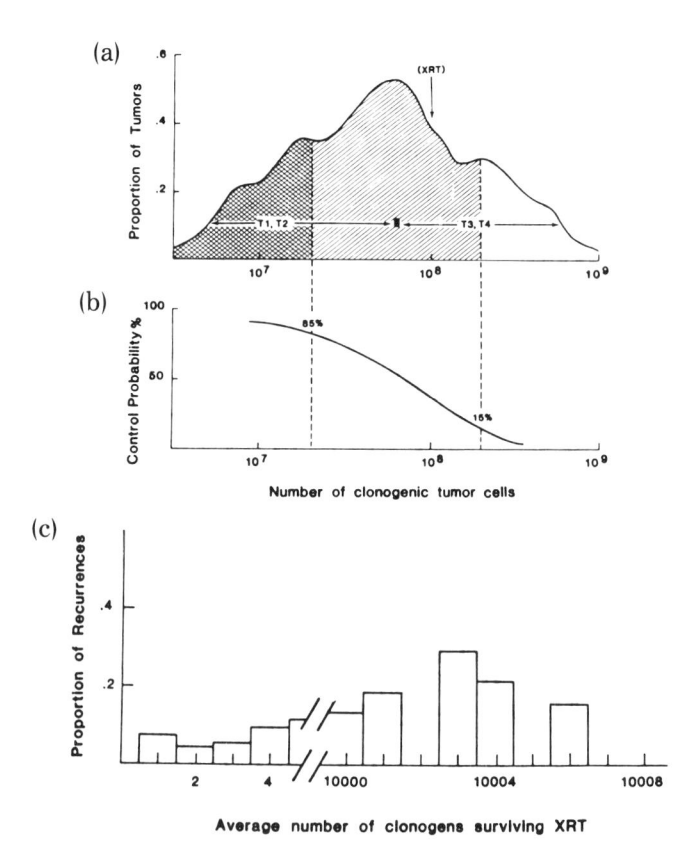

Figure 4.11. Effect of clonogen number on rate of local control and time to recurrence of failures (from Thames et al. 1983). (a) Hypothetical clinical distribution of tumours in terms of initial clonogen number. Vertical lines indicate numbers associated with 85% (left) and 15% (right) control, relative to T-stage of primary. The arrow indicates that radiotherapy reduces survival by the factor $10^8$. The small tumours in the doubly hatched area are controlled with high probability, and control probability decreases with increasing number of clonogenic cells. (b) Proportion of tumours controlled vs. initial clonogen number after a course of radiotherapy that reduces cell survival on average by 8 decades. Vertical lines indicate initial clonogen numbers associated with 85% (left) and 15% (right) local control. (c) Proportion of recurrences vs. number of tumour clonogens that survive radiotherapy. Continuity of the distribution of initial clonogen number suggests that, when control probability is as high as 85% (i.e. when 85% of the tumours have 0 surviving clonogens), a few recurrences would be expected to regrow from very few (1 or more) survivors. If the doubling rate is fairly constant, these would be the last to be detected, while the larger (10 000 or more clonogens) residual tumour masses resulting from geographical misses or improperly defined margins would appear first. (Reproduced with permission of Pergamon Journals Ltd.)

loss were to decrease during a regenerative response, a two to three weeks' reduction in treatment time might result in avoiding more than three or four doublings of clonogens during treatment. Assuming that compensation for each doubling requires approximately $2 \cdot 5$ and $3 \cdot 5$ Gy, it is clear that the success of a course of treatment must depend on its overall time.

*Influence of overall treatment time on local control*
The foregoing is corroborated by clinical experience with the effect of overall treatment time on the outcome of treatment. Although good results with split-course therapy have been claimed by Scanlon (1963) and Holsti (1969), retrospective studies with a much larger number of patients with head-and-neck and cervical cancer, in which the same total dose was used in both split-course and continuously treated groups, showed significantly better results for the continuous course (Parsons *et al.* 1980a,b). This was true both in terms of local and regional control and in patient survival, and suggests repopulation of clonogenic tumour cells during the rest interval. As noted in Section 4.2, there may be accelerated repopulation during extended treatments.

The arguments for a high $\alpha/\beta$ ratio for tumours presented in Section 3.3 lead to the expectation that the size of dose per fraction would not be an important factor determining local control. On the other hand, the previous discussion indicates that overall treatment time should strongly influence treatment results, and this is borne out by a number of studies. Maciejewski *et al.* (1983) analysed the dependence of local control of T3/T4, NO/MO squamous cell carcinomas of the larynx on dose per fraction and overall treatment time. They found that local tumour control depended strongly on overall time and weakly or not at all on fraction size. A decrease in local control of base of tongue tumours was observed after protraction of overall treatment time (Spanos *et al.* 1976). Hliniak *et al.* (1983) found that the recurrence rate of basal/squamous cell carcinomas of the skin depended strongly on overall time, decreasing from 88% to 37% as this increased from 10 to 45 days.

Possible exceptions to the rule that overall time is the most important factor influencing tumour cure may be the melanomas (Overgaard 1986) and liposarcomas (Reitan & Kaalhus 1980). Trott *et al.* (1981), however, found a significant effect for *both* time and fraction size with melanomas.

**Accelerated fractionation**

Accelerated fractionation (reviewed by Peters & Ang 1987) involves the use of overall times shorter than is conventional, achieved by giving two or three doses daily (Suit 1977; Withers *et al.* 1982b; Thames *et al.* 1983;

Trott & Kummermehr 1985). The total dose and fraction size are similar to conventional treatments. The rationale for acceleration is based on the idea that, where clonogenic tumour cells proliferate very rapidly, a gain in local control might be realized by administering radiation in a shorter overall time with a reduced intertreatment interval, since the opportunity for proliferation of tumour cells would thereby be reduced. Acute normal tissue reactions would be exacerbated for the same reason, but provided Elkind repair was complete between fractions, one would expect little or no change in the response of the slowly cycling target cells for late effects.

Modern clinical experience with accelerated fractionation began in the mid-1960s (see, however, the older fractionation schemes described in Chapter 5). The first reported of these later studies was for the treatment of glioblastoma multiforme (Simpson & Platts 1976). A series of prospective randomized trials begun in 1965 was reported in which 134 patients were treated at 8- or 24-hour intervals, 7 days per week. The first series compared 30 Gy tumour dose in 21 fractions given in 3 weeks or 7 days; the next 40 Gy tumour dose given in 28 fractions in 4 weeks or 9·3 days, and the final series 40 Gy in 21 fractions in 3 weeks or 7 days (Table 4.5). In none of the trials was there a significant difference in survival between the groups, probably reflecting the low biological doses given. As would be expected, no evidence of brain necrosis was seen, except in a patient who was re-treated.

Table 4.5. Clinical studies of predominantly accelerated fractionation regimens

| Site | No. of pts. | T(wks) | Fx/ day | Dose/ fx(Gy) | Total dose (Gy) | Reference |
|---|---|---|---|---|---|---|
| Brain | 134 | 1 | 3 | 1·80 | 40 | Simpson & Platts (1976) |
|  | 160 | 4 | 3 | 1·6 | 60 | van der Schueren et al. (1985) |
| Burkitt's | 34 | 2 | 3 | 1·2 | 29 | Norin & Onyango (1977) |
| Breast (inflammatory) | 42 | 4−5 | 2 | 1·3 | 7 | Barker et al. (1980) |
| Head and neck | 22 | 1·5 | 3 | 2 | 48−54 | Peracchia & Salti (1981) |
|  | 59 | 2 | 3 | 1·75−2·3 | 50−55 | Svoboda (1984) |
|  | 321 | 6 | 2 | 1·6 | 64−67 | Wang et al. (1985) |
|  | 53 | 6 | 2 | 1·2−2 | 70−74 | Knee et al. (1985) |
| Neck nodes | 35 | 2·5 | 3 | 1·5−2 | 60 | Arcangeli et al. (1984) |
| Melanoma (brain mets.) | 20 | 1 | 2 | 3−3·75 | 30−37·5 | Choi et al. (1985) |

Modified from Peters & Ang (1987).

Malignant gliomas were treated in a randomized study of the EORTC (European Organization for Research on Treatment of Cancer) Radiotherapy Group (van der Schueren et al. 1985). Treatment was given three times daily for 5 days to 30 Gy, followed by 2 weeks rest and repetition of the first course (4 weeks total). No survival benefit could be demonstrated over the conventional arm (60 Gy/30 fractions/6 weeks).

There have been positive results from acceleration. For example, it has sometimes been observed that neck metastases will grow during treatment, even when 10 Gy per week is given (Fletcher 1980). Since this dose would be expected to reduce survival by at least a factor of 6 (assuming an effective $D_0$ of no greater than 5 Gy for fractionated doses of 2 Gy), a rapid growth of tumour clonogens is implied. Accordingly, the weekly dose was increased by giving a concomitant boost with tangential fields. A superior result was obtained by treating with 15 Gy per week.

Norin & Onyango (1977) reported improved clinical results with accelerated treatment for Burkitt's lymphoma (Table 4.5). Based on the frequency of complete tumour regression, the local effectiveness of radiation improved when three treatments per day were employed and the total treatment time was reduced. Thus, there was only one complete regression of nine treated with daily doses of 2·2 Gy for a total dose of 31 Gy in 20 days, whereas 25 of 34 tumours regressed completely after 29 Gy given in 27 fractions of 1·2 Gy in 13 days.

Barker et al. (1980) reported the results of accelerated fractionation for inflammatory carcinoma of the breast. Two treatments per day were given, to a total dose of 71 Gy in 5·5 weeks. The local–regional control rate was significantly better than in a historical control group.

Accelerated fractionation has been most extensively investigated in head and neck cancer (Table 4.5). Overall time was drastically reduced in three studies, and severe mucosal reactions (sometimes followed by severe late reactions) usually resulted. Svoboda (1984) treated with three daily fractions of 1·75 to 3 Gy to total doses of 50 to 55 Gy in 10–16 days, and found that acute reactions could be tolerated in small, but not in large, treatment volumes, where the dose per fraction had to be reduced to 1·75 Gy (Resouly & Svoboda 1982). Although local control was good, some severe late reactions were encountered. Perrachia & Salti (1981) reported horrendous complications from treating with 3 × 2 Gy daily to 48–56 Gy in 1·5 weeks. A higher response rate in neck node metastases resulted from accelerated treatment (Arcangeli et al. 1984).

Other studies have accommodated severe mucosal reactions by introduction of a rest interval. Van den Bogaert et al. (1985) treated with 3 × 1·6 Gy daily to 48 Gy in 2 weeks, and after 3 to 4 weeks the rest of this treatment was resumed until 67–72 Gy was given in 6–7 weeks (it is questionable whether this meets a strict definition of accelerated fractionation). No advantage resulted relative to the control arm. With a modest reduction of 1·5 weeks treatment time Wang et al. (1985) found a significant improvement over historical controls treated with conventional fractionation (64—65 Gy given in fractions of 1·8 Gy over 7·5 weeks).

The interruption of treatment was avoided by Knee et al. (1985) using a concomitant-boost technique. All patients received 1·8—2·0 Gy daily to about 55 Gy; the boost was delivered as a second daily treatment, 1·2—1·5 Gy, 2—3 times a week for 3—5 weeks. This allowed delivery of about 72 Gy in 6 weeks without interrupting treatment in 50/53 patients.

Brain metastases from malignant melanomas were treated with accelerated fractionation, with the result that median survival time was prolonged from 28 to 50 weeks (Choi et al. 1985). These and other results are discussed in the review by Peters & Ang (1987). From this experience, the following tentative conclusions may be drawn:

1. An improvement in local response and control rates appears possible in certain circumstances.
2. Pure accelerated treatment regimens with large fields cannot be tolerated in the head and neck region because of mucosal intolerance.
3. Although a $3 \times 1·6$ Gy daily schedule can be tolerated with a break in treatment after 48 Gy (cf. Example 10, Section 6.10), the rationale for accelerated treatment in terms of tumour regeneration during therapy is largely neutralized by such a strategy (cf. Section 4.2). When a continuous course is given it is unlikely that large volumes of mucosal membranes in the head and neck region can tolerate doses in excess of $2 \times 1·2$ Gy daily, so that significant acceleration of treatment is impossible in these circumstances.
4. The results of Wang et al. (1985) and Knee et al. (1985) suggest that it is possible to reduce treatment time by one to two weeks without reducing the total dose and without an interruption of treatment.

## 4.4. Residual injury and retreatment

**Experimental evidence**

Regeneration of the stem-cell population following irradiation will concomitantly restore the differentiating and mature cell populations in a tissue, so that it might recover. The recovery would be complete if the proliferative and differentiating capabilities of the survivors after irradiation were unchanged, and if there were no influences on these hierarchical cell populations from the irradiated stroma. Also, if there were complete restitution of the target cells, subsequent irradiations should be equally effective unless their sensitivity had changed. However, in most systems complete recovery does not occur.

In the *bone marrow* of mice, there is almost full recovery of stem-cell numbers in three to four weeks following large single doses (reviewed by Hendry & Lord 1983). Correspondingly, animals reirradiated after this time are able to tolerate the full LD50/30, and there are even examples of periods of induced resistance in mice (Porteous & Lajtha 1966) and in sheep (Hanks *et al.* 1966). Subsequent doses are more effective in impairing haematopoiesis, as shown in Figure 4.12. The complement of stem cells can be reduced permanently to 10–20% of normal (Hendry & Lajtha 1972; Hendry *et al.* 1983a). The mature cell populations are maintained near normal by extra divisions in the proliferative precursor cells and by more rapid cycling of the stem-cell population (Hendry *et al.* 1974, 1983a; Croizat *et al.* 1979), as shown diagrammatically in Figure 4.13.

The mature cell populations are maintained at these levels for many

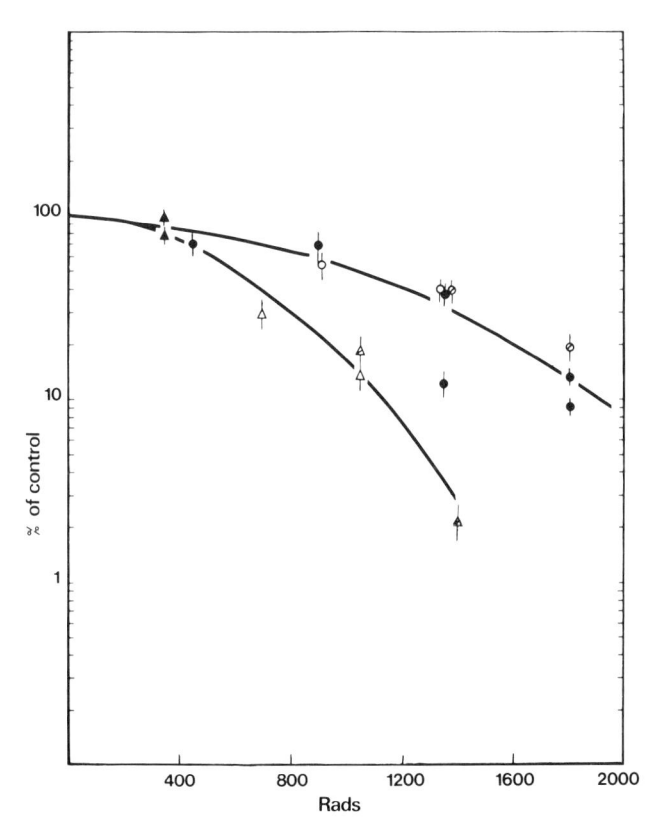

Figure 4.12. Content of haematopoietic stem cells in the mouse femur at 3 weeks after each dose of 4·5-Gy X-rays in a series of 4 doses given at 3 week intervals (circles, top curve), or 3·5-Gy 14-MeV neutrons (triangles, bottom curve). (From Hendry & Lajtha 1972; reproduced with permission of Academic Press Inc.)

months, but not indefinitely, and anaemia develops in the long term (Hendry et al. 1983a). The reasons for the lack of full stem-cell repopulation are unknown, and the effect is surprising in view of the known capacity of stem cells to undergo an enormous number of divisions, sufficient for several mouse life-spans. Possible mechanisms include damage to the stroma and to the regulatory system for proliferation. Grafts of fresh marrow increase the suboptimal plateau, but not to control levels (Hendry et al. 1983a). The stem cells remaining on the suboptimal plateau show little difference in sensitivity from control cells, but the shoulder is reduced (Figure 4.14).

In mouse *intestine*, irradiation of the descending colon using two doses of 12·5 Gy separated by 6 weeks to allow recovery after the first dose persistently reduced the number of crypts when these were assayed 6 weeks or more after the second dose (Hamilton 1979). Also, the sensitivity of the clonogens was smaller by a factor of 1·7. In the small intestine, a similar effect was observed at 6 to 12 months following a single dose of 9 to 11 Gy (Reynaud & Travis 1984). This was shown to be due to induced hypoxia, considered to be secondary to fibrotic changes and subsequent ischaemia. Injection of the radiosensitizer misonidazole before irradiation abolished the induced resistance (Figure 4.15).

In mouse *epidermis*, the tolerance dose for acute reactions is reduced

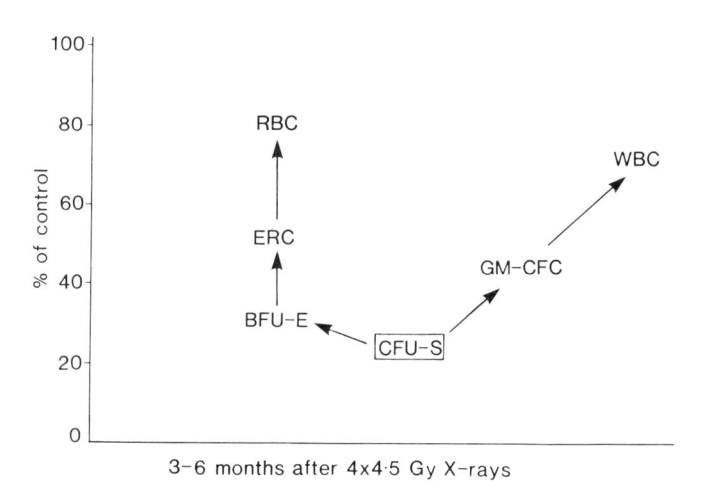

Figure 4.13. New steady-state achieved in the haematopoietic cell hierarchy in mice at 3 to 6 months after 4 repeated whole-body doses (3 week intervals) of 4·5-Gy X-rays (from Hendry 1985a). CFU-S, colony-forming units in the spleen (stem cells); BFU-E, erythroid burst-forming units (early erythroid progenitor cells); ERC, erythropoietin responsive cells (more mature erythroid progenitor cells); RBC, red blood cells; GM-CFC, granulocyte/macrophage colony-forming cells; WBC, white blood cells. (Reproduced with permission of Elsevier Science Publishers.)

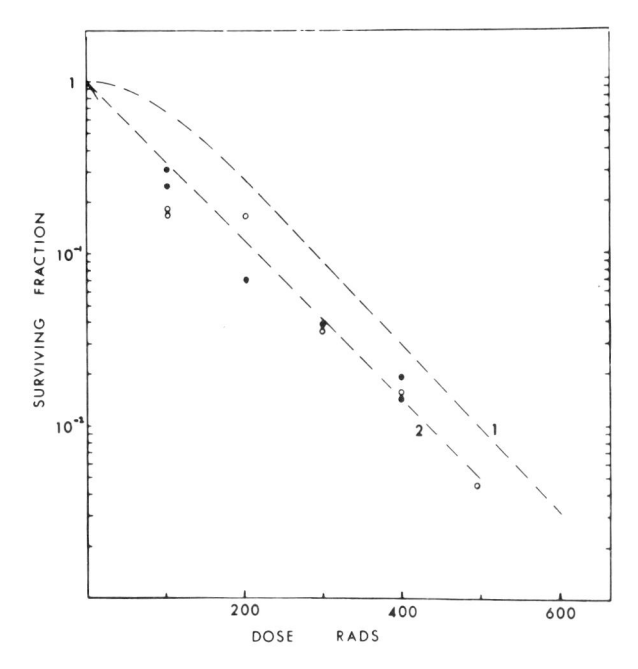

Figure 4.14. Survival of stem cells in the femur (closed circles) or in the spleen (open circles) after γ-rays (from Hendry & Lajtha 1972). Cells taken from mice previously irradiated with 4 repeated doses of 4·5-Gy X-rays (symbols) or control mice (femur, dashed curve 1; spleen, dashed line 2). (Reproduced with permission of Academic Press Inc.)

by about 10% at 6 weeks or more following a first treatment (Denekamp 1975). The effect is also seen following fractionated priming doses (Brown & Probert 1973, 1975). There are macroscopic signs of residual injury at the time of the second irradiation, for example a thin and dry epidermis. There are also microscopic changes, in structural organization and in keratinization (Hendry et al. 1982). The use of microcolony techniques (Chen 1986) has shown that the sensitivity of the colony-forming cells had changed at 6 weeks after a tolerance dose (Figure 4.16). Moreover, there was a greater sparing of the residual injury, assessed by colonies produced after reirradiation, when multifractionated doses were used in the priming treatment which were isoeffective for the acute skin reactions. A similar degree of sparing was found using a skin healing/necrosis endpoint.

The reductions in dose caused by prior irradiation in various normal tissues in mice are summarized in Table 4.6. The dosage changes are expressed as a percentage, being the reduction (negative sign) or increase (positive sign) in the isoeffective test dose given to previously irradiated compared to (aged) control tissues. Induced resistance is found in the intestine and sometimes in the marrow (as noted above), but in lung and

134 *Fractionation in Radiotherapy*

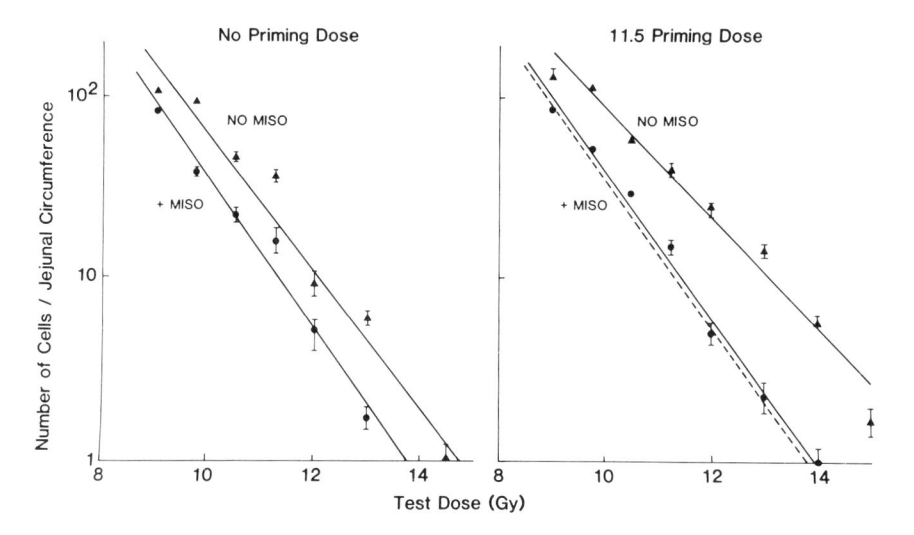

Figure 4.15. Surviving cells per jejunal circumference as a function of a second X-ray dose given alone (▲) or half an hour after misonidazole(1 mg/g) (•) (from Reynaud & Travis 1984). (a) Age-matched control mice not previously irradiated. (b) Mice exposed to 11·5 Gy 4 months previously. The dotted line is the survival curve from control mice given misonidazole. (Reproduced with permission of Taylor & Francis Ltd and the authors.)

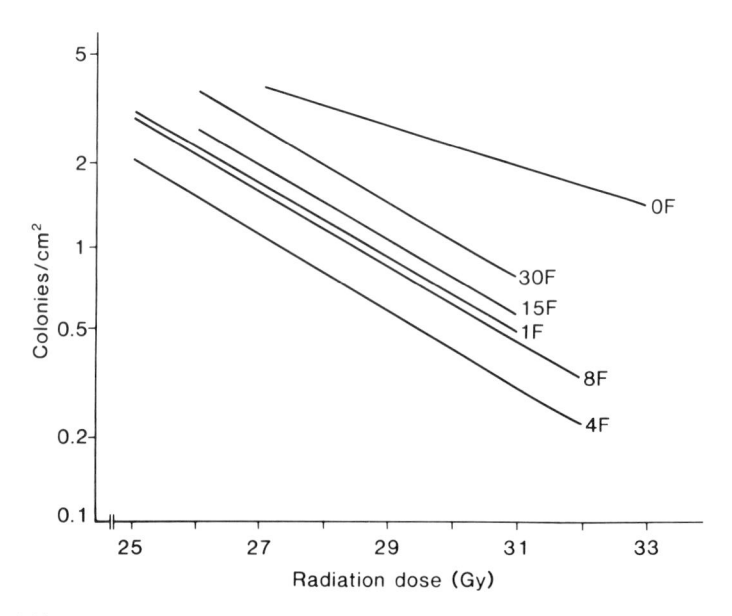

Figure 4.16. Response of mouse tail epidermis to X-rays, assayed using a macrocolony technique (from Chen 1986). Tails reirradiated at 6 weeks after tolerance doses delivered in 1, 4, 8, 15, or 30 fractions. 0F = control.

Table 4.6. Residual injury in different tissues

| Tissue (species) | End point | Priming dose (percentage of dose to give end point) | Time between first and second doses | Dosage change (%) | Reference |
|---|---|---|---|---|---|
| Haematopoietic (mouse) | LD50/30 | 10% | 3 weeks | −10 | Porteous & Lajtha (1966) |
| Haematopoietic (dog) | LD50/30 | 67% | 3 weeks | +13 | Ainsworth & Leong (1966) |
| Haematopoietic (sheep) | LD50/60 | 67% | 1 month | −(22 to 29) | Hanks et al. (1966) |
| Intestine (mouse) | 10 surviving cells per jejunal circumference | 78% | 2 months<br>6 months<br>12 months | +11<br>+15<br>+ 7 | Reynaud & Travis (1984) |
|  |  | 100% | 2 months<br>6 months<br>12 months | +18<br>+24<br>+ 7 |  |
| Skin† (mouse) | ND50 | 70–90% | 6 weeks | −(8 to 11) | Hendry (1978) |
| Lung (mouse) | LD50/80 | 76–85% | 4 weeks | −(15 to 24) | Field et al. (1976) |
| Spinal cord (rat) | White matter-necrosis (ED50) | 80% | 8 weeks<br>16 weeks | −42<br>−26 | van der Kogel (1979) |
|  | Vascular damage (ED50) | 80% | 8 weeks<br>16 weeks | −58<br>−51 |  |
| Spinal cord (rat) | ED50/1 year | 25%<br>50%<br>75% | 14 weeks | − 6<br>−10<br>−29 | Hornsey et al. (1982) |

†Many other values have been published for skin (reviewed by Chen 1986).

spinal cord less dose is needed for the isoeffect. In the cord, the dosage changes are markedly dependent on the size of the initial dose.

**Clinical evidence**

Radiotherapy has been used to treat recurrences or second malignancies in various sites. In the last decade, these include nasopharynx (Yau et al. 1983), brain (Dritschillo et al. 1981), other head and neck sites (Hunter & Stewart 1977; Skolyszewski et al. 1980; Langlois et al. 1985), lung (Green and Melbye 1982), and cervix (Prempree et al. 1984). In general, there is a remarkable recovery of tolerance in irradiated normal tissues. An accurate assessment of the amount of recovery is difficult because of the small number of patients in many series and the differences between series in treatment protocols and in tumour-associated complications. One general feature that emerges is the improved prognosis with longer intervals between courses (Dritschillo et al. 1981; Fu et al. 1975; Langlois et al. 1985; Wang & Schulz 1966; Yau et al. 1983), but there are exceptions to this finding (McNeese & Fletcher 1981). A series of patients treated for malignancies arising up to 30 years after treatments for thyrotoxicosis tolerated radical treatments to larynx remarkably well (Hunter & Stewart 1977).

One interpretation of these results is that late effects occur because of injury to the parenchyma, and that slow regeneration of their renewing populations restores the irradiated normal tissues, making retreatment possible. The kidney may serve as an illustration of the point. The loss of nephrons after injury to the tubular epithelium would be expected to follow a sigmoid dose response to the first treatment. If the damage was such that no loss of nephrons occurred, regeneration of the tubular epithelium would proceed and after a sufficient interval retreatment with the same dose might be possible. If the first treatment resulted in the loss of some of the nephrons, or if the time between treatments was shortened, then the amount of proliferative recovery would be limited and the tolerance of the kidney would be lower.

There is a vascular component to radiation injury, and long-term recovery processes in this tissue component have been reported (Reinhold & Buisman 1973). It is known that there is short-term recovery, and if long-term intracellular repair is a general phenomenon and slow repopulation of survivors occurs, then the recovery of tolerance in the vascular component would be greater than is generally appreciated.

If this model is correct for long-term recovery in late-responding tissues in general, the traditional reluctance to reirradiate may not be well founded.

# Chapter 5
# In hindsight

Forty years after the first recorded use of therapeutic X-rays, the first Congress of Austrian Radiology met in Vienna in September 1936. The founder of radiotherapy, Leopold Freund, was there, as were many of those who had guided the development of various fractionation techniques over the years: Schwarz, a consistent champion of the fractionated method; Wintz, a leading proponent of the concentrated, single-dose method; and Coutard, who achieved the first cures of deep-seated tumours. From these talks the impression emerges that most fractionation techniques that we know of today had been tried in some form by that time, and that the conventional daily treatment techniques then were not very different from what they are today.

What were the factors that guided the various changes in fractionation technique up to 1936? Radiobiology as we know it today did not exist, but some influence was exerted by biological theories of tumour response, based in most cases on data that were biologically remote from clinical application. Of greater influence were two considerations of a purely clinical nature, namely what resulted in long-term cures and what was economically feasible in terms of personnel, equipment, and so on.

In the 50 years since this meeting the time factor has been extensively investigated, and the results of these studies have been conceptualized in various ways. The earliest framework was provided by the power-law models (double-log graphs of log isoeffect dose versus log treatment time) which after various reinterpretations culminated in the Ellis NSD model in the late 1960s. Clinical practice was occasionally influenced by these models. A different interpretation of the time factor was provided by cell-survival models, which came into prominence in the 1970s and 1980s.

The purpose of the present, historically oriented chapter is twofold: first, to outline the evolution of fractionation practices in the early years of radiotherapy, and second, to present a summary in terms of isoeffect models of the interpretations of these early fractionation schemes up to the present time (1986). For the most part our attention will be directed toward the early evolution of fractionation practice, from multiple daily doses in the beginning, then treatment with single doses or a few fractions, and back again to treatment with multiple fractions in the 1920s and 1930s. We cover only selected parts of an enormous literature: Glasser (1959) found 1044 original articles and 49 books on the subject of Roentgenology during its first year, 1896! Subsequent changes in fractionation practice have been less drastic, and we have chosen to discuss these in terms of isoeffect concepts such as the NSD model. Readers interested in more detail can find it in the following sources. For the early Austrian period we recommend Wiess (1966), Wyklicky (1980), Wichtl (1986), and Glasser's (1959) biography of Röntgen. Miescher (1930) and Schinz (1930, 1937) gave accounts of the status of single-dose and fractionated treatments. The early years of the Radiumhemmet at Stockholm were described by Forssell *et al.* (1939). The history of radiology in England is the subject of a recent book by Burrows (1986).

## 5.1. Origins (1896–1940s)

One of the first documented uses of X-ray therapy was by the Viennese dermatologist Leopold Freund (1868–1943) in 1896 (Freund 1897a,b), which followed soon after the discovery of X-rays by Conrad Röntgen (1895). According to Schwarz (1937) the idea occurred to Freund after reading an account by Marcuse (1896) of epilation and skin damage resulting from X-ray exposure; others claimed that he had read such an account in the newspapers (Wyklicky 1980).

In any event, Freund was led to treat the hairy nevus. His technique was to treat daily at the very low dose rate available from the X-ray tubes of that time, until the desired effect had been achieved. This required two or more weeks overall time, and thus the first radiotherapy treatments were given in multiple daily fractions, at low dose rates.

Freund faced numerous difficulties in starting his new method of treatment. It is not hard to imagine the scepticism encountered by a 28-year-old dermatologist barely a year out of medical school, asking for access to an X-ray tube. His interests were promoted by the staff of the Clinic for Skin and Sexual Diseases, where Moritz Kaposi (1837–1902) was a leader; Freund was closely associated with the dermatologist Eduard Schiff there (Wichtl 1986). There were no X-ray tubes in hospitals at the time, and the first therapeutic irradiation took place on 24 November 1896, at the Roentgen Laboratory of the National Institute for Research in Photography and Reproduction Procedures (Röntgen-Laboratorium der k. k. Lehr- und Versuchsanstalt für

Photographie und Reproduktionsverfahren) in Vienna, whose director, J. M. Eder, published an interesting account of these developments (Eder 1922).

Freund believed that X-rays were the active agent in epilation, but many thought the electric field generated by the tubes was more likely to be biologically active, including French researchers in 1898 (Weiss 1966) and the physicist Ludwig Boltzmann; another physicist, Ernst Mach, found Freund's suggestion of a direct effect of X-rays on the skin plausible. However, Freund himself came to doubt his original interpretation, and was only convinced (but slowly) by the later definitive experiments of Robert Kienböck (1871–1954).

Priority in the first treatments with X-rays has been claimed for others, notably E. H. Grubbe, V. Despeignes, F. H. Williams, and G. Voigt (Glasser 1937). Freund (1948), however, in a paper published 10 years after its writing and 5 years after his death, argued rather convincingly that these were one-of-a-kind attempts with little or no rationale and no subsequent follow-up.

The first cures of skin cancer were reported by the Swedish authors Stenbeck (1900) and Sjögren (1901), who used a treatment technique similar to Freund's. In all of this the dose was undetermined, and treatment was guided by day-to-day observation of patient response, that is to say biologically. X-ray tubes of that time, however, were plagued by low (and often variable) output, and when technical improvements led to increased dose rates the advantage of following patient reactions was lost. Robert Kienböck (1900a,b, 1901) showed that the nature and degree of skin injury was proportional to absorbed dose, thus demonstrating the need for exact physical specification of the dose. In response to this need Guido Holzknecht (1872–1931) developed his chromoradiometer; a mixture of salts changed from yellow to green when exposed to X-rays. This change, in proportion to dose, was compared to a colorimetric scale demarcated in Holzknecht (H) units—oddly enough, a dose in the neighbourhood of 1 Gy. The ionization chamber was proposed as a dosimeter a few years later by the French physicist Villard (1908) but it was ignored subsequently. After modifications by other workers it was eventually adopted as the preferred dosimeter at the time of adoption of the standard unit of exposure, the 'röntgen', at the first International Radiology Congress in Stockholm in 1928.

The higher dose rates available to therapists, together with quantitative means of assessing dosage (especially using the Sabouraud–Noiré method of barium–platinum cyanide colour change in conjunction with the Holzknecht colour scale), now led to treatments in one or a few sessions. This change resulted in the loss of the advantage of following patient reactions daily when low dose rates were used, but it was prompted by the fear that a fractionated dose might cause tissue injury because of the hypothesized 'cumulation' of radiation damage. Perthes (1904) recommended treatment in one session or at most a few fractions, with close monitoring of the dose. This method, called the *expedited* or *massive-dose* treatment, led to toxic reactions of unexpected severity. There followed a growing awareness of the *time factor*—the influence of the time during which a dose was delivered on its biological effect. The first clinical demonstration of the diminished effect of a fractionated dose was published by Krönig & Friedrich (1918). An early interpretation of the time factor involved the 'radioimmunization' of normal tissues and tumours (Regaud 1921).

Biological research in the first decade of the twentieth century emphasized the pre-eminent role of proliferative activity in the sensitivity of cells to radiation-induced injury and provided one of the rationales (among many others) for the eventual abandonment of single-dose treatments. Kienböck, in his report (1901) of the first observations concerning the higher radiosensitivity of cell populations with high proportions of mitotic figures, commented that organs in which active cell proliferation occurred were especially sensitive to the effects of radiation. Albers-Schönberg (1903) showed that radiation could induce azoospermia after irradiation of the testicles. Bergonié & Tribondeau (1906) used the same system to develop their law of the proportionality of radiosensitivity to the reproductive activity of cells. This law was later to influence Regaud and his colleagues in Paris in their techniques of radium treatment of uterine carcinoma. Heinecke (1903, 1904) demonstrated the 'explosive' disintegration of the nuclei of lymphocytes very shortly after irradiation—the first report of 'interphase' cell death, as opposed to death at the time of (attempted) mitosis. The importance of the latter was demonstrated in an influential paper by Krause-Ziegler (1906) on the sensitivity of nuclear material.

A more precise linkage of radiosensitivity to degree of proliferative activity was made possible by demonstrations of concomitant changes in both, in the same biological systems. Benjamin *et al.* (1906) showed that intensive irradiation of the circulating blood of the rabbit did not produce aleukia, whereas exposure of the sites of production of leukocytes did. Schwarz (1909) showed that different degrees of sensitivity were manifest depending on the degree of proliferation in the same biological system: dry beans versus sprouting beans. In his studies of the sensitivity of skin exposed to radiation during partial hypoxia, achieved by applying a tourniquet, he found a decreased sensitivity, which he attributed to lowered mitotic activity.

Schwarz (1880—1959), who was one of the first to advance a biological rationale for a therapeutic gain from fractionated treatments, entered Holzknecht's service in Vienna around 1905, a year after the three Viennese pioneers in radiology—Freund, Holzknecht, and Kienböck—

had received standing in the medical faculty. At that time single doses were the rule, although Freund had continued to use fractionated daily doses. It was increasingly appreciated that cells in a state of growth, division, and reproduction were more radiosensitive than those in a resting state; this difference began to influence treatment in some centres. In Paris, Regaud (1870–1940) and colleagues extended the time of application of radium in the treatment of uterine carcinoma to one week; they were mindful of the Bergonié and Tribondeau law (e.g. Regaud & Ferroux 1922) and possibly also of the work of the Austrians. The Regaud method of protraction of radium treatment of uterine carcinoma contrasts with the early Stockholm technique pioneered by Güsta Forssell (treatment in one or a few days) that was used at the Radiumhemmet and at the Finsen Institute in Copenhagen.

In Vienna in December 1914, Schwarz (1914a,b) published some critical observations just after the outbreak of World War I had prevented their dissemination outside Germany and Austria: a mediastinal tumour that had been unsuccessfully irradiated with the single-dose method quickly responded months later to small doses given daily. He concluded: "In the same tumour there will be cells more radiosensitive than others, depending on the phase of the division cycle. Therefore it is not recommended to use one, or a few large doses separated by long intervals, since the most advantageous time for irradiation may be missed entirely or occur during one of the intervals. Instead we recommend a method of small daily doses."†

The view favouring single-dose treatment, which was the more influential one until the 1920s, is illustrated by the arguments of Wintz (1937), as follows (free translation): "The cells of the human body are endowed with variable radiosensitivity and capacity for recovery from radiation damage. It is also reasonable to assume that recovery from radiation injury depends on cellular metabolism, and further that a rapidly growing tumour cell is better able to effect recovery from injury than a connective-tissue cell with its comparatively slow metabolism. Therefore the difference in response will favour the tumour if the cancericidal dose is not applied in the first treatment." Wintz was a leader of the *Erlangen school*, where it was believed that fractionated treatment was decisively inferior, to be judged as "primitive method" and "weak irradiation". Concentrated treatment found most of its followers in Germany, where its most famous practitioners were Seitz and Wintz of the Women's Clinic in Erlangen, and Krönig and Friedrich.

---

†Strandqvist (1944) does not cite these papers (Schwarz 1914a,b), but rather Schwarz (1914c): "Cure of deep-seated carcinomas by external-beam Röntgen-ray therapy". Although widely cited by subsequent authors, the latter article has nothing to do with fractionation, but is rather a critique of a newly developed method of chemical dosimetry.

For a time it also flourished in Austria, however, as evidenced by the following retrospective statement by Freund (1937): "Freund founded Röntgen therapy with a method of the smallest fractional doses; Kienböck developed from this the so-called expedited method with four treatments; and Holzknecht used his chromoradiometer to give the full dose in one treatment. Subsequently, a battle raged for twenty-odd years between the partisans of fractionated doses and those of full (single)-dose treatments."

Thus the controversy between methods of treatment, concentrated or fractionated, continued into the 1920s, each with biological justifications based on an improved therapeutic ratio: in favour of concentrated treatment, the supposition that recovery from injury was more efficient in rapidly growing tumour cells, and in favour of fractionated treatment, that the chance of irradiating cells in the more radiosensitive mitotic phase was higher. This was the situation when Coutard (1876−1950) began his celebrated treatment of head-and-neck tumours with fractionated, low-dose-rate Röntgen therapy in 1919, the year of the founding of the Curie Institute in Paris (del Regato 1986).

Coutard's methods were designed to mimic the radium technique of Regaud, which had led to improved results in the treatment of uterine carcinoma: first, by giving treatment over an extended time and with correspondingly elevated doses, and second, by daily or twice-daily exposures at a low dose rate. Both Regaud (Paris) and Forssell (Stockholm) had been concerned not only with uses of radium in the treatment of uterine carcinoma but also with the treatment of carcinoma of the tonsils, oral cavity, tongue, and lips, using applicators and teleradium (E. Bervens, report at the congress of the German Röntgen Society, Vienna 1929). Coutard circumvented the technical difficulties of using radium to treat these head-and-neck tumours with external beam Röntgen therapy, but maintained similar dosing conditions, i.e. treatment with one or two low-dose-rate fractions per day, extended over at least two weeks, and longer for the larger tumours. In this way he established the first treatment technique capable of lasting cures of deep-seated tumours, particularly of the larynx and tonsil. Oddly enough, this technique was in many respects similar to that originally established and at that time still used by Freund.

As a guideline in his treatments, Coutard aimed for the skin reactions described by Regaud (1927): 'Radioepidermitis', a very intense but fully repairable skin reaction (moist desquamation). He also aimed for a high-grade mucosal reaction (Coutard 1929). Coutard's guiding principle was that the radiosensitivity of the cancer cells was the same as that of the regenerative cells of the tissue of origin (epithelium).

The swing toward fractionated treatments was also occurring in Zurich (Schinz 1930, 1937) and in Vienna, as evidenced by the complaints of Freund (1927), who noted that "Holzknecht, a user of single-dose treatments who had derided his fractionation method for many years, had suddenly switched because of the influence of Schwarz and since that time had been heralded as a pioneer in fractionation." For whatever reason, Holzknecht started a movement in 1921 in Austria against the methods of Seitz and Wintz. According to Schwarz (1937), Holzknecht was a gifted clinician to whom such concepts as the 'carcinoma dose' and 'sarcoma dose' of Seitz and Wintz seemed too formalistic.†

Additional biological evidence accrued for the superiority of fractionated treatments. The increased probability of irradiating cells in a sensitive phase with fractionated doses was confirmed by studies of the sterilization of testicles in the grasshopper (Mohr 1919) and rabbit (Regaud & Ferroux 1927). Nather & Schinz (1923) showed that a certain mouse tumour quickly regressed under the influence of fractionated, but not single-dose, treatments.

Regaud & Ferroux (1927) demonstrated experimentally that more damage was done to the seminiferous epithelium when the same dose was given in four fractions rather than in one. On the other hand, there was less damage to the skin in the four-fraction treatment. They concluded that cells in different physiological states differed in their mitotic activity and in their response to fractionated radiation. On the grounds that cell multiplication in the testis could serve as a model for tumours, a therapeutic benefit was proposed for fractionated treatments.

An interesting variation in fractionation technique, the saturation method, was used in the 1920s and 1930s. It was based on what was perhaps the first mathematical isoeffect model (Kingery 1920; Hoffman & Reinhard 1934). Radiation injury was considered to arise from an accumulation of toxic products, with recovery the result of their removal. It was further assumed that the rate of loss would follow the same first-order (exponential) kinetics as had been observed in chemical and biochemical reactions. Working with low voltage, unfiltered röntgen rays Kingery found that a full dose could be repeated after 14 days, 75% of a full dose after 7 days, and 50% after 3·5 days. The idea behind saturation was that tissues could be kept near the tolerance limit by giving a certain fraction of the first dose each day. For example, if after

---

†A word about the lives of the Austrian pioneers in radiology (Weiss 1966). Kienböck suffered a fracture of the base of the skull in 1910, but after recovering was able to continue working until a partial paralysis forced him to stop. Over the years, Holzknecht suffered radiation burns on his arms and hands, which resulted in a series of amputations; he continued working, however, until his death in 1931. Freund achieved late recognition for his accomplishments, when invited to be a founding member of the Austrian Radiological Society (1934) and keynote speaker at its first meeting (1936). Two years later he was obliged to emigrate after the Anschluss and died impoverished abroad in 1943.

one day 82% of the effects of the first dose remain, then 18% of the full dose might be added daily, and tissues kept at the 'saturation point for radiation effect'. The saturation method was put into clinical practice by Pfahler (1927), but was abandoned in the 1930s because of toxic side effects and the increasing popularity of Coutard's technique.

The conversion to fractionated treatments was widespread and the triumph of Coutard's technique recognized when he reported it at the American Congress of Röntgenology in 1932 (Coutard 1932). This was occasioned as much by evidence of comparative sparing of late complications as by cures of tumours previously thought uncurable. Jüngling (1924) had reported a 23% incidence of severe edema and necrosis after the expedited, single-dose treatment of carcinoma of the larynx, as opposed to the low incidence of these complications in Coutard's material.

An intriguing aspect of the adoption of Coutard's technique was that many centres were obliged on economic grounds to discontinue the low-dose-rate in favour of high-dose-rate exposures. An example is provided by Borak (1937) in his description of the adoption of Coutard's technique at Holzknecht's Institute in Vienna around 1930. Many conditions besides cancer were treated there, and this could not have been continued had they attempted to prolong treatments to 2 hours per sitting at a low dose rate. Therefore, Holzknecht decided to accept the fractionation technique, but not the low dose rate. This decision was justified by the results of later comparisons. Pape (1933) showed that the effect of a four-fold increase in dose rate could be set aside by splitting the dose into halves separated by an interval four times as long as the exposure time at the lower dose rate. Similarly, McWhirter (1935) of the Holt Radium Institute in Manchester showed that dose rate had no influence on the degree of erythema produced by fractionated treatment. Although Schwarz (1930) had shown that after 700 R (R = röntgen unit of exposure) a 1:4; or even 1:3, difference in dose rate could be detected, Borak (1937) found that 4400 R in 200 R fractions caused the same skin reactions whatever the dose rate, i.e. the 1:4 change made no difference. The latter concluded that the important difference was in size of dose per fraction. So also in the beginning Coutard gave large daily doses, especially to the smaller lesions, and it may have been necessary to deliver the large doses at low dose rates for tissue sparing. But this was thought no longer necessary when the daily dose was reduced, and this so-called *simple fractionation* with small fraction sizes was found to give results equivalent to those achieved by Coutard with the *protraction—fractionation* method ('protraction' at that time referred to low dose rate, i.e. protraction from a few minutes to an hour or two per sitting, and is not to be confused with its modern meaning of extended overall time). Indeed, Coutard used large daily doses only on the small tumours, reducing the daily dose and extending the overall time for large field sizes (Coutard 1932, 1934). A comparison of Borak's (1937) results with others using the 'protraction—fractionation' technique is presented in Table 5.1.

This view was shared by Baclesse (1896—1967), who had arrived at the Curie Institute in the late 1920s: "We believe that dose rate plays a smaller role than has been maintained in the past. On the basis of our cures we can state that lowering the dose rate, even to values that threaten the functioning of the X-ray unit, in no way guarantees sparing of injury of skin, once a certain dose has been given. The influence of the daily dose is greater." Beginning in 1928 Baclesse also extended the overall treatment time in developing a technique that avoided the skin and mucosal reactions that had been deliberately kept high with Coutard's method (Baclesse 1949). The purpose was to spare severe reactions, particularly in old and feeble patients.

Baclesse's method was based on avoiding acute reactions, but nevertheless increasing the total dose, which required extension of the overall treatment time and progressive reduction of field size. Doses per fraction were in the range 200—250 R skin dose. Mucositis was avoided on the basis of a 2½ week cycle: if this was avoided at 2½ weeks, then the same dose delivered every 2½ weeks would not result in mucositis. The rhythm for skin was 4—6 weeks, and in the same way if desquamation was avoided after 6 weeks the same dose could be given in the next 6 weeks without desquamation. A dose that avoided moist desquamation at 6 weeks also avoided mucositis at 2½ weeks. Therefore, if these reactions were avoided at these critical times by sufficiently slow treatments, "one could continue with impunity to the next and so on for 8, 10, or 12 weeks, without being hindered by a reaction which would oblige one to stop treatment altogether" (Baclesse 1949).

Coutard's technique was adopted throughout Europe and North America in the 1930s and 1940s. The low-dose-rate fractionation technique was maintained by Schinz and Zuppinger in Zurich, although as a

Table 5.1. Fractionation with low-dose-rate vs. high-dose-rate exposures

|  |  | Low dose rate | High dose rate |  |
|---|---|---|---|---|
|  |  | Coutard (1920—1926) | Schinz (1929—1932) | Borak (1931—1934) |
| Tonsil | Number of cases | 46 | 21 | 13 |
|  | NED after 2 years | 12 (26%) | 4 (19%) | 4 (31%) |
| Larynx | Number of cases | 77 | 15 | 19 |
|  | NED after 2 years | 25 (32%) | 4 (27%) | 8 (42%) |

NED: no evidence of disease.

From Borak (1937)

mixture of simple fractionation and low-dose-rate fractionation (Zuppinger 1941). Simple fractionation (i.e. at high dose rate in each session) was employed in most other places (Borak 1937); e.g. by Chaoul in Berlin, Miescher in Bern, Lenz and Martin in New York, Paterson (1897−1981) in Manchester, and Strandqvist in Stockholm. A survey of results of treatment in tumours of the hypopharynx (Table 5.2, modified from Zuppinger 1960) is of interest here, to reinforce the point of how widespread Coutard's technique had become.

Table 5.2. Hypopharynx tumours: survival after fractionated XRT

| Reference | Years | 3 years determinate | absolute | 5 years determinate | absolute |
|---|---|---|---|---|---|
| Baclesse Paris (1939) | 1921−35 | − | 10·5% | − | 10·4% |
| Coutard/Baclesse Paris (1949) | 1921−42 | − | − | − | 6·4% |
| Ahlbom Stockholm (1941) | 1930−39 | − | − | 7% | 6% |
| Hultberg Stockholm (1953) | 1943−47 | − | − | 14·5% | 12·3% |
| Lederman London (1954) | 1933−51 | − | − | − | 13% |
| Rennaes Oslo (1952) | 1938−47 | − | 13% | − | 6% |
| Oeser/Bade Berlin (1952) | 1926−45 | − | 12% | − | 5% |
| Paterson Manchester (1950) | 1940−44 | − | − | − | 5% |
| Coval/Antoniazzi Milan (1952) | 1928−46 | − | − | 17% | − |
| Harris/Silverstone New York (1954) | 1931−51 | − | − | 16% | − |
| Schinz/Scharer Zurich (1952) | 1929−50 | − | 14·6% | − | 9·7% |
| Zuppinger/Schinz Zurich (1944) | 1929−41 | 20% | 15% | 14% | 10% |
| Zuppinger Bern (1959) | 1947−55 | 23% | 19% | 17% | 14% |
| Wang Boston (1956) | 1931−50 | − | − | 18% | − |
| Garland San Francisco (1952) | 1932−46 | − | − | 15% | − |

From Zuppinger (1960) where the original references may be found.

Marked changes in treatment practice were brought about by World War II, as exemplified by treatments in Manchester. A good example is the evolution of the method of treatment of carcinoma of the cervix using radium. In 1932–33 (Christie Hospital 1939) it was quoted as being "an attempt at fusion of what seemed the best features of the two leading techniques of that time—the Paris technique of Regaud and the Stockholm technique of Heyman. The Manchester technique compromised between the two ideas, incorporating as far as practicable the low intensity factor from Paris and the divided but protracted overall period of treatment from Stockholm. The containers used were modelled on those designed in Paris and gave a similar intensity, but the dose was divided into four applications of 48 hours each. If a course of X-ray therapy was included it was placed between the first two and last two radium applications, the overall time for radium only being 4 weeks, for radium plus X-rays 6 weeks." In 1934–38 (Paterson et al. 1945), treatments using radium alone were reduced to 2–3 weeks. If X-ray treatments were added, these were given over a 3-week period, making 5 to 6 weeks total. In 1939, even shorter treatments were instigated because of restrictions on the use of radium in wartime. At first two treatment periods of 72 hours were used, separated by 3 days. The latter rest period was increased to 4 days when more beds became available, making a total time of 10 days. The working dose level in 1945 was 8000 R at point A for stages I and II, and this became the 'optimum dose' for this type of treatment (Paterson 1952; Cole & Hunter 1985). This remained the situation until radium was replaced by caesium, and dose rates were increased (Cole & Hunter 1985).

Radical small-field X-ray treatments were started in Manchester in 1935, and they increased in frequency, particularly during the war years. In most cases treatments were given 5 days a week over 5 weeks, with all fields being treated on each day (24 treatments were quoted for cancers of the posterior third of the oral cavity; 5500 R to 6000 R in 5 to 6 weeks was quoted for radical whole-neck treatments). Treatments of 10 000 R over 10 weeks were tried. However, many lesions recurred, particularly secondary deposits in the lymph nodes, and these extended treatments were discontinued. With cancers of the mouth, 5-week treatments were used until 1944 (Paterson et al. 1950). Then the pressure on beds and apparatus was so great that 3-week treatments were used, and doses were reduced by 500 R. The success of these treatments, and the increase in the patient load in post-war years, made this the standard schedule for radical treatments and this has remained so to the present day. For example, the basis of present head-and-neck radical practice is 5250–5500 cGy in 15–16 fractions in 21 days (Duthie & Gupta 1985).

What are considered today non-standard fractionation techniques, such as multiple treatments per day, were used in the 1930s. In his closing remarks, Schwarz (1937) underlined this point before the first Congress of the Austrian Radiology Society. Based on his observation of recovery in skin after 2-hour fractionation intervals, he was led to the use of *superfractionation* (this may have occurred in the early 1930s; we are left to guess at the meaning of the words "...seit einiger Zeit..." spoken in September 1936). Appropriate cases were treated at 4-hour intervals three times daily with doses per fraction of 70 R, or 8-hour intervals twice times daily with doses per fraction of 100 R. This was not the only instance, as Coutard had often used two treatments daily, and Zuppinger (1960) reported fewer complications in the treatment of hypopharynx when he used two treatments per day "as recommended originally by Coutard".

The Baclesse technique was brought to the USA by his students, primarily Gilbert Fletcher; there and in Europe, fractionation practices include treatment in 6—7 weeks and differ from those in the UK and the Commonwealth nations where most treatments are with fewer, somewhat larger dose fractions in 3 to 5 weeks, as outlined above.

However, clinical practice was influenced in both schools beginning in the 1950s by various concepts of the time factor in radiotherapy, the first being those based on power-law models, from Strandqvist (1944) to the NSD formula (1967). Much more recently, time-factor concepts have been based on the more biologically oriented survival models (the LQ formalism). We consider next these interpretations and their influence on radiotherapy.

## 5.2. Interpretations: the time factor and power-law models (1930s to 1960s)

The importance of the time during which a dose is delivered in determining biological effect was recognized in the first decade of this century when single-dose treatments began to replace fractionated treatments. In many cases severe complications might have been caused by overdosing, given the primitive techniques of dose measurement at that time. However, it was clear from clinical results that the effect of a dose was diminished by fractionation (Krönig & Friedrich 1918).

**Recovery factors**

In the 1920s and 1930s tabulated recovery factors for fractionated radiation were published, especially those derived for equal daily treatments. Recovery factors multiplied by the biologically effective dose given in a single sitting gave the biologically equivalent dose for treatments given in a specified number of days. Many investigators showed the diminished effectiveness of a dose when it was fractionated (Stenstrom & Mattick 1926; Liechti 1929), but usually with few patients. Reisner (1933) published the first systematic study, using as the biological endpoint a sharp degree of erythema as measured by the 'erythema-ometer' of Schall and Alius (cited by Strandqvist, 1944, p. 73). There were six small fields (2 × 2 cm) on each thigh, of which one received the standard dose (1100 R in air) and the other five fields received various combinations of doses. Reisner concluded: "The results show that, with appropriately chosen total doses, the effect of multiple dose fractions, even very small ones, is in no respect different, in terms of macroscopic skin changes, from that of a single dose."

The recovery factors of Reisner (1933), as well as those of Duffy, Arneson & Edward (1934) and MacComb & Quimby (1936) are set out in Table 5.3. The agreement between these may be considered good, especially in view of the differences in biological endpoint, site, and field size.

Miescher (1935) was concerned that most research dealt only with reactions such as erythema and epilation, whereas the late reactions were of greater concern to radiotherapists. He therefore conducted experiments using the rabbit ear as a model, with the following late endpoints: white hair (depigmentation), permanent epilation, atrophy, necrosis, and hyperkeratoses, and observed that the latency intervals were shorter with the larger doses. Varied were the dose per fraction (200 R, 400 R, 1000 R, and single doses) and fractionation interval (3 hours, 1 day, 4 days, 7 days, 4 weeks).

Miescher (1935) may have been the first to plot tolerance dose against dose per fraction. On the basis of these curves Miescher saw no way to

Table 5.3. Recovery factors for fractionated X-rays[a]

| Reisner (1933) | | | | Duffy et al. (1934) | | MacComb and Quimby (1936) | |
|---|---|---|---|---|---|---|---|
| Brisk erythema (1100 R in single treatments) | | Dry desquamation (1320 R in single treatment) | | Threshold erythema (525 R in single treatment) | | Threshold erythema (525 R in single treatment) | |
| days | factors | days | factors | days | factors | days | factors |
| 2 | 1·3 | 2 | 1·2 | 2 | 1·6 | 2 | 1·5 |
| 3 | 1·5 | 3 | 1·6 | 3 | 1·8 | 3 | 1·6 |
| 4 | 1·6 | 4 | 1·7 | | | 5 | 1·8 |
| 7 | 2·1 | 6 | 2·0 | | | 12 | 2·3 |
| 12 | 2·4 | 9 | 2·3 | | | | |
| 27 | 2·7 | 16 | 2·7 | | | | |

[a] Equivalent dose in $T$ days = recovery factor × equivalent dose in single treatment

distinguish between the response to changing dose per fraction of connective tissues and epithelial tissues. Indeed when the fractionation factors of Reisner (1933) for strong erythema were plotted in Miescher's coordinates, the slope was somewhat steeper than those describing the fractionation response in terms of white hair (depigmentation), atrophy, and permanent epilation.

**The Schwarzschild law**

Similar factors to the fractionation factor were derived for the effect of changing the dose rate of single exposures. Krönig & Friedrich (1918) published findings indicative of stronger erythema when the dose rate was changed from 1·3 to 10·4 R/min. Miescher (1924) found weaker erythema with both 8- and 15-fold decreases of the dose rate. Holthusen & Braun (1933) examined changes in weak-erythema isoeffect doses with dose rate over the range 10−500 R/min (Table 5.4).

Although the single doses were quite different for two dissimilar endpoints, one may still conclude that Holthusen & Braun (1933) found a much stronger dose-rate effect. Other authors were also unable to verify such large protraction factors (Chaoul 1932; Reisner 1933). In any event, from early on many of the researchers (among others, Liechti 1929; Schwarz 1930; Glocker et al. 1931) attempted to link the time factor manifest with changing exposure time in a purely formal way to the Schwarzschild law of photochemistry, which states that the effect of a given exposure of light is proportional to the product of intensity ($I$) and time ($T$) raised to the power $p$, where $p$ is less than 1 (Strandqvist 1944, p.66):

$$I \times T^p = \text{constant} \qquad (5.1)$$

Table 5.4. Recovery factors for low dose rate

| Dose rate (R/min) | Threshold erythema (Holthusen & Braun 1933) | Tumour disappearance (McWhirter 1935) |
|---|---|---|
| 500 | 1·0 | — |
| 50 | 1·56 | — |
| 20 | — | 1·0 |
| 5 | 2·6 | — |
| 2 | −1·43 | — |
| 1·1 | — | 1·65 |
| 0·9 | — | 1·85 |
| 0·7 | — | 2·0 |
| 0·5 | 4·6 | — |

R = röntgen; single dose for threshold erythema at 500 R/min = 480 R; single dose for tumour disappearance at 20 R/min = 2000 R.

This formula indicates that when the exposure time is increased, the effect of the light will be the same only if its amount ($D =$ intensity $\times$ time) is increased (since equation (5.1) is equivalent to $D \times T^{p-1} =$ constant, or $D =$ constant $\times T^{1-p}$). The number $1 - p$ lay between 0 and 1, and therefore this relationship corresponds to a diminished effect with decreasing dose rate ($I$), suggesting some type of 'recovery' in the exposed material. Holthusen (1933) believed that the diminished effectiveness of a dose when dose rate was reduced could be described by the Schwarzschild law, equation (5.1), for all plants and animals. Liechti (1929) surveyed the clinical and experimental data and concluded that $p$ was less than 1, i.e. there was evidence for a dose-rate effect. Glocker et al. (1931) found $p$-values of 0·95 for bean sprouts and 0·96 for axolotl eggs, and further that $p$ appeared constant in the range 5–500 R/min. On the other hand, the data of Holthusen and Braun set out in Table 5.4 indicate that $p$ increases with increasing dose rate (from 0·8 to 0·84 as dose rate increases from 0·5 to 500 R/min), with the implication that the dose-rate effect gradually disappears with increasing dose rate.

To summarize, power-law models were introduced because of the analogy between diminished effectiveness of a light exposure when intensity was decreased and diminished biological effectiveness of a radiation dose when dose rate was decreased. These models predicted a linear relationship between log isoeffect dose and log exposure time.

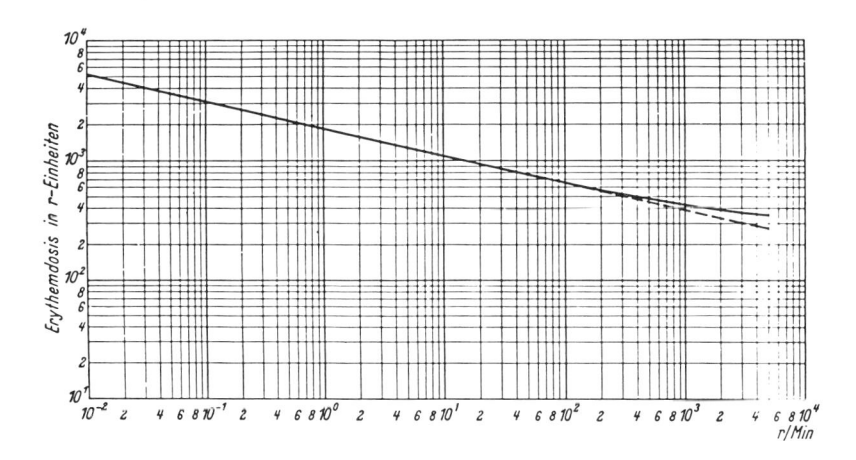

Figure 5.1. Dependence of erythema dose on dose rate, and one of the earliest presentations of isoeffect data on double-log coordinates. The dashed line is an extrapolation of the linear segment at lower dose rates, and indicates that the dose-rate effect for erythema was gradually lost for dose rates higher than about 400 r/min where r = röntgen exposure unit. (Modified from Witte 1939.)

152    *Fractionation in Radiotherapy*

Power-law models

One of the first uses of double-log coordinates was described by Witte (1939), who altered the curve of Holthusen and Hamann (cited by Strandqvist, p. 64) relating erythema dose to dose rate into log erythema dose versus log dose rate and found that the data could be represented by a straight line (Figure 5.1). His presentation of isoeffect dose versus number of treatments, for different dose rates, is shown in Figure 5.2. He pointed out the need for experimental data to test these curves, and in a later publication (Witte 1942) concluded that for higher numbers of fractions dose rate had no effect. In the latter paper, Witte presented the first analysis of log isoeffect dose versus log number of fractions.

Zuppinger (1941) renormalized late-isoeffect doses for telangiectasia to D20 (Dose in 20 days); fractionation factors were larger than those of Reisner for erythema. A parabolic isoeffect curve is shown with his data in Figure 5.3. Zuppinger thought his curves not comparable with Reisner's (1933) because he used a different time point for normalization (20 days), different biological endpoints, and a different dose rate (5 R/min). *Dissociation between early and late reactions* was observed in the treatment of head-and-neck tumours with altered fractionation, with *worse late reactions accompanying larger dose fractions*. This may be the first mention of a phenomenon that has had a decisive influence on experimental and clinical work on fractionation in the 1980s (however see Jüngling 1924).

Others employed the double-log representation for isoeffect doses.

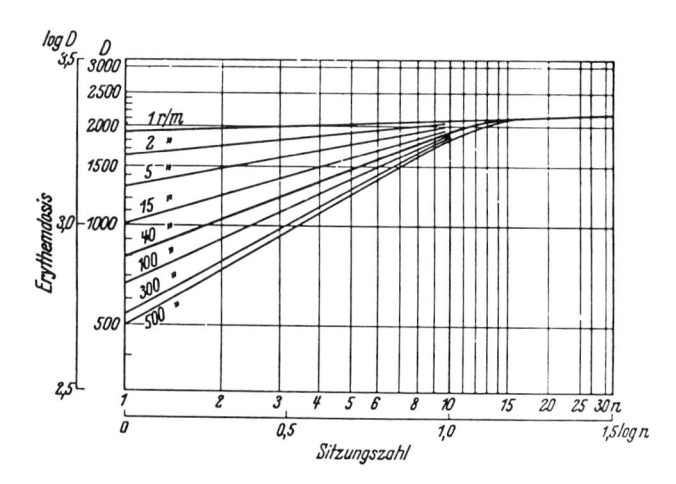

Figure 5.2. Dependence of erythema dose (*D*) on number of treatments (Sitzungszahl) for different dose rates (r = röntgen exposure unit). The dose-rate is gradually lost as the dose is increasingly fractionated. (Modified from Witte 1942.)

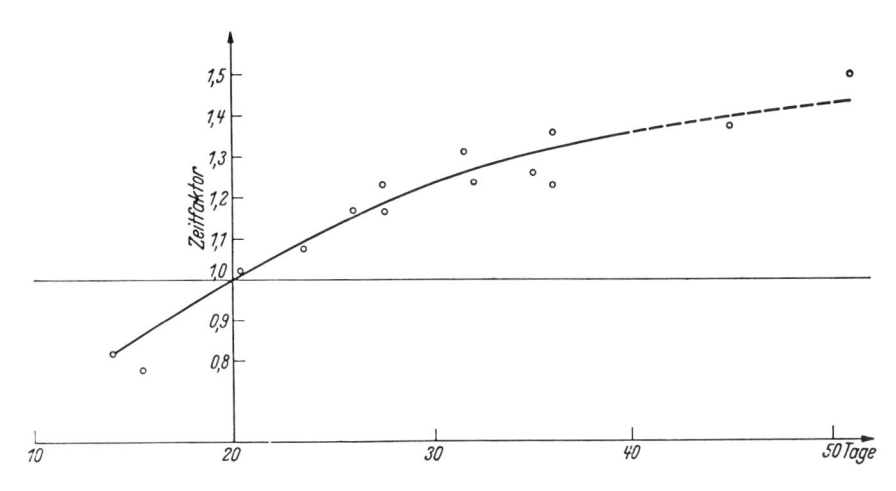

Figure 5.3. The time factor (Zeitfaktor) for late telangiectasia after fractionated irradiation as a function of overall time in days (Tage). Doses have been normalized to the dose given in 20 days, and the circles represent observations. (Modified from Zuppinger 1941.)

Wachsmann (1943a,b), for example, gave perhaps the first presentation of isoeffect relationships showing different slopes for different degrees of skin reaction (Figure 5.4). These were the power-law models used by the authors who influenced Strandqvist's monograph (1944).

### The Strandqvist monograph

Strandqvist's presentation of isoeffect data in double-log coordinates represented a departure from previous practice, since he defined the abscissa in terms of *number of days after the first treatment*, rather than number of treatments. It is worthwhile to review his reasoning, since the change led him to assign a time for a single treatment in a different way, and subsequent authors went back to the practice of plotting in terms of number of treatments when they assigned one day to the time for one treatment. This seemingly trivial matter will be seen to have had significant consequences.

Strandqvist (1944, p.70) made an assumption fundamental to his analysis: "...if not completely definitive on the matter, nevertheless published reports suggest that, within certain bounds, radiation effect depends only on the total dose and overall time. If then the fractions are in the main separated by 24 hours, it is clear that it matters very little if the fractional doses are of variable size, or if somewhat longer intervals occur." This assumption, in accord with the view of Quimby & MacComb (1937), was inconsistent with other evidence pointing toward the importance of size of dose per fraction: Reisner (1933) and Holthusen

154                    Fractionation in Radiotherapy

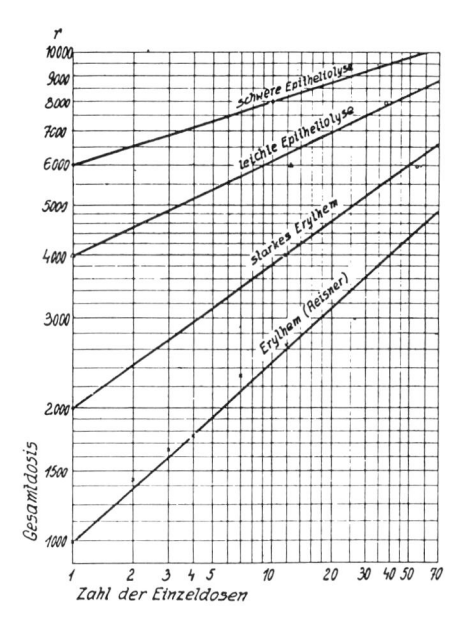

Figure 5.4. Total dose (Gesamtdosis) for equivalent skin reaction as a function of fraction number (modified from Wachsmann 1943a). From the highest to lowest, severe desquamation, light desquamation, strong erythema, and erythema (data of Reisner (1933)).

(1933) felt that, with the same total dose and overall time, lower reactions accompanied the use of smaller fraction sizes, as did Zuppinger (1941).

In addition to the influence that this biological assumption had on his thinking, Strandqvist was influenced by the apparent theoretical value of power-law representations. When he analysed the results of treatment of skin cancer at the Radiumhemmet from 1933 to 1937, in terms of recurrences and complications (skin necroses, not erythema), he found that a parabola could separate these successfully (Figure 5.5). While admitting that recovery probably did not follow a simple curve, Strandqvist appealed to arguments justifying empirical approximations of complex phenomena. These rested on the observation that various pharmacological formulae relating dose and effect (Langmuir absorption formula, Weber—Fechner law, Freundlich formula), whose mathematical representations were respectively hyperbolic, exponential, and parabolic, all lay within 5% of each other over a wide range of concentrations . Strandqvist applied this line of thinking in observing that the diminishing effect of dose with protraction, parabolic in linear—linear coordinates (Figure 5.5), became linear in the double-log coordinates introduced by Witte (1939, 1942). The same was true of the

*In hindsight* 155

Schwarzschild law of photochemistry (equation 5.1), which had been applied to describe dose-rate effects.

Strandqvist chose 0·35 day as the nominal time for treatments conducted in a single sitting based on equivalent late skin reactions after a single dose of 2250 R and 4200 R in 6 days: the line with slope 0·22

Gesamtdosis in r

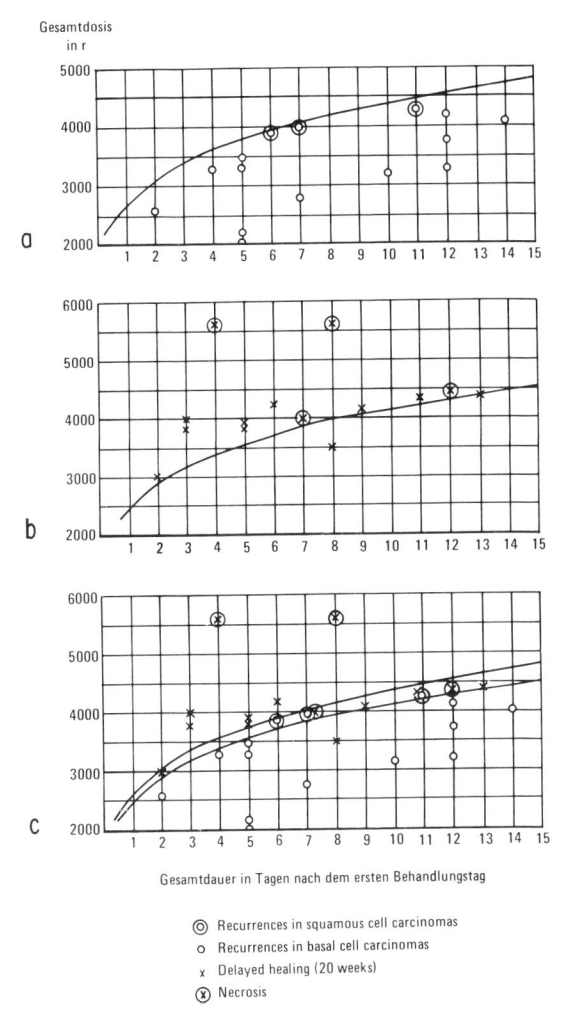

a

b

c

Gesamtdauer in Tagen nach dem ersten Behandlungstag

- ⊚ Recurrences in squamous cell carcinomas
- o Recurrences in basal cell carcinomas
- × Delayed healing (20 weeks)
- ⊗ Necrosis

Figure 5.5. Recurrences and complications at the Radiumhemmet, 1933–37 (from Strandqvist (1944) and Fletcher (1980)). Total dose (Gesamtdosis) as a function of overall time in days after the first treatment day for recurrences within 1 year (circles) and complications (×'s). (a) Curve lying above recurrences; (b) curve lying below complications; (c) boundary zone between the curves of (a) and (b) which separates recurrences and complications with the least possible admixture. (Reproduced with permission of Lea & Febiger and the author.)

intersected the dose axis at time 0·35 days. He also presented the following theoretical argument in favour of this choice (p.225). At moderately high dose rates, the overall time was roughly the sum of interfraction intervals. Therefore it was approximately zero for a single dose, and zero could not be placed on a logarithmic scale. But the single dose could be conceptualized as composed of two half doses, given with a pause short enough that negligible recovery took place during it. Strandqvist considered that the evidence favoured an interval fulfilling this condition of as long as 8 hours. Therefore, the time for a single dose was taken as ⅓ day, i.e. approximately 0·35 day.

Strandqvist was led to the power-law because of the mathematical symmetry between the Schwarzschild relationship for dose-rate effects and power-law representations for fractionation factors on the one hand, and the biological conception of low dose rate as approximated by a series of many, small fractional doses. Thus, in his discussion on the significance of the slope (pp. 232—3), he pointed out that typical $p$-values in the power-law representation of dose rate ($I$) and exposure time ($T$) for isoeffect (equation 5.1) were in the range 0·8—1·0. Then, since $I$ equals dose divided by time ($D/T$), equation (5.1) can be rewritten $D \times T^{p-1} = $ constant, or

$$D = \text{constant} \times T^{1-p}.$$

This has exactly the form of the Strandqvist plot, with $1-p$ approximately 0·2, close to his estimated slope 0·22. He also pointed out the importance of the choice of the time assigned to a single treatment, and that the slope was influenced by this choice.

Figure 5.6 shows the date for recurrences and complications from 1933 to 1937, as Strandqvist first presented them in double-log coordinates, with elapsed time since first treatment as the abscissa. He found the same slope applicable to both recurrences and necroses (0·22) on the double-log plots. Furthermore, he found that *the slope 0·22 resulted in good agreement with the data of Reisner (1933) as well as with those of MacComb & Quimby (1936).*

It is noteworthy that the data of Reisner pertained to strong erythema, and those of MacComb and Quimby to threshold erythema, a reaction whose variability was known to change with its degree. For example, the variability in isoeffect doses was greatest for weak erythema (± 40%, Miescher 1924, ± 30%, Holthusen 1933). For strong erythema it was less (±15—20%, Miescher 1924), and smallest for moist desquamation (Strandqvist 1944, p. 47). In Wachsmann's (1943b) analysis (Figure 5.4), slopes were different for strong and weak erythema. Also noteworthy is the paucity of data on which the slope was based. The data from the period 1933 to 1937 consisted of only 15

*In hindsight* 157

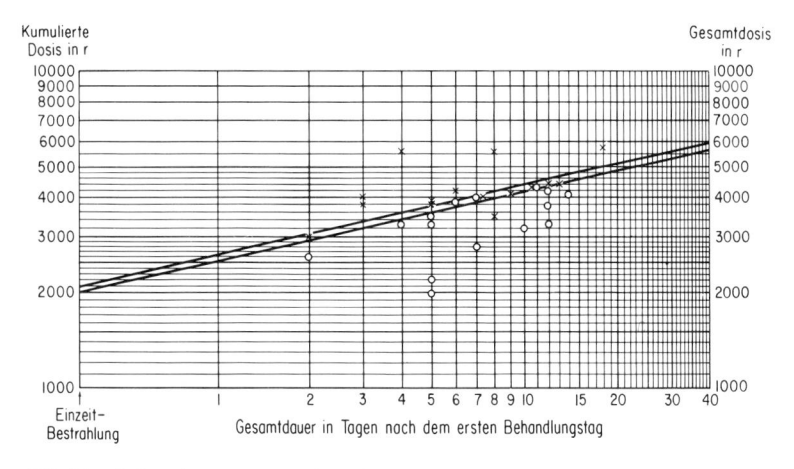

Figure 5.6. Total dose in röntgen units of exposure versus overall time in days since the first treatment day (from Strandqvist (1944) and Fletcher (1980)). The same data are plotted as in Figure 5.5, except that double-log coordinates have been used. Single-dose treatment (Einzeithbestrahlung) was placed at 0·35 days. Recurrences are indicated by circles, and complications by ×'s. (Reproduced with permission of Lea & Febiger and the author.)

recurrences and 14 complications, and *only one patient was treated in a time longer than 14 days*. Of the recurrences, about 25% were squamous cell carcinomas, and the remainder were basal cell carcinomas.

## Normal tissues versus tumours

Cohen (1949b) compared data for normal skin response (single treatment = 1 day) and recurrences of skin cancer (single treatment = '0' days). He deduced that Reisner's data for human skin (strong erythema), Quimby's data (weak erythema), and Ellis' tables (skin 'tolerances') were fitted by a line with slope 0·30, and concluded that "... there can be no doubt that the difference between the Strandqvist exponent 0·22 for squamous carcinoma and the value of 0·30 for normal skin as obtained by three independent observers, is real and significant."

Cohen's analysis (1949b) is illustrated in Figure 5.7. From this and subsequent publications (Cohen & Kerrich 1951; Cohen 1966), there arose the notion that recovery occurred more efficiently in normal skin than in squamous cell tumours, thus explaining the advantage of fractionated radiotherapy.

However, it is unlikely that a difference in fractionation sensitivity of squamous carcinoma and normal skin can be deduced in this way. First, there is the choice of time scale. Strandqvist took pains to point out (pp. 224, 271−2) that his use of 0·35 days for a single treatment represented a departure from the usual practice and that the slope was affected by

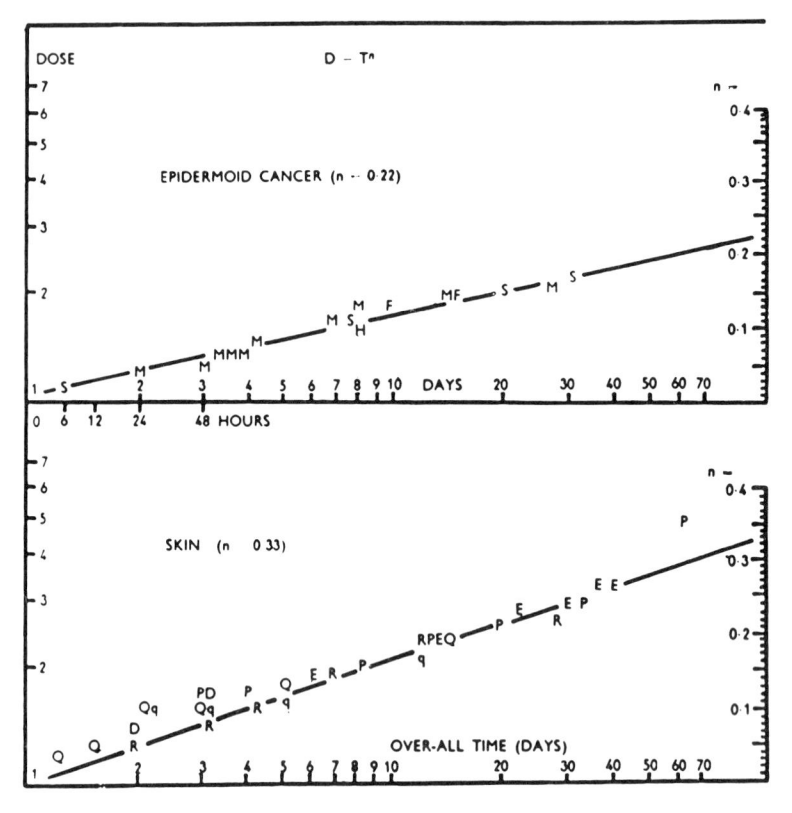

Figure 5.7. Determination of the recovery exponent for skin and skin cancer (from Cohen 1949b). Symbols refer to authors listed in Table I of Cohen (1949b); M = McWhirter (1935), also Ham (1936), and Cowell (1937, 1938); R = Reisner (1933); S = Strandqvist (1944). Note that Strandqvist's convention was followed for the tumours with the result that the recovery exponent was 0·22, while a time of 1 day was assigned for a single treatment for skin reactions (recovery exponent = 0·33). When these are plotted with the same convention for single doses, parallel lines cannot be excluded, as shown in Figure 6.23. (Reproduced with permission of The British Institute of Radiology and the author.)

this choice. Moreover, with the slope 0·22 there was good agreement between his isoeffect data for skin necrosis, those of Reisner (1933) for strong erythema, and those of MacComb & Quimby (1936) for threshold erythema. As pointed out by Fletcher & Barkley (1974, Table II), choice of the time for a single dose has a strong effect on the estimated slope (cf. Figure 6.23). Second, the majority of Strandqvist's patients had basal cell carcinomas, not squamous cell carcinoma. Out of a total of 32 recurrences (15 during the initial time period 1933−37, during which 91 patients constituted the data base for the first isoeffect curves separating recurrences and complications), 8 were squamous cell tumours (including lip carcinoma).

Similar time−dose formulae were applied to different sets of clinical data by various authors in the 1940s and 1950s (Jolles & Mitchell 1947; Cohen & Kerrich 1951; Cohen 1952; Andrews & Moody 1956; DuSault 1956; von Essen 1960). Noteworthy for its effect on subsequent clinical practice was Cohen's (1952) finding that the recovery exponent for breast cancer treated with daily fractions was at least as great as that of normal skin (0·33, the cube-root law). He concluded that "whether there is any advantage, therefore, in prolonged fractionation for this tumour is open to doubt." This principle, when put into practice, led to severe late complications after treatment of breast cancer (Atkins 1964; Montague 1968).

The difficulty of assigning appropriate time exponents to clinical data was illustrated by von Essen's (1960) study of the complications attending treatment of skin cancers. He attempted to determine the position and slope of a line that would separate the majority of successfully treated lesions from necroses. Following Strandqvist, he assigned 0·35 days as the time for a single treatment. He found that a number of slopes and intercepts appeared to achieve equivalent separation for small fields, from $D = 2500 \times T^{0.20}$ to $D = 1400 \times T^{0.34}$; the best separation was found for $D = 1950 \times T^{0.27}$. The small number of necroses resulting from treatment of large fields made it impossible to estimate a slope. This large range of possibilities for slope reflects the considerable scatter in the data, scatter that was typical of most clinical studies.

Thus the time−dose formula, an edifice whose foundations rested on different time scales, few patients, and the concept that overall time but not dose per fraction was important, grew to include the concept that normal tissue recovery differed from that of tumours.

### Number of fractions versus overall time

In all this work, the crucial assumption that varying the number of fractions for the same total dose in the same overall time did not appreciably affect the degree of reaction (Reisner 1933; Quimby & MacComb 1937) was rarely challenged. Evidence to the contrary was provided in 1963, when Fowler et al. published their analysis of experiments on pigskin. This analysis was further supported by Dutreix et al. (1973) from experiments on human skin. Fowler and colleagues were motivated by a theoretical analysis (later published as Fowler & Stern 1960) using 'slow repair' (repopulation) and 'fast repair', which at the time had not been identified. Fast repair was characterized by the experiments of Elkind & Sutton (1959, 1960), which offered a different explanation for the *way in which total isoeffect dose increased with overall time* (or number of fractions), namely the rapid restoration of the original shape of the dose—effect curve ('Elkind recovery', as distinguished from slower tissue repair and repopulation processes).

Fowler et al. (1963) designed experiments on pigskin to distinguish between two competing explanations of recovery: Elkind recovery and slow tissue repair, or repopulation. They knew that the effect produced by 20-Gy X-rays given as a single dose was equal to that produced by 35 Gy in 5 fractions over 5 days or by 55 Gy in 21 fractions over 4 weeks. The critical experiment was to give 5 fractions distributed evenly over 28 days. If 35 Gy were required for the same effect, the important factor would be the number of fractions, because the effect of slow repair and repopulation would be relatively small, and the increase in dose with overall time would be due to the effect of the smaller fractions. If on the other hand 55 Gy were required to produce the same effect, then the overall time of 28 days would be the important factor, and the number of fractions would be irrelevant, whether 5 or 21.

The results showed that 5 fractions over 28 days gave the same skin effect with total doses of about 42 Gy, leading the authors to conclude that overall time was relatively unimportant between 5 and 28 days and that the main effect determining the increase in dose with extended fractionation was the size and number of the individual fractions. The effect of overall time was not negligible, however, as it contributed about one-third of the increase in total dose. The main conclusion was that the use of fewer and larger fractions required a reduction in total dose, in contrast to Quimby & MacComb's (1937) finding.

This late recognition of the importance of fraction size may be attributed in part to the lack of precision in the studies of the time factor using strong (Reisner 1933) and weak (MacComb & Quimby 1936) erythema as endpoints, as well as to questionable isoeffectiveness of the 'tolerance doses' for skin of Ellis (1942) and Paterson (1948). Nias (1963), using a reflectance spectrophotometer and erythema as endpoint on human skin, found a recovery factor of 1·2 instead of the 1·6 of Reisner and MacComb & Quimby. This he attributed to the fact that the 'threshold skin dose' observations could not be accurate, and further that the erythema measurements of Reisner, using a simple colorimeter, were inaccurate. He concluded that none of the early skin experiments could distinguish between fractionation factors ranging from 1.2 to 1.6.

## The Ellis NSD formula

This was the situation in the mid-1960s when the NSD formula of Ellis (1967) was published. At least two key factors influenced its development: first, the perception from the papers of Cohen (1949a,b; 1951; 1952; 1960; 1966) that the recovery exponents for squamous cell carcinoma and acute skin reactions were different; and second, the animal experiments of Fowler and colleagues, which demonstrated that for skin reactions the number of fractions was of greater importance in determining isoeffect doses than time, at least up to 28 days. Ellis interpreted the difference between recovery exponents, $0\cdot33-0\cdot22=0\cdot11$, as the appropriate time coefficient, on grounds that it was justifiable to assume that squamous cell carcinoma was not subject to homeostatic control. Since it could safely be assumed that normal skin was subject to such control, the ground was laid for separation of fractionation and time factors, i.e. the difference between the slopes for normal skin and squamous carcinoma, $0\cdot11$, could be taken as a 'regression' coefficient with time for normal tissue recovery, while the coefficient $0\cdot22$ represented the effect of fractionation. The latter was corrected by R. Oliver for five-times-weekly treatment to $0\cdot24$, and the NSD formula (Ellis 1967, 1969) resulted:

$$\text{Total dose} = \text{NSD} \times N^{0.24} \, T^{0.11}$$

wherein NSD stood for *nominal standard dose*, $N$ = number of fractions, and $T$ = overall time (days).

Ellis (1969) recognized that the NSD could not be considered a realistic single dose, since as such it could not be reconciled with a time measured in days. But he may have been unaware that the separation of time and number of fractions for which his formula is well known was influenced by mixed conventions for the time assigned to a single dose (Figure 5.7), and from the relatively wide separation of $0\cdot35$ and $1\cdot0$ days on a log scale (Fletcher & Barkley 1974; see Figure 6.23). The NSD formula ran into difficulties almost from the beginning and the literature contains many debates on its reliability (e.g. Fowler 1971; Liversage 1971).

Nevertheless, the NSD equation has had a significant impact on clinical practice. One reason was that it established a method for giving fewer than five treatments per week, with obvious potential for reducing the cost and time consumed by treatment. Two-fractions-per-week treatment is still in use in the UK (Bates 1975); but the possibility of reducing the number of treatments to one per week has had perhaps its greatest impact in third-world countries, sometimes with adverse consequences (Singh 1978). The most important reason for the success of the NSD concept was that it allowed for routine adjustments of dosage in the clinic, and the calculation of putatively isoeffective treatment regimens with different numbers of fractions, overall times, etc. (see Examples in Section 6.10).

Various extensions of the formula were developed. Kirk *et al.* (1971) developed the CRE (cumulative radiation effect) system to account for the effect on normal tissues of 'subtolerance' doses. They proposed that for different levels of injury in skin,

$$D = \text{CRE} \times N^{0.24} T^{0.11}.$$

At full tolerance, CRE = NSD, while at lower levels of reaction, families of isoeffect curves could be generated, each with its own CRE. The effects of sequential schedules could be considered, and Kirk *et al.* showed that a particular fractionation regimen achieved a certain CRE, whatever the order of its individual fractions. No experimental justification was given, however, for the concept of partial tolerance. Kirk *et al.* chose their exponents to match those proposed by Ellis, until further information should become available.

Orton & Ellis (1973) introduced the TDF (time, dose, and fractionation) factors, which had the advantage of additivity of partial tolerances (PT), defined (Ellis 1969) as

$$\text{PT} = (n/N)\,\text{NSD}$$

where $N$ = number of fractions of a chosen size to give full tolerance, and $n$ = number of such fractions actually given. The PTs were additive, but very cumbersome for computations. Orton and Ellis noted that whenever the biological effect of alternative fractionation schemes was the same, the NSD cancelled and played no further part in the calculations. Therefore, tables of the factor TDF:

$$\text{TDF} = n.d^{1.538}(T/N)^{-0.169}10^{-3}$$

where $d$ = dose per fraction, could be prepared that were independent of any specific NSD value (see Section 6.10 for practical examples worked out with the NSD or TDF method).

Split courses, in which a rest interval intervenes after the first part of treatment, were accounted for by the correction used by Ellis (1968a) and Winston *et al.* (1969). Kirk *et al.* (1975) proposed an exponential decay factor. The formulae also differed in their treatment of continuous exposure (Kirk *et al.* 1972; Orton 1974). These and other distinctions were discussed in the review by Goitein (1976).

### Critique

The difficulties encountered in the use of the power-law model plague each of these formulae equally, since they all rest on Ellis's original NSD equation. A critique can be presented along three lines of argument. First, misconceptions connected with the origins of the power-law models, which have been discussed already, e.g. the idea that normal tissues, notably skin and squamous cell tumours, were characterized by different time factors, and the mixed conventions for the time scales. A second line of criticism is statistically oriented; that is, given that the power-law models provide approximations to clinical experience over limited ranges of fraction number and time and that the techniques by which the exponents were arrived at were primitive at best, more appropriate modern methods should produce more reliable estimates (Herbert 1986). The possibility of deriving more reliable exponents for clinical use, however, is opposed by the third line of criticism, based on biological reasoning, which suggests that power-law models are inappropriate over any range of time and over extended ranges of number of fractions, particularly with different tissues characterized by different fractionation sensitivities.

The biological case is briefly as follows. First, the use of a power-law representation for the time factor implies that recovery is maximal in the first week or two of treatment and progressively decreases thereafter (Withers & Peters 1980, Table 2.20). But this contradicts biological data, which indicate that proliferation begins only after a certain time lag, becomes rapid, and then gradually returns to equilibrium (or lower, if a large dose has been given). Therefore, no matter how sophisticated the fitting techniques or careful the design of the experiment, no power-law representation of proliferative response can be expected to describe the data adequately. Second, in connection with the number-of-fractions exponent, it is known that tissues differ in their fractionation sensitivity (see Table 2.5 and Figure 2.14). Therefore, no single exponent can describe 'connective tissue tolerance', especially when this has been derived from acute skin reactions. While account could conceivably be taken of these differing fractionation sensitivities by applying different number-of-fractions exponents (Orton 1985), there is the added difficulty that these should depend on fraction size (Table 2.5). Thus, the steepness of the fractionation response should be greatest for the large dose fractions and gradually decrease toward 0 with decreasing dose per fraction, as experimentally demonstrated, for example, by Dutreix and colleagues (1973).

## 5.3. Interpretations: the survival-curve models (1956–1986)

From the early work of Rous & Jones (1916), to the much later work of Puck et al. (1956), technology was developed that permitted the evaluation of the proliferative capacity of individual mammalian cells, in particular after their exposure to ionizing radiation (Puck & Marcus 1956). This development introduced a completely new way of thinking about radiation isoeffect data, namely as manifestations of killing of target cells characterized by specific survival curves (Elkind 1960; Fowler & Stern 1960, 1963; Munro & Gilbert 1961; Lajtha & Oliver 1961). When the recovery effects observed in culture (Elkind & Sutton 1959, 1960) were used to predict tumour and normal-tissue response to fractionated radiotherapy, it was found that the total dose required to reach a given survival level was expected to increase with the number of treatments. This provided a new explanation for the time−dose factor and led to experiments testing the relative influence of Elkind-type recovery (dependence on number and size of fractions) and other factors, such as proliferation, believed to be more dependent on overall time (Fowler et al. 1963).

**Tissue isoeffect and cell survival**

Fowler & Stern (1960) based their approach on the observations of Gray & Scholes (1951) that chromosome breaks in irradiated *Vicia faba* roots increased linearly with dose at low dose rates, and with higher powers of dose as the dose rate increased. Following Read (1958), who concluded that chromosome damage was the most important direct action of radiation involved in tumour elimination, they assumed that biological response depended on a linear and on a dose-squared term. In conformity with the usage of Strandqvist's predecessors, Witte (1942) and Wachsmann (1943a,b), Fowler and Stern plotted data in terms of log dose versus log number of fractions, rather than overall time.

Strictly speaking, this approach was not based on cell survival, as it was in Elkind (1960) and their later paper (Fowler & Stern 1963). It is only in retrospect that we may recognize 'biological effect' as interpretable in terms of log survival, with characteristic downward curvature of the isoeffect plot. This is in contrast to the upward curvature characteristic of isoeffect curves based on the multitarget model (cf. Section 6.4), used by Elkind (1960) and Fowler & Stern (1963). The latter authors in fact stated that they could not reconcile the data with isoeffect curves, unless they used what "culturists of single cells *in vitro*" considered rather large extrapolation numbers. The trouble was that the multitarget model (equation 6.1) always underestimated cell kill at small doses.

The first formulation of the cell population kinetic (CPK) model of Cohen & Scott (1968) built upon these ideas by assuming that survival models derived from *in vitro* cloning studies had predictive value, at constant levels of survival, for tissue isoeffect doses (the same ideas were promoted at the time by Jean Dutreix, as exemplified in his later publication (Dutreix et al. 1973)). The model assumed cell killing by a two-component mechanism (cf. equation 6.3). Regeneration was assumed to occur logistically, as opposed to exponentially. There was no initial time lag, but the initial exponential rate of growth gradually decreased to zero to reflect limited regenerative capacity. The critical log surviving fraction was defined by $Q = -\log S$. Subsequently, there were adjustments for field-size dependency, and slope adjustments to correct for RBE and OER (Cohen 1983). The model was fitted to isoeffect data by assuming that if different treatment schemes were found to yield similar reactions in a tissue, then each must have resulted in the same surviving fraction of target cells. Therefore, parameters were varied until the computed values of $Q$ were approximately the same for the different isoeffective treatment regimens. Cohen and his co-workers compiled tables of parameter values for different normal tissues. Using these, they were able to calculate therapeutic ratios for different fractionation schemes and to select some as 'optimal' for certain normal tissues.

The regenerative response to radiotherapy in most normal tissues occurs after a variable (and possibly dose-dependent) time lag that is longer in the slowly turning-over tissues, an aspect which the model does not accommodate since it describes an immediate response. More serious difficulties arise from the limited data available, and as a result, from the limited meaning that may be attached to the parameters. The salient requirement is wide variation in treatment variables such as time, dose, and dose per fraction. However, in the past such wide variations had led to clinical disasters, such as after large single exposures (Andrews 1965) or a few large fractions (Singh 1978). It is unlikely that such clinical data can now be obtained ethically.

## Low-dose limit of effective fractionation

Dutreix et al. (1973) proposed a new isoeffect formulation based on the concept of increase in spared dose when the dose per fraction $D_s$ was halved ($2D_i$). Thus, they determined the recovered dose $D_r = 2D_i - D_s$ in isoeffective regimens for skin (Dutreix et al. 1973) and gut (Wambersie et al. 1974) injury, when either a single dose $D_s$ was given or two doses $D_i$ were separated by the interval $i$ (cf. Sections 2.3 and 3.5).

When interpreted in terms of survival curves, their results led to several important conclusions. First, little additional sparing in skin and gut could be achieved by further fractionation below 2 Gy per fraction. This result was incompatible with the single-hit, multitarget model and favoured a model with nonzero initial slope, such as the two-component model (equation 6.3). The data were consistent with an inverse initial slope of 4–5 Gy. Second, and as a consequence, the dependence of total isoeffect dose on number of fractions disappeared as the fraction size was decreased. Reactions in skin and gut thus seemed dependent on fraction size up to about 15 fractions, after which protraction resulted in an increased isoeffect dose mainly by virtue of cellular repopulation, amounting to over 1 Gy per day (see also Denekamp 1973).

Their studies were extended to dose-rate effects (Dutreix & Sahatchiev 1975; Wambersie *et al.* 1978; Wambersie *et al.* 1979). Wambersie *et al.* (1978) showed that for the intestinal LD50 endpoint in mice the increase in isoeffect dose when dose rate was decreased from 61 to $2 \cdot 6$ cGy/minute was roughly equal to that achieved by fractionation, and furthermore was in good agreement with the increase expected when taking into account only the repair of sublethal lesions. However, it was concluded that no dose-rate effect was to be expected from the small fraction sizes used in conventional radiotherapy.

The results of both fractionation and low-dose-rate experiments were interpreted in accord with the hypothesis of isosurvival for the LD50 endpoint (cf. Section 2.2). Accordingly the parameters of the two-component model (TC) were estimated as $_1D_0 = 4 \cdot 5$ Gy, $_ND_0 = 2 \cdot 25$ Gy, and $N = 10$ (cf. equation 6.3). These are in fair agreement with those obtained from fractionation experiments (Thames *et al.* 1981): $_1D_0 = 3 \cdot 7$ Gy, $_ND_0 = 2 \cdot 5$ Gy, $N = 11$. The bone-marrow syndrome, assessed through measurement of the LD50/30, was observed to be less dependent on dose rate than the gastrointestinal syndrome.

## The linear—quadratic model

A different survival model was employed by Douglas & Fowler (1976) for interpretation of skin isoeffect doses for fractionated radiation, namely the so-called linear—quadratic (LQ) model. Because log survival is linear in the parameters, an algebraic manipulation permitted simplification of the determination of the coefficients that was not possible with the two component (TC) model. Namely, if equation (6.4) is written for fractionated doses with the assumption of equal effect per fraction:

$$\ln \text{s.f.} = -n(\alpha d + \beta d^2)$$

and minus log survival is relabelled $E$ (for 'full effect'), then dividing by the total dose $nd$

$$1/(nd) = \alpha/E + (\beta/E)d$$

we obtain a linear relationship between dose per fraction and reciprocal total dose. The actual survival parameters $\alpha$ and $\beta$ cannot, of course, be determined unless the constant $E$ is known.

In the 10 years following publication of Douglas and Fowler's work, the LQ isoeffect model has grown in influence, perhaps because of the discovery that the fractionation sensitivity of tissues may be classified according to the ratio $\alpha/\beta$ (Thames et al. 1982; Withers et al. 1982c; Barendsen 1982). There is, however, no reason other than simplicity and convenience to prefer it over other survival-based isoeffect models. For example, the survival response *in vivo* of renewing populations in the murine testis (Thames & Withers 1980), jejunum (Thames et al. 1981), and colon (Tucker et al. 1983) was equally well described by the LQ and TC models. Hethcote et al. (1976) showed that the data of Douglas and Fowler could be well described by either the TC or the LQ models. The multi-target single-hit model, however, was inadequate, as were the power-law models. The key feature is a *nonzero initial slope*, in agreement with the results of Dutreix et al. (1973). As in the case for the multitarget, single-hit model, the NSD formula predicts unlimited increase in isoeffect with dose per fraction (Hethcote et al. 1976; Withers & Peters 1980), which is equivalent to zero initial slope of the cell survival curve of the target cells.

The LQ isoeffect models of the early 1980s arose for several reasons, but primarily because of the importance of specifying the fractionation sensitivity $\alpha/\beta$ separately for each tissue, and of the realization that this ratio of target-cell survival parameters could be estimated from isoeffect data, as described (Figure 5.8) by Thames et al. (1982). The essential point is that the intercept-to-slope ratio is an estimate of $\alpha/\beta$, and the unknown log survival ($E$) cancels out.

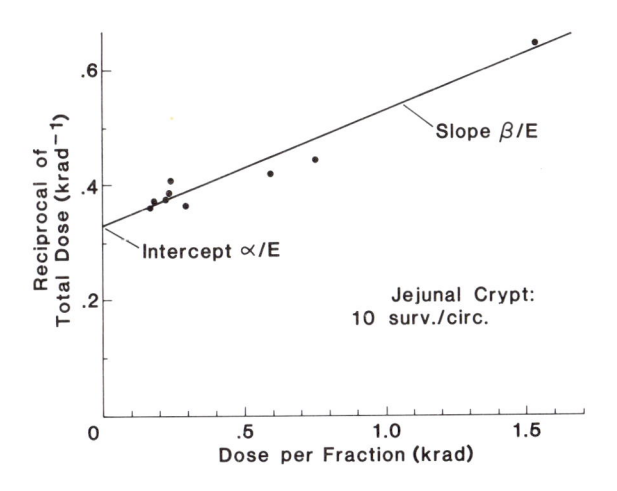

Figure 5.8. Reciprocal total dose for isoeffect as a function of dose per fraction (from Thames et al. 1982). The data points refer to the effect 10 survivors per cross-section of mouse jejunum after fractionated doses. The data lie approximately on a straight line. The ratio of the intercept and the slope of the line is an estimate of the $\alpha/\beta$ ratio. (Reproduced with permission of Pergamon Journals Ltd.)

It is not absolutely necessary to regard $\alpha$ and $\beta$ as survival parameters of the target cells, even though that is the approach we have taken in this book. Fowler (1983) pointed out that for isoeffect calculations the only necessity is that $\alpha/\beta$ faithfully reflect the change in *tissue* response after altered fractionation.

The intercept $\alpha/E$ is the reciprocal of the isoeffect dose given in very many, very small fractions. This dose, $E/\alpha$ has been labelled the extrapolated total dose (ETD) (Barendsen 1982):

$$\text{ETD} = (1 + (\beta/\alpha)d)\ \text{ED50}$$

The model is applicable to late effects tissues where regeneration may be assumed to play a negligible role. A constant dose increment per day, after a variable time lag (each according to tissue), is to be added when the model is applied to acutely responding tissues. Since ETD is related to log survival, it is additive, so that the effects of different partial treatments may simply be added, as with TDFs, to reach the 'tolerance' ETD. An LQ method very similar to Barendsen's, the FDF method for practical dosage calculations, is described in Section 6.10.

Withers *et al.* (1983) have proposed a slightly different variant, derived from simple algebraic manipulation of equation 6.4. If $D_1$ is the reference tolerance dose given in fractions of size $d_1$, then the tolerance dose $D_2$ in fractions of size $d_2$ may be computed from

$$D_2/D_1 = (\alpha/\beta + d_1)/(\alpha/\beta + d_2)$$

where $\alpha/\beta$ is appropriate for late effects in the tissue of interest. Although somewhat easier to compute, practical use of this version is awkward when the effects of partial treatments are to be added.

**Critique**

At the time of writing, there were indications of at least two possible difficulties associated with the use of the LQ model. First, there is an indication from studies of paralysis in the rat spinal cord (Ang *et al.* 1985b) that isoeffect doses may be overestimated when dose per fraction is less than 2 Gy. The same finding was made for kidney by Stewart *et al.* (1987). This could be interpreted as the manifestation of an initial linear part of the survival curve of the target cells, not well approximated by the LQ model at very low doses per fraction, or by incomplete repair during the short intervals that were used (Thames *et al.* 1987a). Although there is some ambiguity about the extent to which these results may be applicable in man, and about the possible influence of the large priming doses used in the experiments, the dangers of overdosing in these tissues is clear.

Second, there is the possibility that repair kinetics in tissues (cf. Section 3.4) may have several components, and moreover may not always be first-order, i.e. that repair rate may depend on size of dose per fraction. There is experimental evidence for such an effect in studies of the role of DNA strand-break rejoining (e.g. Wheeler & Nelson 1987), as well as evidence from tissue repair kinetics *in vivo*. Ang et al. (1986) demonstrated a difference in repair kinetics in the rat spinal cord after 2- and 4-fraction regimens from that observed in 10-fraction regimens. On the other hand, no dependence on fraction size was observed in jejunum, colon, and lung (Thames 1984; Travis *et al.* 1987). Such a difference, if it indeed existed, would have important therapeutic implications since complete repair in late-effect tissues might be possible in shorter interfraction intervals than in the relatively long ones predicted from first-order repair kinetics (Thames *et al.* 1984).

# Chapter 6
# Radiobiological guide for radiotherapists

As noted in the foreword, in this chapter we have presented in a form suitable for trainees in radiotherapy the ideas in the main text of this book, and other topics in basic radiobiology. To do this, we have chosen a format which covers much of the Syllabuses for the Examining Boards of the American College of Radiology (Davis et al. 1985) and the Royal College of Radiology (UK). Some topics not covered in the text were included in order to put the main theme into a broader context and hence to have a wider appeal. However, some topics were excluded, as explained in the Foreword. Reference texts for the latter are cited below (Section 6.12). Following these are texts for further reading on various aspects of the syllabuses.

## 6.1. Interaction of radiation with matter

### Type of ionizing radiations

The types of damage caused in absorbing media exposed to ionizing radiation vary considerably, depending on the nature of the radiations. For example, charged particles interact very strongly with the valence electrons of the material through which they pass. Therefore, it is to be expected that charged particles will lose their energy quickly as they pass through matter (such as mammalian cells) that contains a large number of electrons. The main example of charged-particle beams of importance in radiotherapy is the *electron beam* (beta-particles). *Heavy-ion beams* composed of ions of neon, carbon, or other elements are currently used on a trial basis.

*Photons* (X-rays and gamma-rays) and *neutrons* interact with matter in a different way, since they are chargeless particles. In the case of charged particles, energy is dissipated in a fairly homogeneous fashion near the trajectory of each particle. Photons and neutrons, on the other hand, may be completely absorbed in the first few collisions. In fact, a photon or neutron might lose from zero to all of its energy during the first collision. Electrons and heavier charged particles lose a large part of their energy by a multitude of 'brushes' in which a small amount of energy is lost, and this continues until a charged particle loses virtually all its energy and comes to rest at the end of its *range*. The range is approximately proportional to particle energy and inversely proportional to particle mass, over limited values of these. Thus a 20-MeV electron beam will have about twice the range of a 10-MeV beam.

To summarize, it is reasonable to discuss the interaction of charged particles with matter in terms of range. In contrast, with photons and neutrons the possibility of large energy losses and large changes in direction means that there is no sharply defined distance beyond which none will penetrate, and as a result the distribution of energy from these radiations is exponential along their path.

## Ionization and excitation

When ionizing radiation interacts with the atoms of an absorbing medium, two things can occur. First, the electrons in the valence shells may be excited to higher energy states. The atom is raised to an excited state (*excitation*), and this energy may be dissipated through disruptive dissociations of the molecules that eventually result in biologically observable damage. Second, if the energy of the ionizing radiation is high enough, an electron may be completely ejected from an atom (*ionization*). This process is best conceived of as a collision between a photon and an electron of the outer shell of the atom. In the case of neutrons, *recoil protons* result from the elastic collision of the primary neutrons with hydrogen atoms in the molecule. These facts can now be considered in a description of the main interaction processes of the radiations of most interest in radiotherapy, namely photons and neutrons.

## Absorption of photons

In the interactions between photons and biological materials three major processes are of importance, and their probabilities of occurrence depend on the energy of the incident photon. First, the absorption of the photons by the atom (*photoelectric effect*, which occurs mainly at the lower energies), second, the interaction of the photon with an electron which is ejected as a result of the collision (*Compton effect*, at higher energies), and third, interaction of the photon with the nucleus (*pair production*, at very high energies). For the present purposes only the first two are of importance as pair production occurs only above a threshold energy of 1·02 MeV and does not become a significant interaction until energies of many MeV.

In the photoelectric effect a photon is completely absorbed by the atom, which subsequently undergoes ionization. The ionized atom is in an excited state, and gives up its energy by picking up a neighbouring electron and readjusting electrons to lower, more stable energy states. Fluorescent radiation is emitted in the form of lower-energy photons, which may be X rays, UV, or visible light. The probability of the photoelectric effect increases approximately with the fourth power of the atomic number of the absorbing material ($Z^4$). For low-energy photons and high-Z media, the photoelectric effect is the predominant method of photon absorption. The increase in dependence with atomic number for the photoelectric effect explains its importance in diagnostic radiology, where X rays are preferentially absorbed in high-Z materials (bone) as opposed to those of low atomic number (e.g. soft tissue).

As the energy of the photon increases, the Compton scattering process gradually replaces the photoelectric effect as the most important mode of interaction. The probability for Compton scattering varies directly with the atomic number Z of the scattering medium. Therefore, as the energy of the incident photon beam increases the importance of atomic number decreases. In fact, with beams such as cobalt-60, for many purposes differences between absorption of bone and soft tissue may be neglected. This is certainly not the case for lower-energy X-ray beams, such as 250-kVp X rays.

In a Compton interaction (Figure 6.1), the energy of the incident photon is sufficiently high for the atomic electron with which it interacts to be considered virtually free and the entire process may be regarded as a collision between photon and electrons. The photon transfers part of its energy to the electron, and the remainder to the ionized atom. The scattered photon proceeds on, as does the knocked-out electron, which itself may have appreciable energy, sufficient to induce subsequent ionizations before finally coming to rest.

**Absorption of neutrons**

The interactions of X rays, gamma rays, and charged particles with matter are caused by electromagnetic forces between them (or the electrons they have dislodged) and the electrons in the valence shells of the atoms. In contrast, neutron interactions are completely dependent on nuclear forces. Since these are of very short range and because nuclei are very small compared with atoms, there are only a small number of neutron interactions per path length. Consequently, neutrons can be

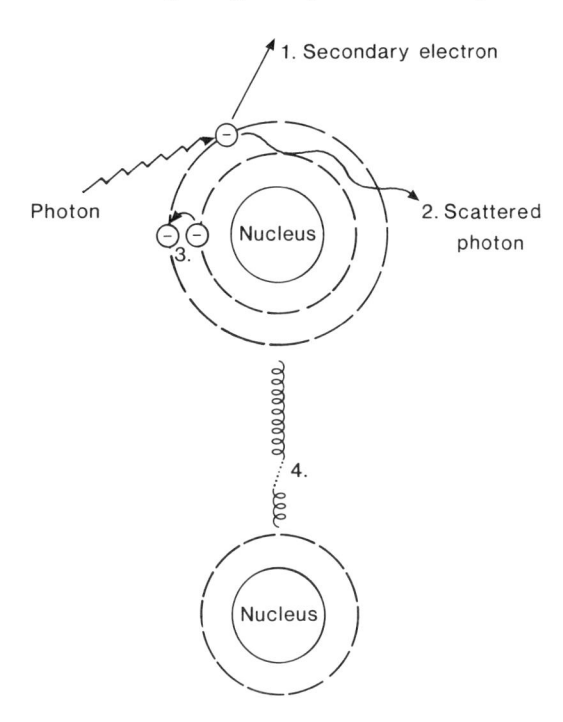

Figure 6.1. Compton scattering. The incident photon collides with a valence-shell electron and *ionization* results. The kinetic energy of the photon is given to (1) the ejected electron and (2) the scattered photon; an additional 30 to 35 eV is dissipated locally as *excitation* energy. Of this about 13 eV is used in producing ionization, so that the majority of the 30 to 35 eV goes into excitations. They can be either (3) *electronic excitation* or (and this is of greater biological significance) (4) *vibrational excitation*. Since 5 eV is sufficient to break carbon—carbon bonds, many dissociative chemical changes can occur for each ion pair produced.

considered a penetrating radiation in the same sense that gamma radiation is, and their absorption will proceed approximately exponentially.

The passage of a neutron beam through matter is similar to that of X rays or gamma rays, in that each interaction removes a neutron from the beam either by scattering or absorption. For the purposes of radiotherapy, *elastic scattering* processes are the interactions of most interest, followed by those that result in the production of charged particles. Scattering is called *elastic* (e.g. a billiard-ball collision) if the reduction in kinetic energy of the neutron is accounted for by a commensurate increase in the kinetic energy of the struck nucleus. For scattering by heavy nuclei, the reduction in neutron energy is small. However, for very light nuclei (hydrogen) the reduction can be a large part of the neutron energy. The struck hydrogen nucleus is removed from the atom and is then called a *recoil proton*. Compared with other interactions the probability of collision with a hydrogen nucleus is high. This accounts for the fact that shielding of neutrons is best achieved by low-Z materials like water.

As the energy of a neutron is degraded by a series of elastic collisions it may eventually be absorbed by the nucleus of an atom. When a neutron is absorbed, the nucleus is excited and subsequently undergoes a reaction in which photons or subnuclear particles are emitted. When a photon is emitted, the absorption process is called an *n—gamma reaction*. Particle-emission reactions result in the emission of particles such as alpha particles or protons or neutrons. Neutron-absorption reactions in which photons are the primary emitted particles are of great interest since they can occur at any energy and generally represent the ultimate fate of neutrons. It is important to understand that matter irradiated with neutrons will suffer damage not only from the neutrons but also from emitted gamma rays. Therefore, a neutron of energy in the 1 to 30-MeV range absorbed in biological material would first undergo elastic scattering reactions, resulting in the production of recoil protons, which themselves induce biological damage in their trajectories.

**Direct and indirect effects**

The basic mechanism for the deposition of energy and production of biological damage by ionizing radiation is *excitation* and *ionization* of molecules by charged particles (Figure 6.1). For X rays and gamma radiations of interest in radiotherapy, where the Compton effect is important, it is possible that for every atom ionized directly by an interaction, thousands may be ionized or excited by the action of secondary electrons (e.g. vibrational excitation and rupture of covalent bonds in Figure 6.1). The same is true of neutrons, for which charged particles or gamma rays are generated when high-energy neutrons are absorbed.

The *energy deposited locally* per ion pair produced is about *30 to 35 eV*. This figure includes energy that goes into producing excitations. The actual energy used in producing ionization in water is 13 eV, so that for each ion pair produced, about 20 eV goes into producing excitation. Therefore, considerable numbers (perhaps a majority) of molecules interacting with ionizing particles are excited, and when it is recalled that 4 to 5 eV are sufficient to break carbon—carbon bonds, it may be appreciated that many chemical changes may occur for each ion pair produced (reaction 4 in Figure 6.1). Such immediate consequences of the local deposition of energy are known as *direct effects* (Figure 6.2).

There are, however, other chemical changes resulting from ionizing radiation and these are thought to result from *free radicals*. The free radical is an entity characterized by the presence of an unpaired electron. In tissues, it is reasonable to consider that the free radicals resulting from interactions of ionization with water are of great importance. These interactions may be summarized as follows (von Sonntag 1987):

Radical production:

$$H_2O + \text{radiation} \rightarrow H_2O^+ + \bar{e} \text{ (ionization)}$$
$$H_2O + \text{radiation} \rightarrow H_2O^* \rightarrow \cdot OH + H \cdot \text{ (excitation)}$$

Radical reactions:

$$H_2O^+ \rightarrow H^+ + \cdot OH$$
$$\bar{e} + nH_2O \rightarrow \bar{e}_{aq}$$
$$\cdot OH + \cdot OH \rightarrow H_2O_2$$

Effect of oxygen:

$$H \cdot + O_2 \rightarrow HO_2$$
$$\bar{e}_{aq} + O_2 + H^+ \rightarrow HO_2$$
$$2\, HO_2 \rightarrow H_2O_2 + O_2$$

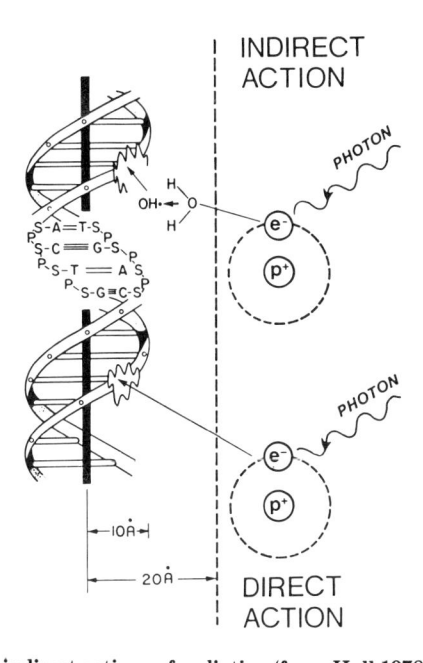

Figure 6.2. Direct and indirect actions of radiation (from Hall 1978). The structure of DNA is shown schematically; the letters S, P, A, T, G, and C represent sugar, phosphorus, adenine, thymine, guanine, and cytosine, respectively. *Direct action*: A secondary electron resulting from absorption of an X-ray photon interacts with the DNA to produce an effect. *Indirect action*: The secondary electron interacts with a water molecule to produce an OH radical, which in turn produces the damage to the DNA. The indirect action is dominant for sparsely ionizing radiations such as X-rays. (Reproduced with permission of Harper & Row Inc. and the author.)

One possible mechanism for the documented increase in biological effect with increasing oxygen concentration (see Section 6.5) is provided by these last reactions, showing that oxygen scavenges H· and thus permits build-up of $H_2O_2$. Other mechanisms include the formation of less-easily-repaired peroxy radicals.

The free radicals and $H_2O_2$ produced in aqueous solutions are available to cause many deleterious effects on biological macromolecules such as DNA. This mode of radiation action has been labelled *indirect action*, in that the molecule ultimately damaged need not absorb energy directly from the ionizing radiation. Instead energy is thought to be absorbed indirectly through transfer of free radicals (Figure 6.2).

Direct-action, whereby a molecule undergoes change by being ionized or excited by direct interaction with ionizing radiation (Figure 6.2), can be conceptualized in terms of *target theory*. In this description, each biological system is thought to have one or many microscopic sensitive volumes (e.g. macromolecules). If an ionization or excitation occurs in any one of these volumes, then damage is produced, perhaps irreversibly. Further it is postulated that ionization produced outside these volumes produces no significant damage. In the multi-target version of this theory, more than one target must be hit to produce significant damage (cf. Section 6.4).

## 6.2. Linear energy transfer (LET)

For all types of ionizing radiation, the absorption of energy at the local level takes place through the agency of ionizing charged particles. This is obvious when the primary radiation consists of charged particles, but is also the case with X rays, gamma rays, and neutrons. Thus, ionizations and excitations attributed to neutrons in energy ranges of interest for radiotherapy are usually caused by recoil protons, the nuclei of hydrogen atoms, and photons, all generated in the interactions. Gamma rays and X rays, on the other hand, produce most of the ionization and excitation attributed to them by means of high-speed electrons knocked off atoms with which they interact.

We conclude that energy is transferred to biological material by means of the *slowing down of charged particles*. In order to quantify this process, the linear rate of energy loss is introduced, which is the magnitude of energy transfer by ionizing particles as they progress down their trajectories. It is given mathematically by the amount of energy lost per unit path length. More precisely, *linear energy transfer* is defined as follows:

> The LET of charged particles in a medium is the quotient of the change in local energy by the path length over which that change occurs, this

energy being imparted to the medium by charged particles of specified energy.

There are limitations to this concept, having to do with expressing what exactly is meant by 'locally imparted'. This may refer either to a given distance from the track of the particle (*track-average LET*) or to a given range of energy loss outside which loss is no longer considered local (*energy-average LET*).

LET is a concept most easily applied to types of radiation for which the primary particles are charged. In these cases, there is a well defined particle trajectory and energy dissipation occurs in close proximity to this trajectory. For photons and neutrons, on the other hand, energy is not homogeneously distributed along the particle trajectory, since in a particular interaction photons and neutrons can lose from none to all of their energy: it is these large statistical fluctuations that give rise to exponential attenuation of these radiations. However, the concept of LET can be used with reference to neutrons, X rays, and gamma rays, but only in an approximate sense and usually only for rough comparisons, such as 'high-LET neutrons' or 'low-LET X rays'.

Even for charged particles there is not a unique value for the LET. Instead the LET is described by a spectrum of values that depends on the energy spectrum of the charged particles and the interactions they undergo. The LET spectrum for indirectly ionizing radiations is given as the LET spectrum for the secondary charged particles generated by the primary radiation. The study of energy transfer at the statistical level necessary to describe these concepts is called *microdosimetry*.

For electrons, the LET is almost constant except at the very low energies typical of the end of the slowing-down process, where the electron velocity becomes very low. Here the energy imparted increases per unit path length, and the LET shows a maximum as the electron comes to a stop. For protons, and other charged particles, the LET is in general much higher than that of electrons. This is because electrons are *sparsely ionizing*, in that individual ionization events are well spaced from each other along their trajectory, whereas heavy charged particles such as alpha particles give rise to a high density of ionizing events along their trajectories and are *densely ionizing*. Neutrons fall between these extremes and are referred to as particles of *intermediate ionizing density*. The LETs of these particles are simply a way of describing in a general way the density of ionization in their tracks; therefore, alpha particles are said to be high-LET, neutrons intermediate-LET, and electrons, gamma rays and X rays low-LET.

## 6.3. Assays of cell survival and tissue injury

*Cell survival* is the term usually applied to the ability of cells to divide many times after treatment with a toxic agent. Cells that survive retain their *reproductive integrity*. When they replicate many times they form a *clone* of daughter cells. The daughter cells will have the same *genotype* (gene complement) and may also have the same *phenotype*, if the same genes are expressed. Alternatively the daughter cells may differentiate and express different genes. When the daughter cells are in close proximity they can be identified as a cluster or focus of *viable* cells. The term viable is applied either to the ability of a cell to form clones or to the healthy morphological appearance of a cell. When a cluster of cells originates from one or more than one ancestral cell, it is called a *colony*. This is the case when clones coalesce or when other cell types (helper cells) are required to assist in the growth of a clone.

### Colony-forming cells

Colonies or clones can be grown when *colony-forming cells* or *clonogenic cells* (the *clonogens*) are sparsely distributed and are stimulated to divide. They can be sown sparsely in culture medium in a Petri dish or flask. Many tumour and normal cell types can now be grown in culture (Potten & Hendry 1985). With these primary cultures the proportion of plated cells forming colonies (the *colony-forming efficiency*) is often low. This can be due to there being only a small proportion of clonogens among the plated cells or to unsuitable culture conditions for the growth of the cell type under study. The colony-forming efficiency can be increased by repeated culture of the cells in order to select for the more undifferentiated clonogens, thus producing cell lines. The culture conditions can also be modified to improve the *plating efficiency*.

Colonies can be grown *in vivo*. In this case the necessary sparse initial distribution of clonogens is achieved by using the cytotoxic agent under investigation to sterilize all but a few clonogens in the tissue, leaving the remainder to proliferate and form discrete colonies. Alternatively, a higher dose of the agent can be used to sterilize all endogenous clonogens, and then a few untreated clonogens in a cell suspension can be injected into the tissue. Even when tissues do not contain endogenous clonogens of the type it is wished to grow, they can in some cases support the growth of colonies of other cell types. Tissues in which assays of colony-forming ability have been developed are listed in Table 6.1. A few examples are given here to illustrate the different techniques.

### Spleen colonies

These can be produced by irradiating donor mice to the whole body with single doses of 4- to 6-Gy X rays. Seven to 11 days later, the mice are killed, the spleens are removed, fixed, and stained, and the colonies are counted on the surface by eye or by using a low-power microscope. The number of colonies is related to the dose of the radiation.

It should be noted that macroscopic endogenous colonies can be produced in other tissues as well (e.g. in gastrointestinal mucosa—13 days in mice after 15 to 22 Gy, and epidermis—12 to 21 days in plucked mouse dorsum after 10 to 30 Gy, 19 to 28 days in unplucked mouse tail after 29—36 Gy). Alternatively, mice are lethally irradiated using at least 8-Gy X rays, injected intravenously with about $4 \times 10^4$ nucleated bone marrow cells, and killed 7 to 11 days later. About 10 nodules will be found on the surface of the spleen; the number is proportional to the number of cells injected. The apparently low colony-forming efficiency is expected because of the low proportion of clonogens amongst the mostly mature cells composing the marrow and because only about 10% of injected clonogens settle and grow in the spleen: the remainder reside in the marrow. The cells can be irradiated in the donor mouse, in suspension, or after injection into the recipient mouse. The number of colonies decreases with an increase in the dose of radiation, and in practice the number of irradiated cells which are injected is increased to maintain the number of colonies at around 5—10 per spleen. Spleen colonies can be produced easily in the mouse, less easily in the rat, and not at all in other species. This is probably related to the fact that the spleen is both a haematopoietic and lymphoid organ in the mouse, but only a lymphoid organ in other species.

### Intestinal crypts

Regenerating crypts are produced by irradiating mice to the whole body with doses from 8 to 16 Gy, and leaving the mice for 3 to 4 days before they are killed. Transverse sections of the gut reveal microscopically that some of the normal number of about 130 crypts around the circumference are regenerating. After high doses, when only a few percent of crypts survive, the chance of two clonogens surviving in a crypt is remote. Hence in this case the reduction in numbers of crypts with increasing dose directly reflects the reduction in numbers of single clonogens. However, after lower doses there is a greater chance of a surviving crypt with two or more surviving clonogens, and a correction is applied to the data to take this effect into account. This mathematical correction is based on the assumption that cells are killed at random. In this case, Poisson statistics can be used to describe the distribution of surviving cells among crypts that normally contain a large number of clonogens. One feature of the Poisson distribution is that if the average number of surviving clonogens per crypt is $m$, the fraction of crypts which are sterilized and contain no surviving clonogens will be $\exp(-m)$. Hence, by counting the number of regenerating crypts in transverse

Table 6.1. Assays of tissue injury (modified from Hendry & Fowler, 1986)

| Tissue | Assays of tissue injury | Likely target cell population | Colony assay |
|---|---|---|---|
| Alimentary canal | | | |
| Mouth | Taste loss | Taste buds/salivary glands | |
| | Mucositis (including tongue and lip) | Mucosa | |
| Oesophagus | Ulceration/fibrosis | Mucosa/stroma | |
| Stomach | Emptying | Neurological/hormonal | |
| | LD50/40 | Mucosa | Crypt microcolonies |
| Small intestine | Surface area, denudation, protein leakage, LD50/7 | Mucosal clonogens | Crypt micro/macrocolonies |
| Colon | Strictures/stenosis | Mucosa/stroma | Crypt microcolonies |
| Skin | Erythema | Capillaries/epidermis | |
| | Hairs/hair follicles | Follicular clonogens | Follicle survival |
| | Pigmentation changes | Melanoblasts | Melanocyte colonies |
| | Skin reactions/ necrosis | Epidermal clonogens | Micro/macrocolonies |
| | Explants and cultures | Fibroblasts and keratinocytes | Colonies *in vitro* |
| | Telangiectasia | Vasculature | |
| | Contraction, atrophy/fibrosis | Dermal components | |
| | Deformities | Epithelial/stromal | |
| Testis | Fertility | Stem cells | Regenerating tubules |
| | Hormonal deficiencies | Sertoli cells/Leydig cells | |
| Haematopoietic tissue | Blood and marrow counts, LD50/30 | Marrow precursor cells | Colony assays *in vitro/in vivo* |
| | Scintigraphy | Erythroid precursor cells | Erythroid colonies |
| | Repopulation of ectopic implants | Marrow and stromal precursor cells | Fibroblastoid colonies |
| Immune system | Immune responses | Lymphocytes, macrophages | Lymphocyte colonies |
| | Responses to mitogens | Lymphocytes | |
| | Analysis of subsets | Precursor + effector cells | |
| | Repopulation | Stem cells/stroma | |

Radiobiological guide for radiotherapists 181

| Organ | Clinical/Functional endpoints | Target cells | Experimental assays |
|---|---|---|---|
| Central nervous system | EEG abnormalities<br>White matter necrosis | Granular and subgranular zones<br>Oligodendrocytes/vasculature | |
| Nerve roots | Paralysis/radiculopathy<br>Telangiectasia/infarcts | Schwann cells<br>Vascular endothelium | |
| Glandular tissue | | | |
| Thyroid | Hormone synthesis, iodine uptake<br>Protein release | Follicular cells | Colonies *in vitro* and in fat pads |
| Adrenals | Weight | Colloid endocytosis/<br>hydrolysis process<br>Cortex | |
| Kidney and bladder | Weight<br>LD50<br>Urinary enzymes<br>Osmolality/electrolyte excretion/filtration rate/plasma<br>Flow/haematocrit/ blood pressure<br>Ureteral blockage<br>Urinary frequency<br>Bladder permeability<br>Bladder capacity:<br>Oedema/fibrosis | Tubule epithelium<br><br><br>Vasculature/tubules<br><br><br><br>Epithelium<br>Epithelium?<br>Epithelium<br>Muscle cells | Regenerating tubules |
| Lung | Surfactant, enzymes<br>LD50/180<br>Breathing rate<br>Blood gases, gas transfer<br>Lung weight, density, oedema, protein leakage<br>LD50/360<br>Fibrosis, collagen synthesis | Type II cells<br><br><br>Type II cells/ endothelial cells<br><br>Endothelial cells/Type II cells | Colonies *in vitro* |
| Liver | Biochemical analysis<br>Adaptive growth | Hepatocytes | Colonies in fat pads |
| Heart | Cardiopathy | Myocardium/capillaries | |
| Musculoskeletal tissue | Growth retardation | Cartilage growth plate | Microcolonies *in vivo* |
| Eye | Cataracts | Anterior lens epithelial cells | |

histological sections, and from this calculating the proportion of nonregenerating crypts, one can deduce $m$. $m$ will of course be dose dependent. The validity of using this mathematical correction has been shown by measuring the distribution of regenerating crypts between sections taken from a single mouse, and between mice.

The principle of this procedure (the *microcolony assay*) is the same as that used to produce spermatogenetic colonies at 35 days after 9 to 15 Gy, and kidney colonies at 420 days after 11 to 16 Gy. After high doses the very few surviving crypts can be left for 13 days to develop into macroscopic colonies, but this is possible only if the irradiation has been localized to a loop of the intestine. Otherwise the animal would die in the first week as a result of severe denudation of all the mucosa (see below). It is likely that at 13 days these macro-colonies represent the survivors of the more resistant crypts that reside over Peyers (lymphoid) patches.

**Fat pad assays**

Fat pad assays involve the use of regions of fat on the back of the rat or mouse, in the axillary or inguinal regions. The method has been developed for mammary, thyroid, and liver cells, where the appropriate stimuli for growth of the test cells are treatment respectively with hormones inducing mammary gland growth and lactation, a goitrogen, or a 2/3 partial hepatectomy of the recipient animal. The appropriate treatment is given before the test cells are injected in up to 12 sites in the fat pads. At least 200 mammary cells, 10 thyroid cells, or 2000 liver cells are required to give growth in 50% of the injected sites. Growth is detected by removing the fat pads, dissolving the fat, staining the colonies appropriately, and viewing them using a low-power microscope. Again using Poisson statistics, if $m$ clonogens are injected, the probability that 50% of sites will have no clonogens is $0 \cdot 5 = \exp(-m)$. Hence, $m = -\ln 0 \cdot 5 = 0 \cdot 693$. Hence the proportion of sites with no *takes* is related to the mean number of clonogens injected. If the cells are irradiated either in the donor animal or in suspension, more cells will be required to achieve the same probability of a take, and hence the survival level of the irradiated clonogens can be deduced. The approximate period for growth of the colonies is 20 days for all the fat pad techniques.

Techniques with tumour cells make use of the same principles. The number of injected cells required to produce leukemia or a solid tumour in 50% of animals is determined. Another method involves the intravenous injection of leukemic cells which lodge and grow to form colonies in the spleen, or cells from solid tumours which produce colonies in the lung. Colony production in the lung is enhanced by prior lung irradiation with at least 5 Gy.

### Normal tissue endpoints other than survival

Many radiation-induced changes in normal tissues that are of clinical interest cannot be studied using cell survival assays of response. However, there are endpoints that relate to functional changes in these tissues. A commonly used endpoint is the probability of inflicting some dramatic change such as necrosis, paralysis, or death. This is called a binary, quantal, or all-or-nothing type of endpoint, since either the change occurs or it does not. The dose range over which these changes occur is normally small, and commonly the dose that elicits a 50% response is defined using probit and logistic analysis techniques. The second type of functional endpoint involves gross reactions or physiological changes, such as degree of skin damage, change in renal function, etc. These can be measured over a wider range of dose, because nonlethal injury can be quantified over a very wide range of severity. The different normal tissues and endpoints that have been used to study the effect of ionizing radiation are set out in Table 6.1.

The third column of Table 6.1 lists possible target-cell populations associated with normal-tissue injury. These have been suggested by direct observation of morphological and kinetic changes *in situ* or assaying colony-forming ability to examine the correlation of radiation doses necessary to produce tissue injury with those required for survival of clonogens in the tissue when the dose and the conditions of dose delivery (fractionation, dose rate, LET, etc.) are changed (cf. Chapter 2).

## 6.4. Survival curves

Ionizations produced in biological material by sparsely ionizing radiation, either gamma rays emitted from isotopes or X rays produced by machines, are distributed at random. The inactivation of single molecules (for example proteins or viruses) by these ionizations also occurs at random. Because generally the number of inactivations is infinitesimally small compared with the number of molecules available for inactivation, the chance of inactivating a molecule is independent of previous inactivations. In other words, each increment of dose inactivates a constant proportion of molecules (Figure 6.3). This *proportional* (note, not linear) decline in unaffected molecules with a *linear* increase in dose is equivalent mathematically to an *exponential* decline. An important consequence of this mode of decline is that there is no dose at which *all* molecules are inactivated in *every* sample, because some very small proportion will remain unaffected no matter how high the dose.

An exponential decline is described by a Poisson distribution (cf. Section 2.1 for a more detailed presentation). If there are $m$ events per

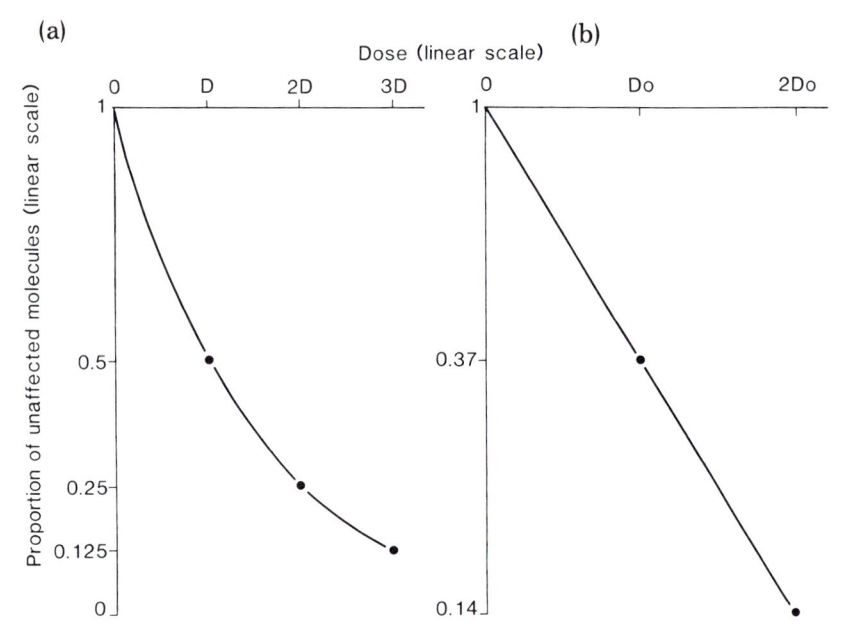

Figure 6.3. Proportion of unaffected molecules versus dose. (a) Linear y-axis shows characteristic exponential curve never reaching zero, with equal depletions caused by equal increments of dose. (b) Logarithmic y-axis shows a *constant proportion* of unaffected molecules after each of two doses delivered in sequence with no time interval between them. A dose $D_0$ results in an unaffected fraction of $1/e = 0\cdot37$, and a dose $2D_0$ $(1/e)^2 = 0\cdot14$.

unit volume, where $m$ is proportional to dose, the proportion of unit volumes containing no events is $\exp(-m)$. Following a further $m$ events (making a total of $2m$ events), the new proportion of volumes containing no events is $[\exp(-m)] \cdot [\exp(-m)] = \exp(-2m)$. This description can be continued with $3m$ and $4m$ events, etc.

It follows that when the inactivation of a molecule means the breaking of a critical bond in the DNA, which leads to a chromosomal lesion preventing successful cell divisions, then cell survival $= \exp(-m)$ where $m$ is the number of lethal events per cell. $m$ is proportional to dose, so that $m = kD$. It should be noted that after low doses, most cells can often divide once or twice, but not much more. Hence if the criterion for survival were set at colonies comprising 2 cells, or 4 cells, more irradiated cells would survive than if the criterion was set higher, and thus $k$ would be lower. By convention, the criterion is set at around 50 cells, which is 5 to 6 divisions (i.e. $2^5 = 32$, $2^6 = 64$). Cells which have undergone this number of divisions successfully are usually capable of many more, and hence these are the true survivors (colony-forming cells). After high doses (20 Gy), sterilized cells in culture do not divide at all, and after very high doses (200 Gy) they may lyse in interphase. After high doses *in vivo*

(20 Gy), it is not clear if doomed cells can do one or two divisions. These divisions may provide more differentiated cells for a tissue, but they would not be colony-forming cells.

By convention, for the colony-forming cells $k = 1/D_0$ where $D_0$ is the dose resulting on average in one lethal (sterilizing) event per cell. Hence at this dose $m = 1$, and $\exp(-1)$ or 37% of cells will not receive a lethal event and so will survive (Figure 6.3). $D_0$ is defined as the *mean lethal dose*, and it is the dose that will just sterilize a cell. Because of the random nature of dose delivery, after delivery of the dose $D_0$ a cell has a 37% chance of not receiving one lethal lesion and correspondingly a 63% chance of receiving one or more lethal lesions (cf. Section 2.1 and Figure 2.3). A dose $D_0$ will reduce survival to 37% of its previous value anywhere on the exponential survival curve, e.g. from B to A or B' to A' in Figure 2.4.

An exponential curve describing the rate of cell depletion with increasing dose is not very common for mammalian cells. It is observed for several types of haematopoietic cells and for human skin fibroblasts (reviewed by Hendry 1985c). For most other cells it is observed only for low doses. At high doses cells become more sensitive and there is curvature in the semi-logarithmic plot. This effect is commonly ascribed to the *accumulation of sublethal injury* into lethal injury (cf. Section 3.1).

The mechanism of accumulation of sublethal injury is not fully understood. Clearly there are repair enzymes, e.g. DNA polymerases, which can repair some of the injury caused by ionizing events. With increasing doses, the repair system becomes increasingly ineffective. This is either because (1) accumulation of injury occurs faster than the operating time of the repair system, (2) there is misrepair of injury, (3) the repair system is limited in size and saturates with increase in injury, or (4) the repair system is itself radiosensitive. The first two reasons are considered the most likely. At doses where the repair system becomes ineffective, the sensitivity will approach a maximum. Hence the curvature in the semi-logarithmic plot will tend to straighten out. These features of the common shape of survival curves are observed for many types of cells, and an old but still used set of parameters for describing this shape is shown in Figure 6.4. The parameter $D_0$ has been defined already. The parameter $N$ is the *extrapolation number*, and this is the point of extrapolation of the linear portion of the curve on the $y$-axis (the ordinate, i.e. log surviving fraction) of the semi-log plot. The parameter $D_q$ is the *quasi-threshold dose*, which is the dose at which the linear portion of the curve crosses the $x$-axis (the abscissa, i.e. dose). The equations which relate these parameters to the surviving fraction (s.f.) are as follows:

$$\text{s.f.} = 1 - (1 - e^{-D/D_0})^N \qquad (6.1)$$

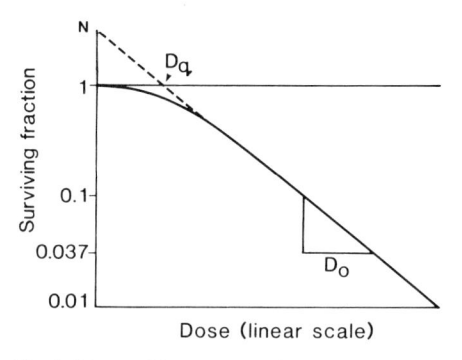

## Figure 6.4. Single-hit, multitarget survival curve, where $D_q = D_0 \ln N$.

and $$D_q = D_0 \ln N \tag{6.2}$$

Equation (6.1) is known as the *single-hit multitarget* equation for cell survival. It may appear quite complex, but it can be constructed from its component parts easily using the ideas of *target theory*. An understanding of this is necessary if other descriptions of the shape of survival curves, and their relevance, are to be understood.

Target theory was developed by Lea (1946). It was postulated that there were a number ($N$) of targets in the cell, all of which had to be inactivated in order to kill the cell. One or more unaffected targets would rescue the cell. On this basis, equation (6.1) was constructed as follows. The term $\exp(-D/D_0)$ is the probability of a single target surviving after an average number ($D/D_0$) of lethal events have been delivered to each cell. The term $[1 - \exp(-D/D_0)]$ is therefore the probability of the target being inactivated (cf. Section 2.1). When the cell contains $N$ targets, the probability of all of them being inactivated, and hence of the cell being killed, is $[1 - \exp(-D/D_0)]^N$. Thus the probability that one or more is not inactivated, and hence of the cell surviving is $1 - [1 - \exp(-D/D_0)]^N$, which is the same as equation (6.1).

Equation (6.2) follows because $D_0$ is the dose required to inactivate one target. When a cell has $N$ targets, $D_q$ is the dose required to inactivate all but one of them. Therefore $D_q$ theoretically has no killing effect, but with an additional dose $D_0$ the last target is inactivated, so $D_q$ is a quasi-threshold dose in the sense that the response to doses higher than $D_q$ is exponential with slope $D_0$. $D_q$ is defined as the *x*-intercept of the asymptote to the survival curve; the slope of the latter is $1/D_0$ which must be the change in ordinate ($\ln N$) divided by the change in abscissa ($D_q$), i.e. $D_q = D_0 \ln N$. Note that in practice there is some cell killing at dose $D_q$ (Figure 6.4) — hence the denotation *quasi*-threshold dose.

Equation (6.1) describes the curve that has no decrease in survival at very low doses (when $N$ is greater than 1) i.e. when there is no *initial slope*. However, many cell types demonstrate such an initial slope, and so equation (6.1) was modified by using a further exponential term as follows:

$$\text{s.f.} = e^{-D/_1D_0}[1 - (1 - e^{-D/_ND_0})^N]. \tag{6.3}$$

Equation (6.3) is known as the *two-component multitarget* equation. The parameter $_1D_0$ describes the sensitivity of the cells to very low doses, purported to be caused by a fraction of the dose which inactivates all targets simultaneously or which inactivates a different target that is then lethal to the cell. This fraction has been hypothesized as a high-LET component of low-LET radiations such as photons, consisting for example of secondary electrons near the ends of their ranges.

Equations (6.1) and (6.3) are still useful for describing and comparing the shapes of survival curves, but the target theory on which they were based has no biological basis. We know that the most common form of cell death after irradiation is mitotic death, and that fast repair processes act to correct radiation-induced damage. Further, even one unrepaired or misrepaired genetic lesion that expresses itself in terms of a gross structural change in a chromosome can prevent the successful completion of mitosis (Revell 1983). Hence many (unrepaired) lesions are not required. However, there are many potential sites at which this lesion can occur, and hence target theory can still be applied but in a different way. The essential difference is that only *one target* of many has to be inactivated in order to kill the cell, in contrast to the foregoing type of target theory where *all targets* had to be inactivated to kill the cell. The mathematical construction of the survival curve equation is slightly more complicated than in the case of equation (6.3), but the same principles are applied. It is based on the inactivation of a target pair by a single event or by two interacting events, leading to a break in the double-stranded DNA. It is likely that the potential number of sites where this break can occur is very large, and in this case the survival curve equation can be well approximated by the following equation:

$$\text{s.f.} = e^{-\alpha D - \beta D^2}. \tag{6.4}$$

This is known as the *linear–quadratic* (LQ) equation for cell survival (Figure 6.5). It can be constructed simply by proposing that the mean number of lethal events is $(\alpha D + \beta D^2)$ and comprises a linear term, where the number of events is proportional to dose, and a quadratic term, where two sublesions (each produced in number proportional to dose) interact to produce a lethal event. Hence the fraction of cells without a lethal event is $\exp - (\alpha D + \beta D^2)$. When the potential number of sites

188                    Fractionation in Radiotherapy

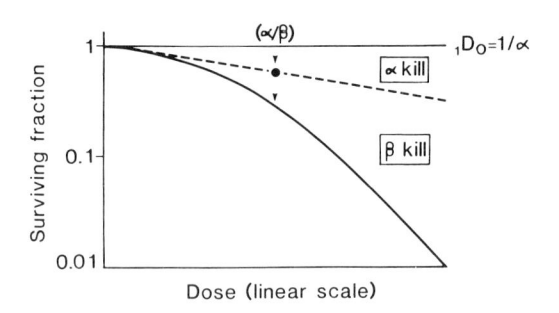

Figure 6.5. *Linear–quadratic* survival curve, showing that $(\alpha/\beta)$ is the dose at which the components of cell killing from the $\alpha$ and $\beta$ modes are equal. Note also that $\alpha = 1/{_1}D_0$.

where the lethal event can occur is relatively small, the linear–quadratic equation is an approximation to a more complicated equation which has an exponential final slope (Gilbert et al. 1980). Hence it should be recognized that exponential survival curves can be interpreted using the modern form of target theory, as well as by using the original form.

By comparing equations (6.3) and (6.4) it can be seen that $\alpha$ corresponds to $1/{_1}D_0$, which is the *initial sensitivity* or initial slope of the survival curve. As a consequence of the term $\beta D^2$ sensitivity increases with increasing dose. The ratio $(\alpha/\beta)$ is a measure of the relative importance of the $\alpha$ and $\beta$ terms, i.e. the amount of curvature in the survival curve. Also, taking equation (6.4), it can be seen that when the surviving fraction is expressed as s.f. $= \exp(-\alpha D) \times \exp(-\beta D^2)$, equal survival levels from both factors are produced when $\alpha D = \beta D^2$, i.e. when $D = \alpha/\beta$. Hence, $(\alpha/\beta)$ is the dose at which the components of cell kill from the $\alpha$ and $\beta$ modes are equal (Figure 6.5).

The linear–quadratic equation is now widely used, in particular for application to fractionated doses. Another biological basis to its construction is not in terms of target theory, but rather of repair phenomena. With *repair models* it is thought that radiation damage occurs linearly, or very nearly linearly, with dose (Figure 6.3(b)). If no repair took place, the survival curve would be straight exponential with slope $(1/D_0)$. This damage is potentially lethal (as opposed to sublethal, cf. Section 6.5) since if unrepaired it leads to cell death. As lesions are repaired, however, the biological effect of a dose is progressively reduced, and the curve swings upward (Figure 3.5). Now if the repair efficiency were the same at all doses, the ultimate result would be a straight-exponential survival curve with slope equal to $(1/{_1}D_0)$. But the curve bends downward at higher doses on account of a reduced effectiveness of repair at higher doses (see Figure 3.5 for the parameters describing the shape of the survival curve). This is assumed to result from a variety of factors, including damage fixation, misrepair, exhaustion of factors essential for repair, and saturation of the repair process. Thus the survival-curve shoulder is thought of as a result of temporally dependent repair processes coupled with fixation, saturation, or misrepair effects at higher doses.

Other survival-curve equations have also been postulated. However, these are generally more complicated and their biological basis is less sound than for those described here. Interested readers can find many of these described elsewhere (Elkind & Whitmore 1967; Proceedings of the 6th L. H. Gray Conference 1975).

## 6.5. Biological and chemical modifiers of cell survival

### Repair of potentially lethal damage

Cell survival is usually measured by irradiating cells and immediately inducing them to proliferate so that the survivors form colonies. At the time of the irradiation the cells may already be in the cell cycle and proliferating, or alternatively they may be out of cycle and in a nonproliferative state. In the latter case the cells could be induced into proliferation at any time after irradiation. If there is such a time delay, *repair of potentially lethal damage* (PLDR) is likely to occur (cf. Section 3.1). This process stops when the cells are induced into cycle, e.g. when they are induced to proliferate and form colonies. PLDR increases the level of survival (Figure 3.3). The initial phase of repair occurs over a period of 4 to 8 hours. With many cells in culture, the increase in survival is dose dependent, so that there is an apparent decrease in sensitivity. With some normal cell types assayed in fat pads, the increase in survival is by a constant factor so that the shoulder is increased but the sensitivity is unchanged. Also, with bone marrow stem cells a *decrease* in survival by a constant factor is observed for doses above $0\cdot5$ Gy. A possible reason for this is differentiation induced by the irradiation. Another possibility is differentiation occurring naturally during a period of mitotic delay, but in this case a dose-dependent decrease in survival would be expected which generally is not observed. A summary of measurements of PLDR in normal cells is given in Table 6.2.

PLDR continues for very long times if cells remain nonproliferative after irradiation. This has been observed in terms of a loss of chromosomal lesions in hepatocytes and thyroid cells. Also, an increase in cell survival was demonstrated with clonogenic endothelial cells *in vivo* and with hepatocytes, where the increase was dose dependent.

Whether assayed using cells in culture or *in vivo* using animal tumours, PLDR seems to be minimal or nonexistent after high-LET radiation. This point is illustrated in Figure 3.7, which shows results of

Table 6.2. Effect of PLDR on survival parameters for various cell types

|  | Immediate assay | | Assay delayed for 24 hr | |
|---|---|---|---|---|
|  | N | $D_0(Gy)$ | N | $D_0(Gy)$ |
| Mammary cells | 5·0 | 1·3 | 23·0 | 1·2 |
| Thyroid cells | 4·0 | 2·0 | 12·0 | 2·0 |
| Hepatocytes | 0·9 | 2·7 | 2·3 | 2·7 |
|  | 1·6 | 2·5 | 1·7 | 3·3 |
| Bone marrow | 2·4 | 0·7 | 1·1 | 0·7 |

(From Hendry 1985c; Fisher & Hendry 1987).

experiments in which lung carcinomas were irradiated *in situ* and then were excised at various times thereafter, single cells separated out, and survival of these assayed. While survival after gamma rays was enhanced by the delayed removal of the tumours (PLDR), there was little evidence of such an effect with neutrons.

### Repair of sublethal damage

According to this concept cells that survive irradiation nevertheless sustain some radiation injury. This injury is *sublethal* but it can accumulate and become lethal. This was inferred from the increasing sensitivity of cells at higher single doses (Figure 6.4). Sublethal injury can be repaired (SLDR), and this can be demonstrated by separating two (or more) doses by increasing intervals of time and measuring the resultant increase in level of survival (*split-dose recovery*). An example of the time course of split-dose recovery is shown for clonogenic cells in mouse intestine (Figure 6.6). For most cell types half of the increase in survival is reached in about 1 hour, and virtually the total increase is achieved in 2−4 hours. After this time the surviving cells respond to the second dose as if they had not been irradiated before.

The amount of the increase in survival resulting from SLDR is dependent on dose. At low doses where little sublethal injury is induced, there will be little effect of splitting a dose into two parts. This is in the region of dose where the killing of cells described by the $\alpha$ component is much in excess of that due to the $\beta$ component (Figure 6.5). As the dose increases, surviving cells will contain a greater amount of sublethal injury, and hence a greater increase in survival is demonstrated by splitting the dose into two parts (Figure 6.7). It had been thought that an exception to the greater increase in survival with high split doses occurred 'off the shoulder', at doses high enough for survival to be exponential. It is now known, however, that in tissues the general rule is for more sparing effect from SLDR, the higher the dose, because the

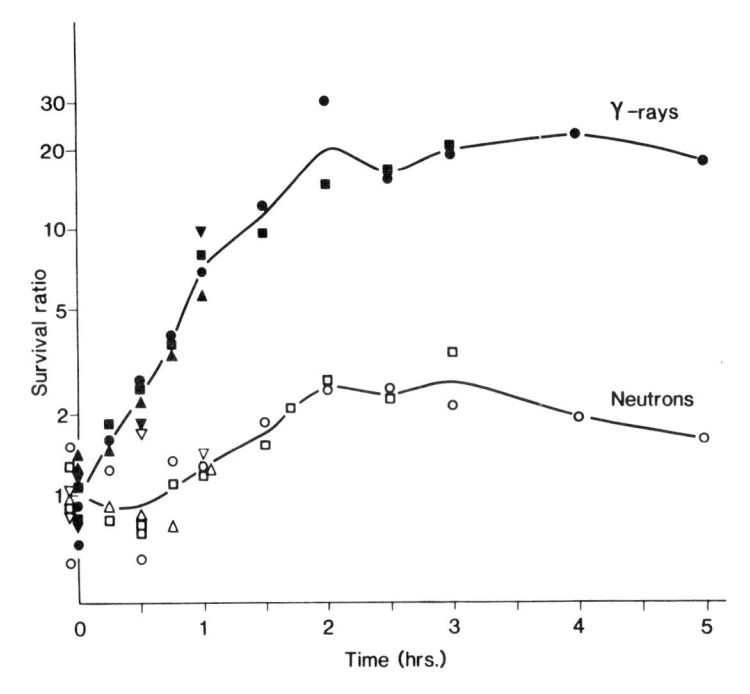

Figure 6.6. Response of intestinal clonogens to split-doses of γ-rays (6·5 Gy + 6·5 Gy) or 14·7-MeV neutrons (3·25 Gy + 3·25 Gy) (Hendry 1984a). Different symbols represent separate experiments. Survival ratio = ratio of numbers of clonogens given split-dose/single dose.

survival curve is bending for the renewing populations in the tissues whose depletion results in tissue injury (*target cells*, cf. Section 1.3).

It is common experience that the increase in survival caused by splitting doses into two parts separated by 4 hours is predicted from the shape of the survival curve measured using single doses. In other words, the shape of the single-dose survival curve is repeated in full when the surviving cells are re-irradiated. When more than two doses are given, the effect of SLDR in many systems is repeatable (cf. Figures 2.7 and 3.1). This has been demonstrated directly using up to 70 fractions of 1 Gy delivered to hepatocytes *in vivo*. Also, the repeatability is compatible with the response *in vivo* of several types of epithelial clonogenic cells to fractionated doses (see below).

Both PLDR and SLDR may occur at the same time. The distinction between them is operational, and the same enzyme system may be responsible for both types. SLDR is demonstrated by measuring the response to a second dose of radiation, which is not needed for assessing PLDR.

Lastly, it should be noted that many simpler biological systems such

192　　　　　　　　　*Fractionation in Radiotherapy*

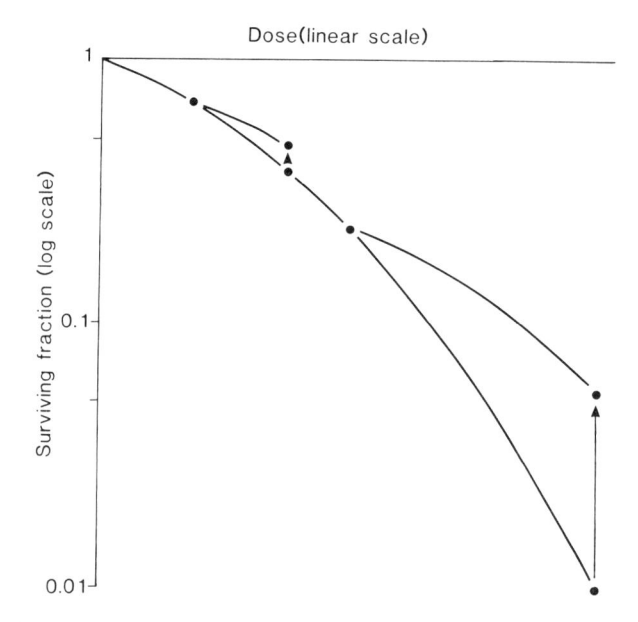

Figure 6.7. Split-dose effects, showing a greater increase in surviving fraction when larger doses are split into two equal parts.

as yeast and plant cells have repair systems that are stimulated by irradiation. In these cases the increases in survival are much greater than predicted from the survival curve measured using single doses, but definitive evidence for such effects has not been reported in mammalian cells.

### Effect of LET on the survival curve

High-LET radiation is *less* efficient than low-LET radiation for the inactivation of single molecules, because of wasted energy in the densely ionizing particle tracks. However, less injury is repaired after high-LET radiation, making these radiations *more* effective for cell killing. Equivalently, the ratio of direct to indirect action is greater for high LET, and injury induced by direct action is less modifiable by agents that modify indirect action, such as oxygen (see below). The increasing steepness and loss of curvature of survival curves with increasing LET are shown in Figure 6.8. These features were described using the old form of target theory by the greater ability per unit dose of densely-ionizing radiation to inactivate all targets simultaneously or a separate (lethal) target, and using the modern form by the greater ability to produce one (unrepaired) lethal genetic lesion. Repair-type models invoke less repair after high-LET radiation, for reasons that include the

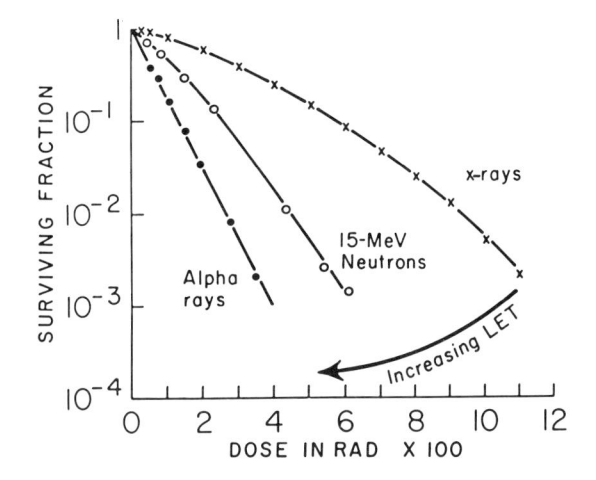

Figure 6.8. Survival curves for cells exposed to 250-kVp X-rays, 15-MeV neutrons, and 4-MeV alpha-particles (from Hall 1978). As the LET of the radiation increases, the slope of the survival curves gets steeper and the size of the initial shoulder gets smaller. (Reproduced with permission of Harper & Row Inc. and the author.)

idea that 'clean' breaks in the DNA double-strand are more difficult to repair correctly than the 'staggered' breaks characteristic of low-LET radiation.

### Relative biological effectiveness (RBE)

Different biological effects require different degrees of ion density to bring them about. Equivalently, the same doses of ionizing radiations of differing LET do not produce the same biological effect. This being the case, it is desirable to have some measure of the doses required from different beams to elicit particular biological effects. The concept of the *ratio of doses that produce the same biological effect* is termed the RBE. A more precise definition is as follows. The RBE of a test radiation compared with a standard radiation is defined by the ratio $D_s/D$, where $D_s$ and $D$ are, respectively, the doses of the standard beam and the test radiation required for equal biological effect.

Before continuing with the discussion of the RBE it is necessary to introduce the concept of *dose-modifying factor* (DMF). We would say that in the presence and absence of a dose-modifying factor the *ratio of doses for equal cell kill is constant*, independent of level of cell kill (i.e. dose), and that the agent was therefore *dose-modifying*. In terms of the survival curves measured in the presence and absence of a response-modifying agent, this would be a DMF if the ratios of initial (low-dose) and final (high-dose) slopes ($D_0$s) were the same. On the (LQ) model, this would be described by saying that the ratios of the $\alpha$'s equals the square root of the ratio of the $\beta$'s.

The RBE is affected by a number of factors. To illustrate these it is worthwhile to proceed with an example of how the RBE is determined in a particular case. It may be seen in Figure 6.9(A) that the ratio of equally effective doses (doses that result in the same level of survival) is 3 at a level of survival around 60%, and about 1·5 at 1% survival. So first the RBE in general *changes with increasing dose* and is highest at small doses and decreases progressively thereafter. Second, different cells in various tissues are characterized by different survival responses to various radiation beams, and hence the RBE is *different in different cells and tissues*. Third, the RBE may be modified by changing the LET of the test beam. Finally, changes in radiosensitivity with position in the cell cycle (see Section 6.6) are more pronounced for low- than for high-LET radiation, and so RBE should *change with phase of the cell cycle*, and this has been confirmed experimentally (Gragg et al. 1978).

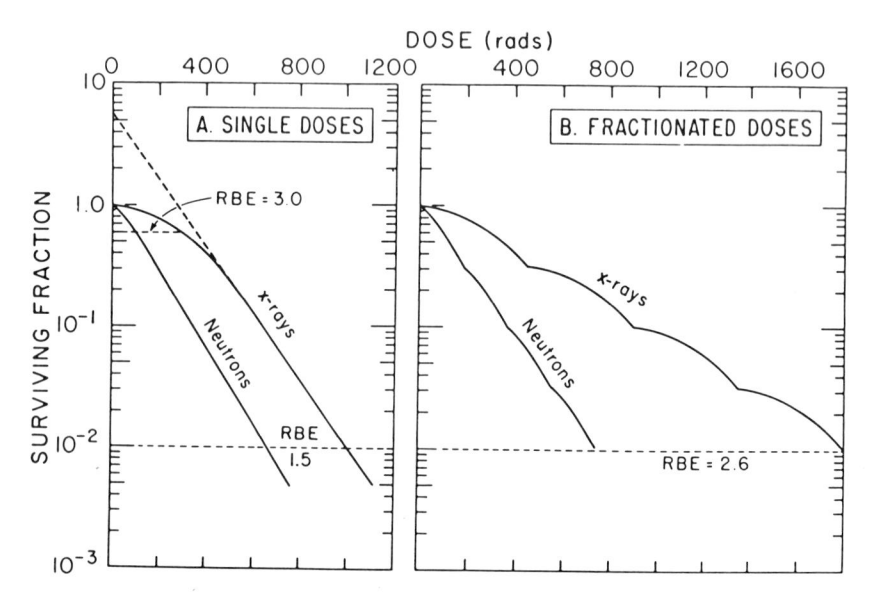

Figure 6.9. Typical survival curves for mammalian cells exposed to X-rays and fast neutrons (from Hall 1978). A. Single doses. The survival curve for X-rays has a large initial shoulder; for fast neutrons the initial shoulder is smaller and the final slope steeper. Because the survival curves have different shapes, the RBE does not have a unique value, but varies with dose, getting larger as the size of the dose is reduced. B. Fractionated doses. Illustration of the effect of giving doses of X-rays or fast neutrons in four equal fractions to produce the same level of survival as in (A). The shoulder of the survival curve is re-expressed after each dose fraction; since the shoulder is larger for X-rays than for neutrons, this results in an enlarged RBE for fractionated treatments. (Reproduced with permission of Harper & Row Inc. and the author.)

It has been found experimentally that the same biological effect will be produced by either heavy or light charged particles provided their energies are chosen so that both have approximately the same average LET. This leads to the conclusion that the *RBE is determined to a large extent by LET*. The variation of RBE with LET is shown in Figure 6.10. RBE increases with LET, and reaches a peak at about 100 keV/$\mu$m. There is a decline in RBE at very high LET, considered to result from over-production of primary lesions with very densely ionizing radiation.

From Figure 6.9(A) it was clear that the RBE varied with size of dose, and it is thus not surprising to find that the *RBE changes with size of dose per fraction* in a fractionated radiotherapy schedule (Figure 6.9(B)). Here we intend comparisons between such beams as high-energy neutrons and cobalt-60 gamma rays or X rays. Since the RBE increases with decreasing dose, it may be expected that with decreasing dose per fraction (or increasing fraction number), the effectiveness of neutrons would increase relative to that of X rays. It may be appreciated that the relative change in RBE with changing size of dose is primarily a function

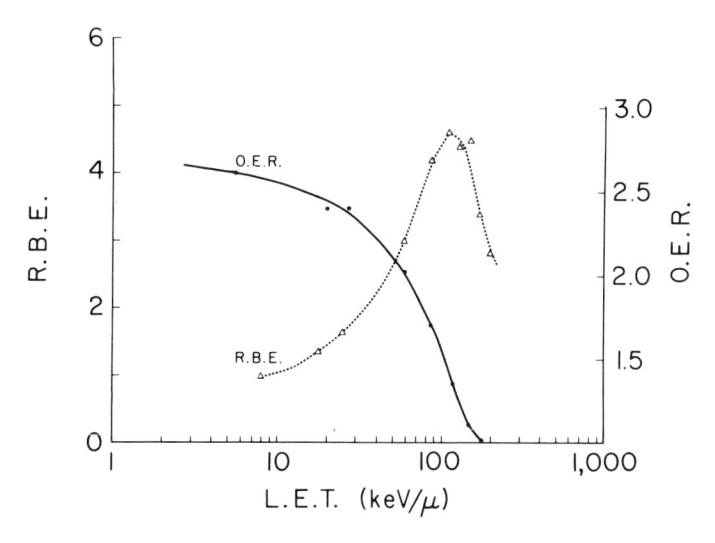

Figure 6.10. The RBE and OER as functions of radiation quality (from Withers & Peters 1980). The data plotted are for monolayer cultures of human kidney cells exposed to monoenergetic particles of different energies. Both OER and RBE values are relative to 250-kVp X-rays and the RBE values are for 10% survival. Note that the efficiency of cell killing (RBE) increases with increasing LET (ionization density) up to 100 keV/$\mu$m and then decreases again as the probability of each cell's receiving more than one lethal 'hit' (overkill) increases. OER decreases progressively with LET. The OER for fast neutron beams suitable for radiotherapy is 1·6–1·7; monoenergetic heavy charged-particle beams have very low OERs in the distal Bragg peak, but their OER increases significantly when the Bragg peak is widened sufficiently to be of clinical use. (Reproduced with permission of Lea & Febiger and the authors.)

of the shape of the low-LET dose survival curve, which determines the slope of the response to fractionated doses (Figure 3.1). Consequently, *the higher RBE that has been observed for late than for acute effects results at least in part from the preferential sparing of late-effects tissues with small dose fractions* (see Sections 3.3 and 6.10). Since this higher RBE for late effects reflects peculiarities in the low-LET survival response, rather than in those of high-LET response, it is likely to be found in a comparison of X rays with all high-LET beams and is not an inherent characteristic of the latter (Withers et al. 1982b).

## Radiosensitivity and the cell cycle

The radiosensitivity of cells depends on their position in the cell cycle (described in Section 6.6 below) at the time of irradiation. The common finding is that cells in mitosis or at the $G_1/S$ boundary are most sensitive and those in late S are most resistant. The radiosensitivity can vary by as much as factor of 3 among the phases of the cycle. As with split-dose

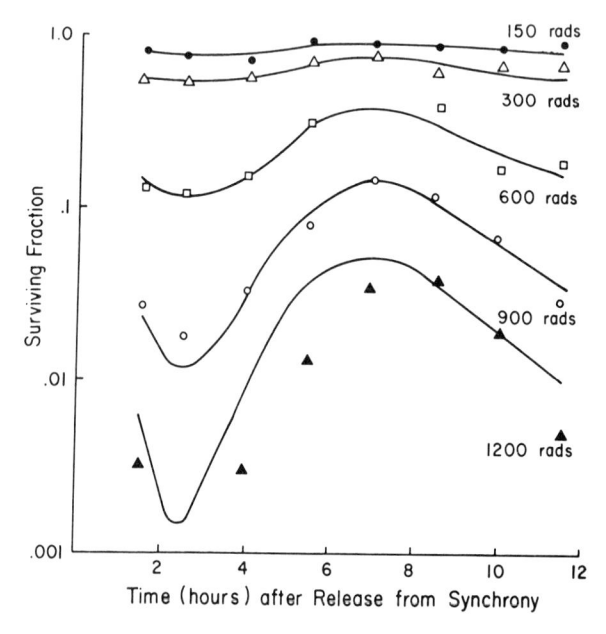

Figure 6.11. Variation in radiosensitivity with position in the cell cycle of Chinese hamster cells after synchronization at time 0 by mitotic shake-off (Section 6.6) (from McLarty 1976). Data (Sinclair 1969) were extracted graphically from plots and fitted using a mathematical model that accounted for variable radiosensitivity through the division cycle (McLarty 1976). At high doses survival increased to a maximum in late S, but at doses of 1·5 to 3 Gy there was negligible variation in sensitivity. (Reproduced with permission of the author.)

repair (SLDR), there is more variation in sensitivity, the higher the dose, and one possibility is that the phenomenon is a result of variable repair capacity in the division cycle. A generalized picture of these features is shown in Figure 6.11. There are a few exceptions to this general rule, even cases showing almost the reverse changes in sensitivity.

The variation in radiosensitivity through the cell cycle is much less with neutrons, and less still with very high-LET radiations such as alpha-particles, than with high doses of low-LET X rays as shown in Figure 6.11. Much of the peak-to-valley changes in radiosensitivity are lost with low doses of X rays. Since clinical radiotherapy is highly fractionated, with doses per fraction in the range 1−3 Gy, variations in radiosensitivity through the division cycle (including any circadian variations) will not have nearly as pronounced an effect as the high-dose data might have suggested, thus largely undercutting what had once been thought of as a rationale for high-LET radiotherapy.

Radiosensitivity does not depend markedly on the proliferative state (resting or growing) of the cells at the time of irradiation provided that cells are proliferative shortly after irradiation. This has been shown for hair follicles, bone marrow stem cells, and intestinal clonogens. This appears to conflict with an old 'law' of radiobiology, namely that radiosensitivity varies in proportion to proliferative activity (Bergonié & Tribondeau 1906), but it does not. The latter described the differential sensitivity of rapidly versus very slowly proliferating cell systems where proliferative stimulants were not applied. Hence the genetic injury remained latent in the virtually quiescent cell systems, and it was repaired (PLDR), so that the injury was not expressed in mitosis.

## Sensitizing agents

There are two classes of chemicals which sensitize cells to irradiation. The first of these are the halogenated pyrimidines, such as 5-bromodeoxyuridine, which are incorporated into DNA in place of the DNA precursor thymidine. This substitution sets up stresses in the DNA and makes it more liable to injury. Large amounts of incorporation make the cells more susceptible to X-ray damage. This effect has not yet been employed successfully in therapy.

The second class of sensitizers, which are *electron-affinic*, sensitize the cells by making the radiation more efficient. More radicals are produced in the initial radiolysis products in the cell (cf. Section 6.1). One of the most efficient sensitizers of this type is free molecular oxygen. When the oxygen is removed from cells by gassing with nitrogen or argon, cells are two to three times more resistant. The effect was thought to be dose modifying, but it is now known that the *OER is reduced at lower doses*, to about 2−2·4 for clinical doses (Palcic and Skarsgard 1984). There is a tendency in many cases for the extrapolation number to be reduced. Cells are more responsive to radiosensitizers when they are depleted of their natural radioprotector, glutathione.

Two chemicals that have been used clinically as oxygen replacements are metronidazole (Flagyl) and, more extensively, misonidazole (Ro-07-0582). These have been used in clinical trials but have been found to be too neurotoxic at the dose levels required for marked sensitization of cells in man (Dische et al. 1985; Fowler 1985). Other variants are being tried that are less neurotoxic and more electron-affinic, e.g. Ro-03-8799.

Very little oxygen is required to sensitize cells, and cells that are at about 1/2 percent oxygen ($PO_2 = 5$ mm Hg) already show about half the maximum change in sensitivity from 0 to 100% $O_2$ (Figure 6.12). The level of $O_2$ that results in half-maximal sensitization is known as the $K$ value, and corresponds to about 5 mm Hg in the examples shown in Figure 6.12. The shape of the curve showing the relationship between radiosensitivity and $O_2$ concentration can be described by the equation:

$$\frac{S}{S_n} = \frac{m[O_2] + K}{[O_2] + K}$$

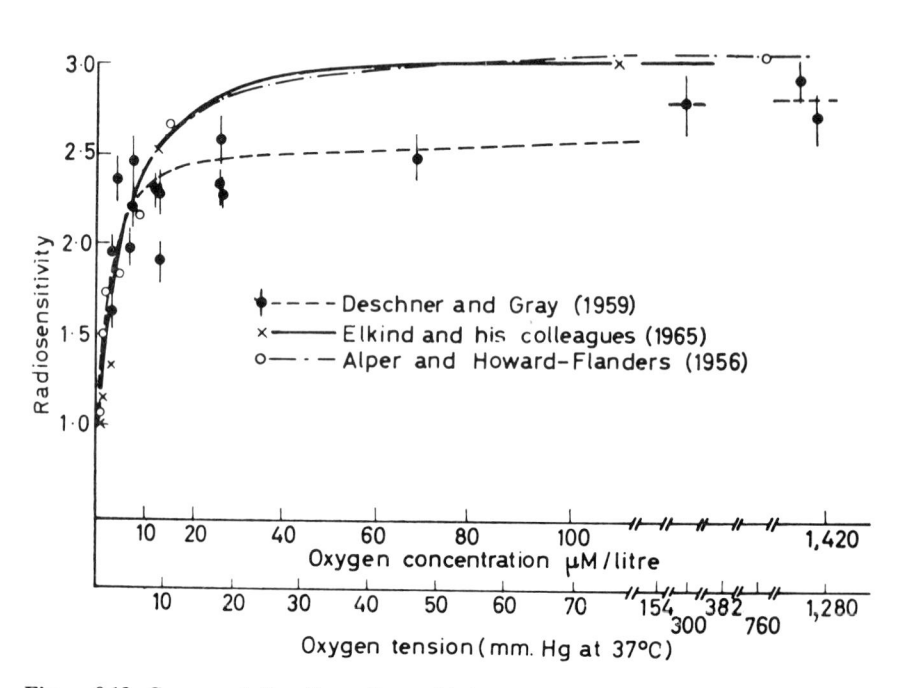

Figure 6.12. Curves relating the radiosensitivity of cells in arbitrary units to the oxygen concentration in their environment at the time of irradiation. (Taken from Thomlinson 1967 where the references can be found; reproduced with permission of Butterworths and the author.)

where $S$ is the sensitivity (i.e. $1/D_0$) at any value of $O_2$ concentration, $S_n$ is its value at 0% $O_2$, and $m$ is the maximum ratio of $S/S_n$ at high concentrations of $O_2$.

Many cells in the body are at venous oxygen tensions (40 mm Hg or ~4% $O_2$) and hence are on the virtual plateau of maximal sensitivity. Exceptions to this are the hypoxic fraction of cells in many tumours (see below), avascular cartilage, the oesophagus (in mice), and skin where blood flow is markedly reduced (by cooling or compression).

The oxygen enhancement ratio (OER) varies in an important way with LET of a radiation beam. As shown in Figure 6.10, with increasing LET the OER falls slowly at first until the LET reaches about 60 keV/$\mu$m, after which the OER falls rapidly towards 1 as the LET passes 100 keV/$\mu$m. Possible reasons for this are the lesser ability to modify injury resulting from direct action, which predominates with high LET, and the generation of oxygen in the densely ionizing tracks.

## Protective agents

There are chemicals that act as radical scavengers, making the indirect action of radiation less efficient. The best known are the sulphur-containing thiols or *sulphydryl compounds*. These compounds do not protect anoxic cells, but rather protect best those cells containing oxygen at concentrations around the $K$ value. They are less effective for fully oxygenated cells. There are *naturally occurring radioprotectors*, such as *glutathione*, containing a sulphydryl group.

The fact that sulphydryl compounds protect against radiation injury has been known for a long time. However, the toxicity of these compounds discouraged interest in their use until the 1970s, after the introduction of WR-2721 ($\beta$-mercapto-ethylamine derivative) and experiments suggesting selective protection of normal tissues from radiation damage. The following hypotheses were put forward to explain this: differences in cellular metabolism and drug absorption characteristics between tumours and normal tissues, deficient blood supply to tumour cells, and relatively poor protection of severely hypoxic cells. The latter two were considered most likely.

More recent experimental results have clouded the picture. Substantial protection of several rodent tumours has been demonstrated. Also, variable oxygen concentration, and thus variable protection, has been demonstrated among normal tissues. Phase I clinical trials have demonstrated that the maximum tolerable dose of WR-2721 is about 250 mg/m$^2$ when given 4 times weekly up to 6 weeks (Brown 1985), but it is not known whether this dose level will yield a significant degree of protection.

## 6.6. Cell and tissue kinetics

The cell cycle comprises the physiological events that occur in the cell from the time of its birth after the division of its parent until it undergoes mitosis (M) to form two daughter cells. The duration of this cycle is known as the *cell-cycle time*. The cell cycle is divided into four phases based on the nature of the physiological activities in those phases. The DNA synthetic phase (S phase) is the time during which the cell actively synthesizes DNA to duplicate its genetic material. There is an interval between the birth of the cell after mitosis of its mother and the beginning of DNA synthesis in S phase; this interval or 'gap' is known as $G_1$. After the completion of DNA synthesis in S phase, there is a second time interval before mitosis called $G_2$.

The duration of these phases differs according to cycle type and degree of commitment to the division cycle. The variability in cell-cycle time is mostly attributable to variability in the $G_1$ phase. When cells divide very slowly, a fifth phase, $G_0$, is used to indicate that for a period of time they are not committed to divide, but may be recruited into the cycle after an appropriate stimulus.

The technique of *autoradiography*, developed by Howard & Pelc (1953), is based on introducing radioactive label into newly synthesized DNA by feeding the cells radioactively labelled DNA precursors. The label commonly used for this purpose is *tritiated thymidine*, an emitter of short-range beta-particles (electrons). This is given to a growing cell population for a short period of time (*pulse labelling*), and those cells in the population in S phase at the time of the labelling incorporate the label into their DNA. After completion of pulse labelling, usually of the order of 20 to 30 minutes, the radioactive thymidine is washed from the system and the cells are fixed and stained for ease of viewing. They are covered with a very thin layer of photographic emulsion. Beta-particles from the incorporated radioactive label create a latent image in the emulsion. This is subsequently developed and fixed, and the areas through which beta-particles have passed appear as black spots which serve as a marker for the cells that were actively synthesizing DNA when the label was available.

Populations growing in log phase are distributed asynchronously through the cell cycle, and cells may be found in each of the four phases of the cycle. For many applications, however, it is desirable to use cells known to be in particular phases of the cell cycle, i.e. *synchronous cultures*. The basic idea is that cells can be blocked at different parts of the cycle. For example, they can be obtained in mitosis by a technique known as *mitotic harvest*. This exploits the fact that when cells are near mitosis they round up and become loosely attached to the surface of containers. If at this stage the medium in which they are growing is subjected to gentle shaking, the mitotic cells detach and float in the medium. This medium is then removed from the culture vessels and plated out onto new dishes, and the population consists almost entirely of mitotic cells. Other techniques for synchronization of cultures involve the use of drugs.

The relative lengths of different phases of the cell cycle can be studied using a technique known as *percent labelled mitoses* (PLM) or fraction

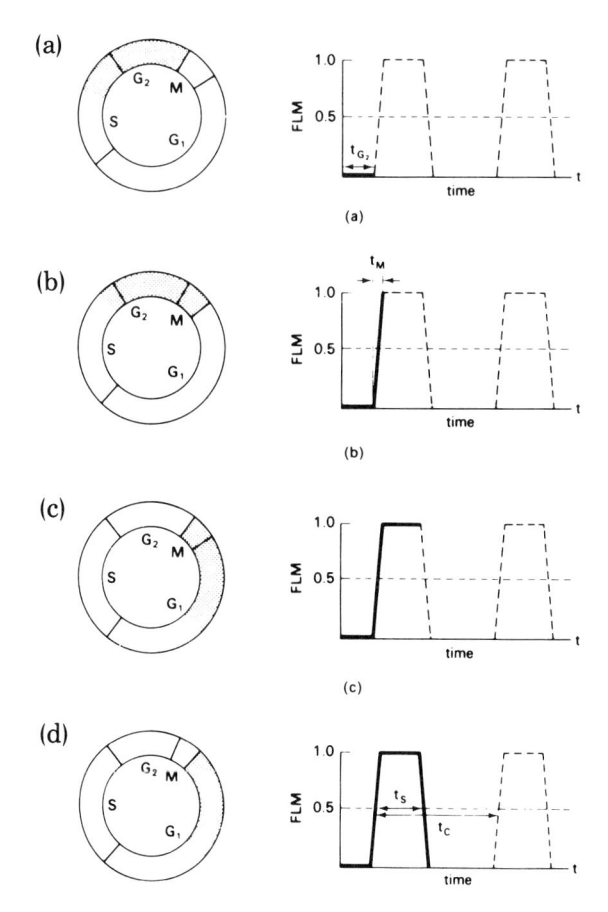

Figure 6.13. Analysis of PLM experiments (from Aherne *et al.* 1977). (*a*) A pulse label of tritiated thymidine has been taken up by cells that were in S phase, some of which have progressed through $G_2$; no mitotic figures are evident yet. (*b*) The leading edge of the labelled cohort has completed mitosis, and almost all mitotic cells are labelled. (*c*) The trailing edge of the labelled cohort completes mitosis, after which (*d*) the number of mitotic cells with label falls to zero. The width of the peak is an estimate of the time spent in S phase, and the distance between the leading edges of the two peaks (the second a manifestation of the reappearance of labelled cells in the mitotic 'window' after a complete cell-cycle traverse) is an estimate of the cell-cycle time. (Reproduced with permission of Edward Arnold Ltd and the authors.)

labelled mitoses (FLM). The principle is to apply a pulse label of tritiated thymidine. Cells in S phase take up the label, whereas those in other phases of the cycle do not. The excess label is then washed out, and the cells continue their progression in the division cycle. At regular times after administration of the label, samples of the population are removed, fixed, and stained for autoradiography. After development and fixation, the percentage of mitotic cells that carries a radioactive label is determined, and this is the PLM.

The analysis of the results of PLM experiments is illustrated in Figure 6.13. The labelled cohort of cells that was in S phase at the time of pulse labelling moves through the $G_2$ phase. During the next few hours autoradiographs show no labelled mitotic figures (Figure 6.13($a$)), but when the first of the labelled cohort reaches mitosis the leading edge will appear as mitotic figures with label (Figure 6.13($b$)). The percentage of figures that are labelled will then reach a maximum of close to 100% as the cohort passes through mitosis (Figure 6.13($c$)), and then will drop as the cohort leaves mitosis (Figure 6.13($d$)). For the next few hours all mitotic figures will be lacking label, until the leading edge of the labelled cohort again reaches mitosis. This occurs after the labelled cohort has gone through the entire division cycle and comes back to mitosis, and then this pattern of events is repeated.

Therefore, theoretically waves of labelled mitoses would be expected, but in practice, because of variability in the *transit times* through the different phases of the cycle, the second peak is usually considerably

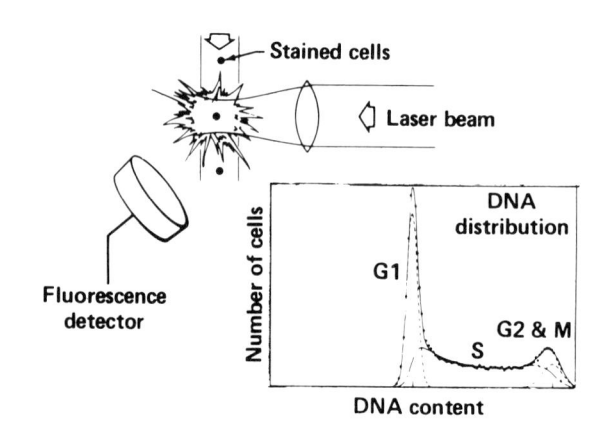

Figure 6.14. Schematic illustration of the principles of DNA distribution analysis by *flow cytometry* (from Gray et al. 1986). Suspensions of fluorescently stained single cells flow one at a time through a light beam whose wavelength is adjusted to excite the fluorescent dye. The fluorescence stimulated in each cell is recorded as a measure of that cell's DNA content. Thousands of cells can be measured each second and the results accumulated to form a DNA distribution like that shown in this figure for asynchronously growing CHO cells. (Reproduced with permission of Taylor & Francis Ltd and the authors.)

smaller than the first. Nonetheless, the distance between the peaks is clearly an estimate of the cell-cycle time and the width of the first peak an estimate of the duration of S phase.

Cell-cycle analysis can also be accomplished by *flow cytometry* (reviewed by Gray et al. 1986). In this method, single cells are stained with a DNA-specific fluorescent dye. The cells in suspension are passed one-by-one through the machine at several thousand per second. The dye is stimulated to fluoresce using a laser, and the amount of fluorescence is a measure of DNA content (Figure 6.14). The profile of the DNA distribution among the cells shows two peaks, one in $G_1$ and the other in $G_2 + M$, where there is double the amount of DNA. S phase is represented by the continuum between the two peaks (Figure 6.15).

Cell-cycle traverse can be studied by incorporating bromodeoxyuridine (BrdUrd) into the cells and then measuring its quenching effect on the fluorescence from the DNA-specific dye Hoechst 33258. Alternatively, monoclonal antibodies can be used against BrdUrd incorporated into DNA so that the BrdUrd-labelled cells fluoresce weakly. This is

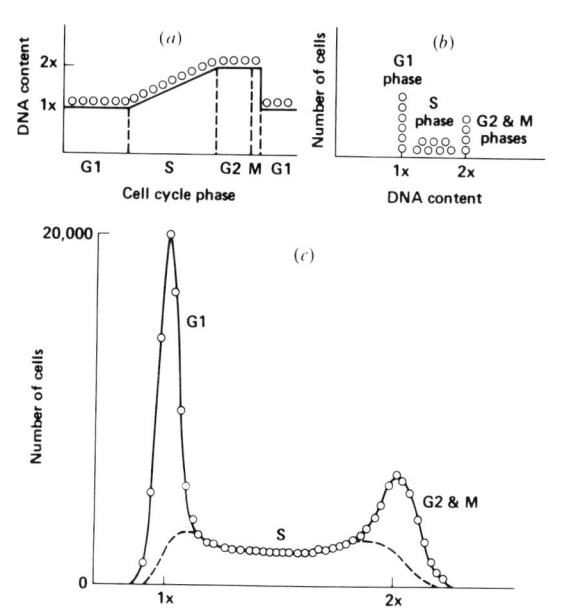

Figure 6.15. Schematic illustration of the relation between the distribution of cells around the cell cycle and the DNA distribution (from Gray et al. 1986). (a) DNA content vs. position in the cell cycle. (b) The DNA distribution expected for this hypothetical population. (c) A DNA distribution measured for an exponentially growing population. This distribution illustrates the broadening of the $G_1 -$ and $G_2 + M$ phase peaks produced by variation in the cell preparation and measuring process. (Reproduced with permission of Taylor & Francis Ltd. and the authors.)

equivalent to a measurement of the labelling index. Simultaneous measurement of DNA content and amount of incorporated BrdUrd can be done, using two dyes that fluoresce at different wavelengths. The method can be applied to the study of kinetic changes in perturbed cell populations and discrimination and sorting of subpopulations of cells.

## 6.7. Radiobiology of renewing normal tissues

### Proliferative organization of normal renewing tissues

The more rapidly renewing tissues in the body include haematopoietic tissue supplying the various types of blood cells, and various epithelia such as the gastrointestinal mucosa, the epidermis and its associated hair follicles, and testicular tubules. All of these so-called *hierarchical tissues* have a common underlying pattern of proliferative structure (Figure 6.16). This comprises a virtually quiescent *stem-cell* population, a rapidly dividing population of *differentiating proliferative cells* which amplifies the number of progeny (sometimes called transit cells), and *maturing/mature cells* which are the functional end-cells of the particular lineage. The large but almost quiescent stem-cell population has the advantage that these cells normally are used at slow rates, and they are required to undergo only a limited number of divisions before maturation. Hence the risk of genetic errors introduced at mitosis is limited, and there is relatively more time for repair of any genetic injury during the quiescent phase ($G_0$).

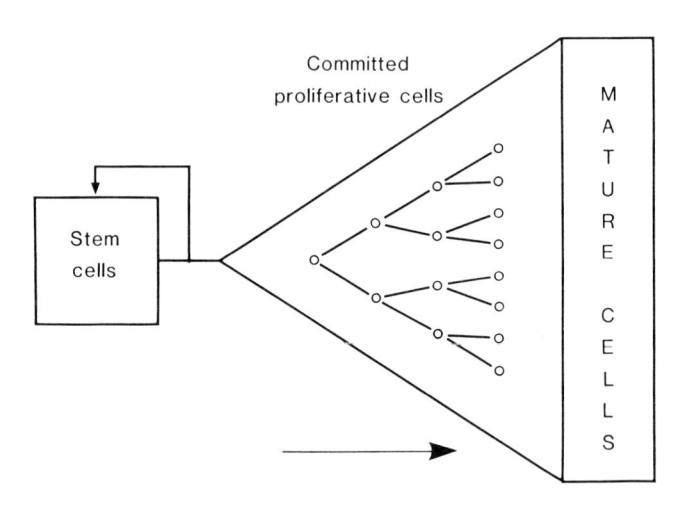

Figure 6.16. Proliferative organization of hierarchical tissues.

The number of amplifying cell divisions varies among tissues. It is three to four in epidermis and gastrointestinal mucosa, and up to at least eight in haematopoietic tissues. The spatial distribution of these populations of cells is shown diagrammatically in Figure 1.2.

### Response of renewing tissues to irradiation

Hierarchical-type tissues respond to radiation in a very characteristic way which is related to the resistance of the nondividing mature cells and the sensitivity of the stem cells when they are stimulated into proliferation (cf. Section 1.2). Following high doses of radiation, there is a continual loss of mature cells at the normal rate since these are typically nondividing and for the most part unaffected by radiation (but there are important exceptions, mature cells that can undergo interphase death, e.g. small lymphocytes and the serous cells of various glands, see Section 1.2). However, there is little cell production because the stem cells will be sterilized and the existing transit cells may undergo only one or two divisions. Hence the mature-cell population will decline at a rate characteristic of each particular tissue. The decline will stimulate proliferation in the stem-cell population to compensate for the reduction in mature cells, and this induced proliferation will express the lethal injury in the stem-cell population. The decline in mature cells will continue until a critical level is reached, resulting in tissue failure.

The duration of the decline in functional, mature cells correlates well with the *latent interval for expression of tissue injury*. It has been shown that the times to denude fully the epidermis (15−30 days for different sites) and the intestinal mucosa (3 days) in mice corresponds to the transit times through the amplifying- and mature-cell populations. Another example is the testis, where in man the decline in sperm counts and hence fertility is noticeable at 46 days, which is the transit time from the radioresistant preleptotene spermatocytes to spermatozoa. The times of death of mice from the GI syndrome (4 to 7 days) and the bone marrow syndrome (10 to 30 days) are related to the transit times of the maturing-cell populations. A clear example of the relation of cell kinetics to time of death was observed for gut death in mice, with a prolonged latency period as expected for germ-free mice where the transit time is longer (Tsubouchi & Matsuzawa 1973). Also, as might well be expected, the time course of denudation is independent of dose in the high-dose region, since additional dose increments will have no effect on an already sterilized population (cf. Figure 1.5).

After low doses, where sufficiently many stem cells survive, there will be regeneration of the mature-cell populations from surviving stem cells. The time for full recovery is dose dependent, i.e. dependent on the level of survival of the stem cells. The *rate of recovery* of the mature cells depends on the cycle time of the progenitor cells and the rate of differentiation into the amplifying-cell populations. The *doubling time of the stem cells* during regeneration will be longer than the cycle time because of differentiation of stem cells at each division. The doubling times of stem cells during regeneration in epidermis, intestinal mucosa, and bone marrow are reasonably similar at about 24 hours. In bone marrow, this results from a cycle time of about 6 hours, and a 40% rate of differentiation at each division.

Dose−response curves for these tissues can be obtained in terms of the severity of response versus dose, for assessments made at given times after irradiation. These curves generally show a threshold region of dose where injury is minimal and unimportant regarding the continued function of the tissue, followed by an increasing severity of injury after higher doses. This pattern is described as a *nonstochastic effect*. This contrasts with a *stochastic effect*, where the incidence, but not the severity, increases with increasing dose. For example, leukemia is a stochastic effect, arising from a single transformed cell. The endpoint is the same at all doses, but of course the incidence increases with increasing dose at low doses. On the other hand, skin desquamation is a nonstochastic effect, arising from the combination of the same effect (death) occurring in many cells. The number of similarly affected cells increases with dose, and hence so does the severity of the desquamation. Nonstochastic effects are illustrated diagramatically in Figure 6.17.

Alternatively, dose−response curves can be presented using the proportion of tissues where the injury is less than a specified level. This level could be, for example, death following irradiation of a critical organ such as bone marrow, gut, or kidney. In this case the dose−response curve is S-shaped or sigmoid on a linear plot, showing a threshold region, then a range of dose where the proportion of affected samples increases rapidly from 0% and tends to 100% after high doses when all samples are affected (Figure 2.2). In the ideal case, the sigmoid curve would have 'sharp corners', because a dose would be reached where all samples would be similarly depleted below the critical level, and the curve would promptly increase to 100%. However, this never happens in practice. The reason is that there is always some *heterogeneity* which smooths out the curve to some degree.

There are various reasons for this heterogeneity. First, it can be introduced by the cytotoxic agent itself, in other words when all cells do not receive a lethal lesion. This is indeed the situation with radiation, where lethal events occur at random (cf. Sections 2.1 and 6.4). Hence if the specified level of injury is directly related to the number of surviving stem cells in a tissue, and each such cell contributes equally and independently to the repopulation of the tissue, then the steepest dose−response curve that will be seen will be determined directly by $D_0$,

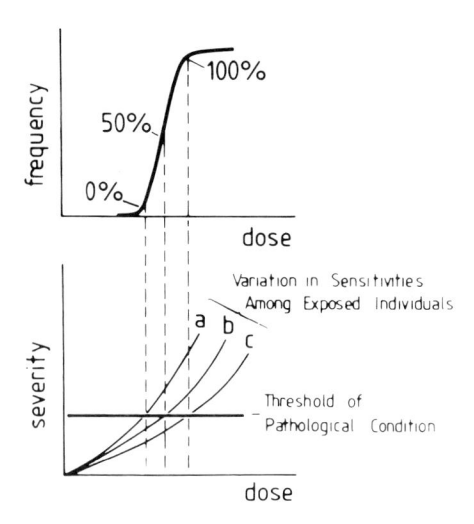

Figure 6.17. *Nonstochastic effects* increase in severity as well as frequency with increasing dose (from Field & Upton 1985 and ICRP 41 1984). Since the mechanisms of nonstochastic effects include cell killing and other stochastic effects which may in themselves be observable at incipient stages, delineation of the dose—response relation for any given type of nonstochastic effect depends on the stage and severity at which the effect is scored. The upper and lower figures illustrate how the frequency and severity of a nonstochastic effect, defined as a pathological condition, increases as a function of dose in a population of individuals of varying susceptibilities. The severity of the effect increases most steeply in those of the greatest susceptibility (lower figure, curve (a), reaching the threshold of clinical detectability as a pathological condition at a lower dose in this subgroup than in less susceptible subgroups (curves (b) and (c)). The range of doses over which the different subgroups cross the same threshold of severity is reflected in the upper curve, which shows the frequency of the pathological condition in the entire population, and which reaches 100% only at that dose that is sufficient to exceed the defined threshold of severity in all members of the population. (Reproduced with permission of Taylor & Francis Ltd and the authors.)

the (inverse) sensitivity of the 'target' cells. Second, if their contribution to repopulation and rescue is not independent, but increases with an increase in the surviving number, then the chance of rescue will decline faster with increasing dose. This would steepen the dose—response curve. Third, if there is a large variation between the initial samples in either content or sensitivity of stem cells, the composite dose—response curve will be shallower. In addition to these factors there is another steepening influence, namely two potential target-cell populations, e.g. parenchymal and vascular, which have different sensitivities and are depleted to critical levels over ranges of dose which overlap.

In experimental systems where variations between samples can be minimized, it has been shown that the $D_0$ value for the target cells measured using colony techniques is the major determinant of the steepness of the dose—response curves (cf. Section 2.1). With human material, where there is more variation between samples, the dose—response curves are often shallower.

Dose—response curves for tumours and for normal tissues, if they were known, would form the basis for optimal treatments in radiotherapy, where patients are treated to tolerance and cure rates are determined. Unfortunately, there are few dose—response curves for human tissues in the literature where doses are not presented in transformed units, e.g. values of NSD (cf. Section 6.10). The steepness of the dose—response curve for normal tissues determines the accuracy with which doses must be prescribed. The position and steepness of the curve for tumours determines first the cure rate at the tolerance dose, and second, the degree of benefit that can be achieved by changing the doses slightly or by using sensitizing agents.

## 6.8. Radiobiology of tumours

**Proliferative organization of tumours**

Tumours are tissues in which the rate of cell production has become greater than the rate of cell loss. This gives a net increase in growth of the cell population, a situation that normally also occurs in fetal life but not in adult tissues.

Tumours can arise from single transformed cells, and the initial stages of growth may be exponential. This is the case when all divisions produce two clonogens, or on average a given fraction of two clonogens, if some fixed rate of differentiation is retained from the tissue of origin.

The growth of solid tumours, in contrast to leukemias or lymphomas, is limited by their blood supply. A tumour clone can continue to grow as a single cluster of cells until it reaches about 300 $\mu$m across, when it contains about $10^4$ cells. With further growth, necrosis will develop in the centre because of the lack of nutrients (particularly oxygen) at distances of about 150 $\mu$m from a capillary, unless blood vessels penetrate the tumour. The latter occurs because of *angiogenesis*, mediated through *tumour angiogenic factor* produced by the tumour. A network of blood vessels becomes established inside the tumour as it grows. Nonetheless, there is still necrosis in the interstices between capillaries when the capillaries are more than about 300 $\mu$m apart. This *microscopic necrosis* can take two structural forms. First, as an outer sleeve around a capillary, forming the *tumour cord*, and second, as a central focus of necrosis at approximately the same distance from several surrounding capillaries.

As the tumour grows, primarily by the growth of new blood vessels, *macroscopic necrosis* develops. This occurs largely because of the poor perfusion pressure from the source of the new capillary network. The source is not the arteriole end of the supply, as it is for normal tissues, but it is the low-pressure capillary system of the pre-existing normal tissue in which the tumour arose. A necrotic core can develop inside tumours, leaving a thick shell of mostly viable tumour on the periphery.

The *volume doubling time* of tumours can be correlated with their cell kinetics. The correlation changes from simple, as in the case of very small tumours, to complex for large tumours. In the former, all cells may be dividing and differentiating at a fixed rate, whereas in the latter it is usually only a fraction and the rate of division and differentiation may be influenced by the nutritional status in the growing tumour. It is clear therefore that in the large tumour, in which only a fraction of the total cell population is actively proliferating, the volume doubling time of the entire tumour can be considerably longer than the cell-cycle time of the renewing populations.

There are three parameters that are useful in describing the growth of tumours: the *cell-cycle time*, the *growth fraction* (GF), and the rate of cell loss or the *cell-loss factor* (CLF). Thus, when all the cells in a tumour are dividing (GF = 1), as in very small tumours, the tumour volume doubling time would be equal to the cell-cycle time. If, however, the GF is less than 1, the doubling time of the population will obviously be longer than the mean cell-cycle time. This difference in the actual as opposed to the potential doubling time of tumours may be caused by a variety of factors, such as nutrient deficiencies. It is quantified by the concept of the *potential doubling time* ($T_{pot}$), which is the population volume-doubling time that would be measured in the absence of cell loss. The relationship among the CLF, the $T_{pot}$, and the observed tumour volume-doubling time ($T_{vol}$) is given by

$$\text{CLF} = 1 - T_{pot}/T_{vol}$$

Thus, if $T_{vol} = T_{pot}$ then CLF = 0, i.e. there is no cell loss (by either death, differentiation, or out-migration) and the tumour volume doubles at the maximum rate. If, on the other hand, the CLF is not 0, then $T_{vol}$ is greater than $T_{pot}$. $T_{pot}$ can be estimated from the duration of S phase ($T_S$) according to

$$T_{pot} = T_S/\text{LI}$$

where LI is the *labelling index*, i.e. the fraction of labelled cells.

While most rodent tumours grow quite rapidly, with tumour-doubling times in the range of 1–3 days, most human tumours grow much more slowly. Although tumours of epithelial origin (carcinomas) can show rapid growth, they tend to be more slowly growing, with volume-doubling times of 3 to 7 days in the mouse and about 100 days in the human. The most rapidly growing tumours are those of mesenchymal origin, i.e. lymphosarcomas or soft tissue sarcomas. These are also the tumours with the lowest CLFs.

The cell-cycle times in rodent tumours are considerably shorter than would be indicated by the $T_{vol}$, with most of the former lying in the range 10 to 20 hours. Similar short cycle times are found in a majority of the rapidly growing sarcomas, which have volume-doubling times in the rodent of around 2 days or less. In some slow-growing sarcomas, however, the cell-cycle time is considerably longer, and this is consistent with the cycle time and the growth fraction being the principle determinants of $T_{vol}$ when the CLF is relatively small. By contrast, in the carcinomas, where the CLF is large it appears to be the main determinant of the overall growth rate ($T_{vol}$). As might be expected, the $T_{vol}$s of sarcomas correlate much better with the cell-cycle time of tumour clonogens than do those of carcinomas, which have high CLFs (Figure 6.18).

### Response of tumours to irradiation

The *responsiveness* of a tumour depends, as does that of a normal renewal tissue, on the radiosensitivity of the dividing cells and the unperturbed kinetics of cell turnover. For example, tumours where cell renewal is governed by high CLFs should shrink rapidly after irradiation, as demonstrated for carcinomas (in contrast to sarcomas) in mice (Denekamp & Fowler 1977). Seminomas also have high CLFs and are responsive tumours.

In contrast to responsiveness, the *curability* of tumours is determined

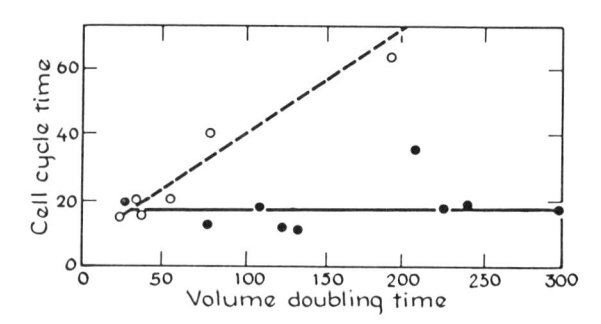

Figure 6.18. Cell-cycle time (hours) for 15 experimental tumours (from Denekamp 1970). The carcinomas (closed circles) show little variation in cell-cycle time over a tenfold variation in growth rate; the sarcomas (open circles) show a longer cell-cycle time in the slowly growing tumours. (Reproduced with permission of Waverly Press Inc. and the author.)

by the content and the sensitivity of repopulating cells. For small tumours, the proportion of repopulating cells is high in undifferentiated tumours, and low in tumours which retain some or many of the differentiation characteristics of the tissue of origin, e.g. squamous carcinomas and seminomas. In large tumours, the proportion of the total volume consisting of repopulating cells becomes lower because of the development of necrosis, the development of the tumour stroma (including blood vessels) and the infiltration of the tumour by host cells (macrophages), as discussed in detail by Moore (1983).

Estimates of the radiosensitivity of the repopulating cells can be obtained by taking cells out of the tumour and growing colonies in culture. In general, the sensitivity of tumour clonogens assessed in this way is much greater at low doses of a few gray than has been deduced from nonmalignant clonogens in their normal tissue of origin. However, this is still open to question, because of the difficulties in making exactly comparable measurements. For example, clonogens with particular sensitivities or capacities for PLDR may be selected in culture, and *in vivo* the sensitivity to low doses is deduced in many cases for the clonogens which survive high doses, i.e. for the resistant clonogens in the population. An assay for tumour clonogens *in situ* has been reported (Kummermehr 1985), but this is possible only for tumours that contain epithelial 'nests' of cells, analogous to an intestinal crypt.

A common feature of the survival curve for cells in tumours, assessed by growing colonies in culture, is the presence of a resistant 'tail' to the curve (Figure 6.19). This indicates heterogeneity in sensitivity among the clonogens, so that the sensitive fraction is killed by low doses, leaving the resistant fraction at high doses. This resistance is conferred primarily by hypoxia. Extrapolating the tail region back to the $y$-axis provides an estimate of the fraction of cells that is particularly resistant. For many experimental tumours this is about 10% although there are estimates from 0 to nearly 100% depending on the size and type of tumour. The ratio of the slopes of the two portions of the curve is in the range 2 to 3, as expected if the resistant cells are severely hypoxic.

Hypoxia is associated with microscopic necrosis and also with the generally poor blood supply to tumours. The classical picture of hypoxia and reoxygenation derives from the work of Thomlinson & Gray (1955). With microscopic necrosis, some cells on the periphery of the tumour cord are anoxic and destined to die and move into the necrotic region. Irradiation kills the viable oxic cells preferentially, and some of the doomed but resistant anoxic cells may be rescued and hence repopulate the tumour. Another feature described recently is that some cords inside tumours are much narrower than others, suggesting that the oxygen tension inside these capillaries is much lower than elsewhere so that whole cords may be radioresistant (Moore *et al.* 1985). *Chronic hypoxia*

212    *Fractionation in Radiotherapy*

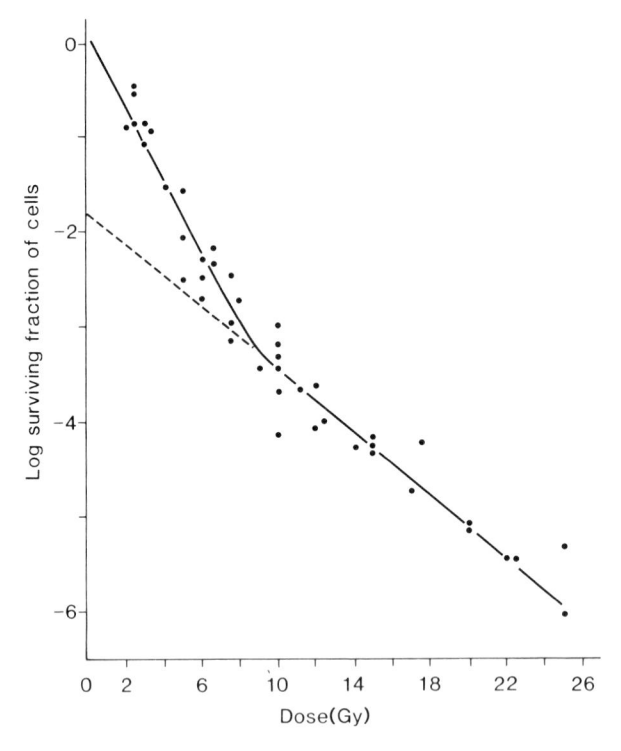

**Figure 6.19.** Survival of 6C3HED mouse lymphosarcoma cells irradiated *in vivo*. The response at doses higher than 10 Gy is determined by the hypoxic cells. (Redrawn from Powers & Tolmach 1963).

refers to the persistent low oxygen concentrations experienced by cells for long periods on the periphery of cords or in whole cords. *Transient hypoxia* refers to that associated with the rapid opening and closing of blood vessels. The latter would also give a radioresistant tail to the survival curve.

Another method that can be used to deduce the sensitivity of tumour clonogens *in situ* is based on *tumour growth delay*. In this case, the growth curves after irradiation are displaced further to the right, depending on the dose (Figure 6.20). When these curves are extrapolated back to the y-axis, an estimate of the surviving fraction of repopulating cells can be made for each dose. Hence a survival curve can be constructed. One of the difficulties in this method is that radiation induces in many cases a *tumour-bed effect*, whereby the irradiated vasculature grows at a slower rate than without irradiation. In this case, the growth rate of the tumour for volumes greater than the preirradiated volume may be reduced, and this would tend to overestimate the level of survival.

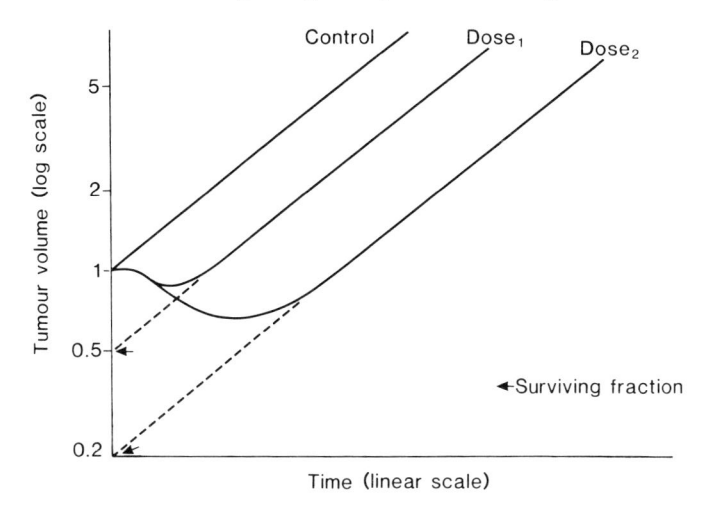

Figure 6.20. Increase in tumour volume with time after irradiation with Dose₁, Dose₂, or sham-irradiated, as measured by *growth delay*. Estimates of the surviving fractions (arrows) are given by the back extrapolate of the growth curves on the *y*-axis.

Clonogen sensitivity can be deduced from the steepness of dose−response curves, where the response is the proportion of tumours sterilized (cured). This is analogous to the deduction of clonogen sensitivity from animal lethality data (cf. Section 2.1). In the ideal case, the deduced value will represent the sensitivity of the clonogens over the range of dose where the probability of tumour cure is changing most rapidly. These will be the radioresistant hypoxic cells in most cases. However, in practice there is heterogeneity in tumour sizes so that the deduced value of sensitivity is only a lower limit. In special experimental situations, for example when similar-sized balls of tumour cells (*spheroids*) are irradiated, the sensitivity can match the value assessed by growing colonies from the cells in culture. Again, extrapolation of the deduced survival curve to zero dose gives a measure of the number of resistant clonogens in the tumours, and this determines whether or not cure will be achieved. This number generally represents less than 1% of the total number of morphological viable cells in tumours *in vivo* (Moore et al. 1983).

When doses are fractionated, the phenomenon of *reoxygenation* can occur (cf. Section 6.10). When oxic cells are preferentially killed by the first dose, oxygen is made available to hypoxic cells. Estimates of the time course of this effect after a large single dose are shown in Figure 6.21 for several animal tumours. The time course varies depending partly on the renewal characteristics of the tumour, which as noted above are related to tumour shrinkage. Similar data are not available for human tumours.

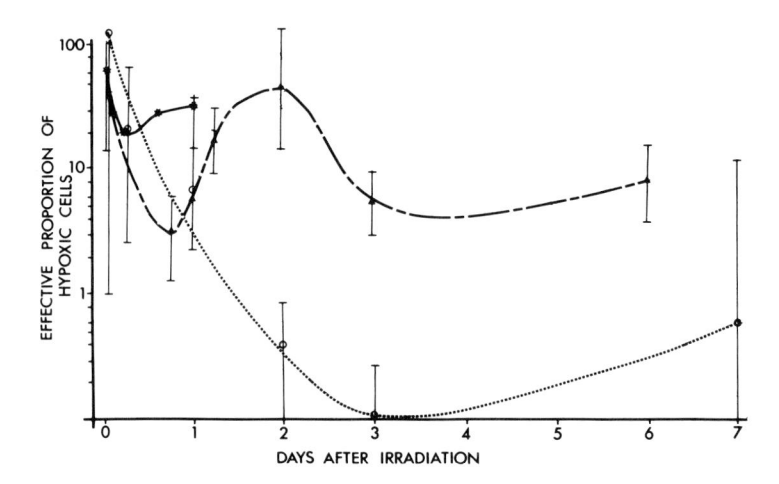

Figure 6.21. The effective proportion of hypoxic cells in a tumour alters between radiation doses (adapted from Moore 1972, where original references may be found). The proportion is made high by a priming dose of radiation, and changes in this proportion are seen which are dependent on the time interval before the second dose.

The classical idealized picture of the life history of the oxygen status of tumours before and after a large single dose of radiation is shown in Figure 6.22. After reaching a level characteristic of the tumour (C) the proportion of hypoxic cells nears 100% because of the higher radiosensitivity of the oxic cells, then falls when cells begin to divide and die (F), providing increased availability of oxygen for the survivors. The tumour may ultimately regain its characteristic balance between hypoxic and oxic cells (J).

With multifractionated irradiation, reoxygenation will occur during the treatment, not just after its completion. It is thought that in many human tumours reoxygenation occurs during treatment, and that this removes this particular potential source of resistance in tumours. Changes in average oxygen tension in tumours have been obtained from oxygen electrode measurements during treatment (Kolstad 1964).

Methods to overcome any remaining resistance due to hypoxia have included tourniquet hypoxia (to equalize oxygen concentration in normal tissue and tumour), hyperbaric oxygen or radiosensitizing chemicals (to reduce tumour resistance due to hypoxia), and neutrons (to reduce the differential in sensitivity between oxic and hypoxic cells). Some of these methods have given an improvement in cure rates, e.g. hyperbaric oxygen (Henk et al. 1977; Henk 1986) and misonidazole (Overgaard 1986). However, the lack of clear-cut improvement in many other studies suggests that hypoxic cells in tumours are not a general problem in tumour cure using multifractionated treatments.

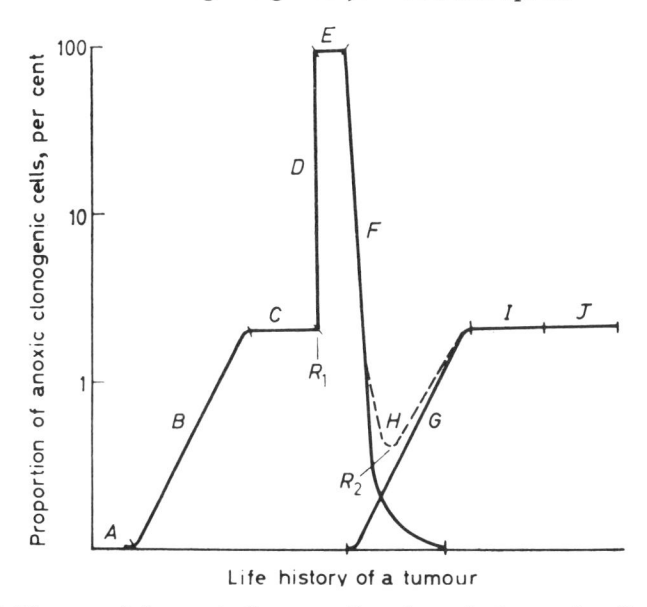

Figure 6.22. Diagram of changes in the proportion of anoxic clonogenic cells in a tumour (from Thomlinson 1967). A, when a tumour is very small there are likely to be no anoxic cells; in some tumours they probably never occur. B, if any anoxic cells are produced they appear as the tumour grows. C, the proportion becomes limited to a level characteristic of the type of neoplasm, dependent on its growth rate, degree of differentiation, and site. D, if a dose of radiation be given, $R_1$, the proportion of anoxic clonogenic cells amongst the survivors of radiation injury rises, perhaps to 100 per cent. E, the proportion remains high until cells divide after irradiation. F, when cells divide irradiation injury leads to cell death, cessation of metabolism, and relative increased availability of oxygen; the anoxic proportion therefore falls, at a rate dependent on the cell-cycle time of the tumour and the number of injured cells. G, surviving clonogenic cells regrow in the tumour at a rate dependent on the cell-cycle time in the postirradiation environment. H, the mean proportion of clonogenic cells reaches a minimum at a time dependent on the type of tumour and its growth rate; this time is optimal for a second dose, $R_1$. I, the characteristic level is restored. J, late irradiation ischaemia is not likely to alter the anoxic proportion greatly unless it were previously zero. (Reproduced with permission of Butterworths and the author.)

Of more significance for tumour curability by fractionated radiotherapy is the phenomenon of *regeneration*, and this is described in terms of the *cycle time* ($T_c$) of the clonogens and their self-renewal probability ($p$) (see Section 1.2). The self-renewal probability is 50% in rapidly turning-over normal tissues, and is likely only a little higher than this in some tumours (e.g. squamous cell carcinomas) prior to treatment. Acceleration of growth after the start of treatment may occur by means of a decrease in $T_c$ or an increase in $p$, but the latter is of far greater significance in increasing the tumour-curative dose. There is abundant clinical evidence of the adverse effect on tumour cure of increasing the treatment time (cf. Section 4.3), and this may possibly indicate an acceleration of growth.

## 6.9. Radiobiology of tissues and organs at long-term risk

The principles and some examples of the organization and acute response of renewing cell populations were described in the previous two sections. There are many other tissues in the body that are unresponsive to irradiation in the short term but which may express radiation injury after a very long latent period. These tissues include many of the organs, e.g. liver, kidney, and thyroid, and structural tissues, e.g. dermal and musculo-skeletal tissues. The proliferative organization of these tissues is considered very different from that of rapidly renewing tissues, which have a hierarchical-type organization (cf. Section 1.1 and Figure 1.1). Proliferation is extremely slow in the normal steady-state (homeostasis), and it is governed by the rate of loss of cells, which in turn is determined by the finite but long metabolic lifetime of functional cells. This contrasts with rapidly renewing tissues, where the lifetime can be determined, for example by the rate of abrasion of cells from the epidermis or GI tract. Although it is difficult to prove whether such slowly proliferating tissues contain a hierarchy of cells with differing proliferative potential, it is generally assumed that all cells of a given quiescent type have the ability to undergo division occasionally. Furthermore, there is evidence for some organs that most cells go into DNA synthesis and undergo a few divisions following resection or direct hormonal stimulation. This is seen following partial hepatectomy, unilateral nephrectomy, or goitrogen treatment of the thyroid, and such tissues are called *conditional renewal* or *flexible tissues*.

Flexible tissues respond to radiation in a characteristic way (Michalowski 1981). They are unresponsive to radiation within a few weeks after irradiation, because of their quiescent nature. The injury is expressed only when cells divide (except in the special cases of serous salivary parenchyma and certain lymphocytes which die in interphase, and minority cell populations in tumours and in normal tissues that die by apoptosis, cf. Section 1.2). Hence the depletion of the cell populations will occur at a very slow rate even after high doses, and this provides a long latent period before the injury is noticeably expressed. When the depletion has reached a level that impairs the function of the tissue, there may be a regenerative response in the remaining cells, which attempt to divide and thereby increase the number of functional cells. Increases in labelling index at long times after irradiation have been measured, for example, in the bladder, spinal cord, and lung (cf. Figure 1.3). It is possible that after high doses the rate of expression of the injury could accelerate and produce an avalanche effect leading to rapid tissue failure. Such an effect should give labelling indices up to around 50%, if all cells come into cycle, but as yet there have been no observations reported of such high values immediately prior to failure of any flexible tissues.

Another characteristic aspect of the response of these tissues is that the rate of decline of the cell population due to mitotic failure will be dose dependent because the proportion of cells affected is related exponentially to dose (cf. Section 6.4). This indicates that the time required to reach a given level of cell depletion, the *latency period*, depends on the dose. This is shown diagrammatically in Figure 1.6. Recovery mediated by repopulation is possible in some tissues, as demonstrated for conditional-renewal tissues (see above), and this will begin later after low doses (Figure 1.6).

Two important points to note concerning the response of these slowly proliferating tissues are as follows.

(*a*) Successful first and second divisions of cells after irradiation could play an important role in the overall response of the tissue. For example, one successful division of all cells would double the latency period. (This is not the case in hierarchical tissues, where one extra division would increase the latency period by only one cell lifetime in the series of many which determine the latency period). Although it is generally assumed that after doses higher than 6 Gy sterilized cells cannot undergo more than one division, there is no direct evidence concerning this ability after high doses *in vivo*.

(*b*) Because of the virtually quiescent nature of these cell populations, there is the possibility of continued PLDR before the cells divide. (In liver it has been shown that this continues for up to at least a year.) It is a dose-modifying effect, so that there is a greater change in effect after high doses. This effect would reduce the dependence of latency period on dose, and would increase the latency period after high doses.

Dose—response curves for these tissues can be expressed as the increase in response versus dose. Alternatively, the decrease (with increasing dose) in the proportion of samples where the injury has not reached a specified level, can be plotted as described above for acutely responding renewal tissues. An extra consideration in the case of late-responding tissues is that the injury is progressive over a long period of time, and hence the shape of the dose—response curve depends on the time at which the assessment is made. Also there are considerations of the interpretations of the steepness of the dose—incidence curve that are not yet resolved. These are as follows.

(*a*) Structural units of renewing tissues, e.g. intestinal crypts and testicular tubules, can be repopulated by single surviving stem cells. However, in such units constituting late-responding tissues, e.g. lung alveoli, it may be the case that several surviving cells are necessary to reconstitute the unit because of the limited division potential of the relevant cell types, or because different cell lineages may be required for different epithelia in the organ. This would have the effect of steepening the dose—incidence curve.

(b) With the bone marrow, the testis, and the gut, all rapidly renewing tissues and all responding rapidly to irradiation, mature cells are fed into a common pool or onto a common surface to provide the functional component of the tissue. Hence it is likely that the contribution of the respective progenitor cells to tissue rescue is independent of their position in the tissue. By contrast, in a linear tissue like the spinal cord, if a middle segment is inactivated survival of other segments will be ineffective in maintaining cord function, and paralysis will occur. This effect would steepen the dose—response curve, particularly for large field sizes where many such segments are irradiated. This effect may also apply to acute necrosis in large areas of skin and to late strictures in the (linear) intestine. The relative shapes of dose—response curves for early- and late-responding tissues is considered in Section 3.3.

(c) There are *tumour-related late complications*, resulting from too-rapid regression of the tumour or from associated destruction of the stroma. This is likely to depend at least in part on the stage of the primary tumour, so that, for example, radionecrosis of the mandible might develop more readily after the same dose given to a large than to a small tumour. First, a larger tumour is more likely to invade the mandible and tumour eradication in this case would result in necrosis. Second, there is a tendency to give higher doses to larger tumours. Other examples are rapid regression of large neck nodes in close proximity to the carotid artery and lymphomas of the bowel wall.

The *pathogenesis* of radiation injury expressed in early-responding tissues (bone marrow, gut, and skin) and in late-responding tissues (lung and spinal cord) is discussed in Section 1.3. *Residual injury* and *re-treatment* are described in Section 4.4.

## 6.10. Normal tissue tolerance: time, dose, and fractionation

### Single-dose versus fractionated treatments (cf. Section 5.1)

The first documented, successful use of radiotherapy was for the treatment of a hairy nevus by the dermatologist Leopold Freund in 1896, soon after the discovery of X rays by Conrad Röntgen in 1895. The output of these first X-ray tubes was very low and consequently the first radiotherapy treatments were highly fractionated, with one or two low-dose-rate treatments given each day until the desired effect had been achieved (loss of hair). Soon, however, the development of higher dose rates led to treatments in one or a few sittings. This change was motivated by comparison with radical surgery, as well as the fear that fractionated doses might cause tissue injury because of 'cumulation' of radiation damage. It was also felt that tumours might become resistant to radiation because of an immunological response. Soon after this change to single-dose, 'massive' treatments it was recognized that the effect of a dose depended on the time during which it was given, and the *time factor* was thus introduced into radiotherapy.

There developed at this time (1910−20) two different approaches to the treatment of cervical carcinoma using radium insertion, namely the Paris and Stockholm schools. At the Curie Institute in Paris Claude Regaud gradually extended the overall time over which radium treatments were given up to one week, whereas at the Radiumhemmet in Stockholm Gusta Förssell concentrated radium treatments in one or a few days. Now the massive single-dose technique (Erlangen School) for external-beam X-ray therapy had been unsuccessful in treating deep-seated tumours, and Henri Coutard, who began work at the Curie Institute in 1919, decided to adapt the Regaud technique to the treatment of larynx tumours. Thus, one or two low-dose-rate treatments were given each day, and treatment was protracted from one to two weeks or more. Doses were adjusted so that a brisk epithelial response accompanied treatment. The first successful treatment of these tumours resulted.

In Vienna, a similar change to fractionated treatments had begun to occur by 1920 (although Freund, despite considerable criticism, had persisted with fractionated treatments). Gottwald Schwarz had reported in 1914 that a mediastinal tumour had been unsuccessfully irradiated with the single-dose method responded much later to small doses given daily. He concluded that the fractionated treatments were better on grounds of higher radiosensitivity of mitotic cells, and a higher probability of irradiating these with fractionated doses. These results, published in 1914, were unknown outside Austria on account of the First World War. By the 1920s, however, the success of Coutard's technique became widely known, and groups in England, Austria, the United States and elsewhere began using fractionated doses. By the late 1930s the treatments were given at high dose rates at almost all centres, because of the conviction that low dose rates had no additional sparing effect in fractionated treatments.

**The NSD concept** (cf. Section 5.2)

These clinical developments led to heightened experimental activity aimed at quantifying the time factor in the 1930s. The principal biological endpoint was *skin erythema* in the experiments of Reisner, Quimby and MacComb, McWhirter, and others. The recovery evident with protracted treatment was conceptualized at that time by invoking the Schwarzschild law of photochemistry, which states that the effect of a given exposure of light is proportional to the product of intensity and time raised to a certain power $p$, where $p$ is less than 1. This led to the double-log plots of erythema dose versus number of treatments by Emil Witte, Felix Wachsmann, and subsequently Magnus Strandqvist in his monograph in 1944. Strandqvist, however, departed from previous practice in defining the abscissa in terms of *number of days after first treatment*, rather than *number of treatments*. Thus there was some uncertainty about the time to be assigned to a single dose, and Strandqvist chose the value $0 \cdot 35$ days. With this choice for the time for a single treatment, he found that both recurrences and necroses (not erythema) could be represented by the slope exponent $0 \cdot 22$ on the double-log plots (see Figure 5.6). Isoeffect doses for skin response were later compared with skin cancer data (doses that lay between recurrences and cures), but with a mixed time convention that assigned 1 day to a single treatment for normal skin and $0 \cdot 35$ day to a single treatment for recurrences. This confusion of the time assigned to a single treatment (and the relatively wide separation of $0 \cdot 35$ and 1 on a log scale) led to different slopes for tumours and normal tissues, and to the deduction that the difference between the Strandqvist exponent $0 \cdot 22$ for skin cancer and the value $0 \cdot 33$ for normal skin could explain the therapeutic gain from fractionated radiotherapy.

It is not generally recognized that the difference between these exponents is dubious, and arose from the use of different conventions for plotting single doses on a logarithmic time scale (which has no zero). This can be seen from the comparison set out in Figure 6.23, where the convention $T = 1$ day has been adopted for a single treatment ($a$) as opposed to $T = 0 \cdot 35$ day for a single treatment ($b$). When the same choice is made for both tumours and normal tissues, there is no difference between slopes.

Thus the time−dose formula, an edifice whose foundations rested on different time scales and few patients, grew to include the idea that normal tissue recovery differed from that of tumours. In all this work, the crucial assumption that varying the number of fractions for the same total dose and the same overall time did not appreciably affect the degree of reaction was rarely challenged. However, the experiments of Jack Fowler and colleagues with pig skin, and Jean Dutreix and colleagues with human skin, conclusively demonstrated the importance of number of fractions, in addition to overall time. This led Frank Ellis to interpret the difference between recovery exponents for normal tissues and tumours as the appropriate time coefficient, on the grounds that it was justifiable to assume that squamous cell carcinoma was not subject to homeostatic control. The time exponent deduced by Strandqvist was taken (after modification for 5 versus 7 treatments per

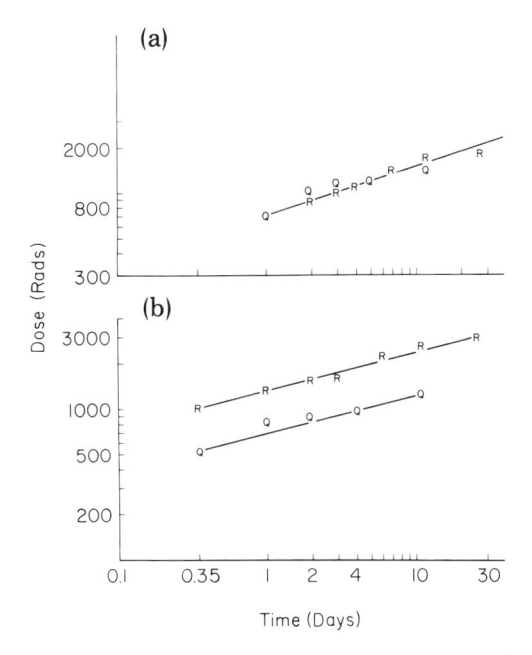

Figure 6.23. Effect of definition of the time for a single dose on the isoeffect exponent (from Withers & Peters 1980). The data plotted are those of Quimby & MacComb (1937) for 'threshold erythema' in 70-cm fields (Q), and of Reisner (1933) for strong erythema in 4-cm fields (R). In (b), the raw data are plotted as a function of the time *between* the first and the last doses, with the single dose points being plotted at $T = 0.35$ days, the convention used by Strandqvist. These isoeffect curves have an exponent of $0.22$. In (a) the data are plotted according to Cohen (1949b), who normalized the doses to a 10-cm diameter field, and defined $T$ (in days) as being numerically equal to the number of daily fractions, i.e. single doses are plotted at $T = 1$ day. This curve has an exponent of $0.33$. This marked difference is a consequence of the use of a logarithmic scale for time in which the interval between 0.1 day and 1 day is the same as that between 1 and 10 days or 10 and 100 days, etc. (Reproduced with permission of Lea & Febiger and the authors.)

week) as the number-of-fractions component of recovery. Thus followed the NSD concept:

$$D = \text{NSD} \times N^{0.24} T^{0.11}$$

where NSD stands for *nominal standard dose*.

This equation, and its variants (CRE or cumulative radiation effect, TDF or time dose factor) have remained in use, despite their foundation on sparse clinical data and mixed conventions for the times assigned to single doses, and despite documented cases of their failure to predict correct isoeffect doses for tumours (e.g. Byhardt et al. 1977) and normal tissues (e.g. Kim et al. 1975). This may be because in most clinical applications the changes in dosage are minor, and practically any mathematical formula predicting increased tolerance dose with increasing fractionation ($N$) and time ($T$) would be satisfactory over small ranges of $N$ and $T$. The documented failures for normal tissue tolerance have mostly involved changes to fewer, larger dose fractions, when the NSD equation led to overdosing of late-effects tissues because of its failure to account for variable fractionation sensitivity among tissues (Example 1 below and Section 3.3). The time factor is also dubious, since it implies that proliferative recovery is maximal in the first week or two of treatment and progressively decreases thereafter. This is in contradiction of the biology, since proliferation begins only after a time lag, becomes very rapid and then returns to equilibrium levels.

## The 4 R's of radiotherapy

Fundamentally different interpretations of the time factor in radiotherapy arose after the work of Puck and Marcus in describing the survival curve for retention of clonogenicity of cultured mammalian cells after their exposure to ionizing radiation. This development introduced a completely new way of thinking about radiation-isoeffect data, namely as a manifestation of killing of target cells characterized by specific survival curves. In 1959 Elkind and Sutton published the first split-dose recovery curves, indicating that the total dose required to reach a given survival level would be expected to increase with the number of treatments. This provided a biological explanation based on target-cell survival for the time factor, and led to experiments testing the relative influence of Elkind-type recovery and other factors, such as proliferation.

The factors that influence the response of cell populations to fractionated treatment were summarized by H. Rodney Withers as *the 4 R's of radiobiology*: (1) repair, (2) repopulation, (3) redistribution, and (4) reoxygenation. An updated version of these, in order of likely importance in fractionated radiotherapy, is as follows:

(1) *Repair*: Cells can absorb some radiation damage as sublethal damage, and it is only if large enough doses are given that this is converted into lethal damage. This sublethal damage is repairable if the cell is left for some hours before the rest of the dose is administered (Elkind & Sutton 1959). Therefore, survival curves show lower efficiency of killing at lower doses, before exponential cell killing is demonstrated at higher doses, and thus they are characterized by a *shoulder*. With sufficient recovery time between doses, this shoulder is re-established when the dose is fractionated, probably as a result of enzymatic intracellular repair during the interfraction intervals. This leads to increased isoeffect doses with increasing fraction number. The increase in isoeffect doses is steeper for the late responding tissues than for early responding tissues

and most tumours (Chapter 3), as quantified by a smaller ratio $\alpha/\beta$ in the late-responding tissues. Potentially lethal damage and its repair (PLDR) can modify the fractionation response, on the grounds that the shoulder of the survival curve may be interpreted on the basis of *repair models*. According to these, the response to radiation is initially single-hit, or exponential, with modification thereafter because of repair. The extent of PLDR, then, would determine the shape of the shoulder and consequently the fractionation sensitivity of the tissue. A *slow repair* process has been identified in mouse lung and in mouse capillaries. The time scale for this repair (about one week) is very much longer than that typical of Elkind-type repair (one to two hours). It has also been seen over a much longer time scale for repair of chromosomal injury and for cell survival in hepatocytes. Slow repair would constitute a small component of the increase in isoeffect dose with increasingly fractionated treatment.

(2) *Repopulation*: In normal tissues, radiation injury is followed in acutely responding tissues by a homeostatic response that results in compensatory proliferation to increase the rate of cell production. This may occur in three ways: from a shortening of the *cell-cycle time*, from an increase in the *growth fraction*, for example, by recruitment of resting stem cells into the division cycle, or by a lower rate of loss of cells along differentiation pathways, i.e. a decrease in the *cell loss factor*. In tumours the rate of production of cells exceeds the rate of loss, and the response to radiation injury may also involve any of these three. The onset of proliferation is fastest in the intestinal mucosa, occurring within a day or two of injury in the mouse, and it is slower in skin. In rodents the response occurs in skin after about 2 weeks, and in humans between 3 and 4 weeks. The mucosal response is somewhat faster, and reactions are seen after 10 to 14 days of daily treatment. The response of tumours is highly variable, and it is possible that these can show an accelerated proliferation after injury as is the case in normal tissues. Consequently a rest period during a course of fractionated radiotherapy is accompanied by efficient repopulation in tumours, which has been shown from clinical data (Parsons *et al*. 1980a,b).

(3) *Redistribution*: After a first dose of radiation, cells are partially synchronized because of two effects. First, *variable radiosensitivity* in different phases of the cell cycle, and second, blocks in the cell cycle, predominantly the pre-mitotic $G_2$ block. The timing of subsequent doses would be affected by the situation of the cell population after the first dose. However, these seem to redistribute themselves into the different phases of the cell cycle fairly rapidly, and attempts at therapy strategies based on synchronization have failed. Another aspect of redistribution was pointed out by H. R. Withers, namely that in rapidly cycling populations, progression of the partly synchronized population will

result in a reassortment of cells into more sensitive phases of the cycle (these having been depleted by the previous radiation dose). In slowly cycling populations the cells remain in their resistant state between doses. This effect could result in apparently higher resistance of the slowly dividing normal tissues relative to tumours, and to a therapeutic gain from fractionated radiation (see however Figure 6.11).

(4) *Reoxygenation*: Hypoxic cells in tumours arise because of imbalances between the rate of production of new cells and the vascularization of the tumour. The proportion of hypoxic cells is highly variable, and in animal tumours many of the values are in the range from 5 to 30%. Because of the relative resistance of hypoxic cells, more of these are likely to survive a dose of radiation. After large radiation doses (10 Gy or greater), hypoxic cells may comprise the vast majority of surviving tumour cells (see Figure 6.19) whereas after doses per fraction typical of clinical treatment (1 to 2 Gy) hypoxic cells will comprise a considerably smaller proportion of the surviving cells, because the protective effect of hypoxia is lower at these low doses. In any event, hypoxic cells may gain access to improved oxygen supply and nutrients and may thus become *reoxygenated* and thereby become more radiosensitive (see Figure 6.21). While this increases their net radiosensitivity, it also increases their potential for regeneration. However, clinical experiments with hyperbaric oxygen and in selected tumours with radiosensitizers (misonidazole) leave no doubt that hypoxia might play a role in limiting tumour cure.

## Dissociation between acute and late effects with altered fractionation

When conventional radiotherapy treatment schedules have been altered to fewer fractions with larger doses per fraction, the changes in dose were guided by the early effects of radiation that were manifest during treatment. When these were matched in the two schedules, however, an increase in late complications often ensued (cf. Tables 3.4 and 3.5). These examples of dissociation between acute and late effects with change in dose per fraction have been confirmed in numerous studies with experimental animals. They can be conceptualized in terms of the steepness of change in isoeffect dose, as shown in Figure 3.12. If proliferation is not a factor, isoeffect doses increase with decreasing fraction size (increasing fraction number) on account of repair, and this increase will occur faster, the curvier the survival curve of the underlying target cells (Thames et al. 1982), as illustrated in Figure 3.9.

## Non-standard fractionation in radiotherapy

The response of tumour clonogens is more likely to resemble those of target cells of acutely responding normal tissues. Therefore, in cases where late injury is dose limiting, a therapeutic gain would be expected from *hyperfractionation* (cf. Section 3.6), i.e. by a marked decrease in the size of dose per fraction and increase in the total dose. This is illustrated in Figure 3.20.

The opposite strategy, *hypofractionation*, would be called for in treatment situations where the tumour is known to have a large repair capacity, e.g. melanomas and liposarcomas. Here fewer, significantly larger dose fractions are used to exploit the higher fractionation sensitivity of these tumours *vis-à-vis* normal tissues, both early- and late-responding.

A third strategy is based not on repair but on regeneration characteristics of tumours, namely *accelerated fractionation* (cf. Section 4.3). The rationale is based on the idea that rapid tumour clonogen regeneration might offset the cell kill achieved by treatment, and that this effect would be minimized by reducing the overall treatment time.

In practice, pure accelerated and hyperfractionation are not possible. This results from the fact that meaningful acceleration of treatment, or reduction in size of dose per fraction with increase in total dose, require treatment two or three times daily. For this reason, with accelerated fractionation, acute tolerance usually requires a reduction in fraction size and with hyperfractionation the tolerance dose may be reached in a somewhat shorter overall time.

## Practical use of isoeffect relationships

The difficulties with variable fractionation sensitivity among normal tissues can be circumvented by use of the linear–quadratic (LQ) model, with different $\alpha/\beta$ values for the different tissues. The NSD and the LQ approaches are best illustrated side-by-side, in their application to practical treatment problems such as those set out in the book by Hall (1978). First, however, we outline the main features of each approach.

### Use of the NSD concept

The principal application of the NSD equation is in calculating dosages for treatment regimens that will be biologically equivalent. These calculations are greatly simplified by the use of TDF (time–dose factor) tables (Orton & Ellis 1973), for two reasons. First, NSD values apply to full normal-tissue tolerance, and values calculated for different parts of a treatment cannot be added. Second, NSD values for tissue tolerance are variable among radiotherapy departments. Use of the TDF tables circumvents these difficulties since (*a*) they are additive, and (*b*) they do not depend on any particular NSD values.

Convenient TDF tables may be found in Hall's (1978) book, from which the following illustration of their use is drawn.

**Example 1** (Hall, 1978, p. 287): In a centre where a protocol consisting of 30 doses of 2 Gy, given 5 times weekly, is considered to represent normal tissue tolerance, design of a comparable course of therapy is required, but based on 3 fractions/week and a daily dose of 3 Gy. How many fractions are needed?

*Solution (using TDF tables):* We use Table 14-5 (Hall 1978) for 5 fractions/week. On the line corresponding to 2 Gy, in the column for 30 fractions, the TDF factor is 99. Any treatment pattern, in any of the Tables 14-1 through 14-5, which results in a TDF of 99 will be equivalent as judged by the NSD concept. To solve this specific problem, we use Table 14-3, which corresponds to 3 fractions/week; for 3 Gy/fraction, between 16 and 18 fractions are needed. Since a whole number of fractions must be used, it is necessary to interpolate in the dose column to obtain an exact solution; 18 fractions of 2·94 Gy will result in a TDF of 99.

*Use of the LQ model: fractionation−dosage factor (FDF) method*
The FDF formulation set out below is equivalent to that of Barendsen (1982), but is perhaps intuitively clearer in its application. The biological effect of a fractionated course of radiotherapy may be quantified in terms of two factors. The first is the *fractionation factor*, obtained by adding the $\alpha/\beta$ ratio for the tissue of interest to the size of dose per fraction, $d$:

$$\text{fractionation factor} = \alpha/\beta + d$$

which is similar to the relative effect (RE) in Barendsen's treatment. The second is the *dosage factor*, which is the total dose given in $N$ fractions of size $d$:

$$\text{dosage factor} = D = N \times d$$

Then the total effect (TE) of a dose $D$ given in $N$ fractions of size $d$ to a tissue whose fractionation sensitivity is characterized by $\alpha/\beta$ (derived by simple algebraic manipulation of equation (7.12)) is

$$\begin{aligned}\text{TE} &= (\alpha/\beta + d) \times D \\ &= \text{fractionation factor} \times \text{dosage factor}\end{aligned}$$

The thinking behind the FDF method may be paraphrased nonmathematically as follows. The injury received from a blow to the head depends on two factors: the hardness of the object hitting the head and the force with which the blow is applied. The former is analogous to the fractionation factor, and the latter to the dosage factor. A hammer will usually inflict more injury than a sofa cushion (fractionation effect), unless the hammer is lightly touched to the head and the sofa cushion is whipped against it with great force (dosage effect).

When the treatment schedule involves a change of fraction size, say from $d_1$ to $d_2$, the partial effect (PE) of each part of the treatment may be added to get the total effect (TE):

$$\begin{aligned} \text{TE} &= \text{PE}_1 + \text{PE}_2 \\ &= (\alpha/\beta + d_1)D_1 + (\alpha/\beta + d_2)D_2 \\ &= (\text{fractionation factor 1} \times \text{dosage factor 1}) \\ &\quad + (\text{fractionation factor 2} \times \text{dosage factor 2}). \end{aligned}$$

Any number of PEs may be added.

The FDF method can be considered to apply to late-responding normal tissues, where the effect of time may be neglected. For tumours and acutely responding tissues, however, special adjustments must be made unless the times in the two schedules under comparison are equal and time may be ignored (neglecting any dependency of proliferation on fraction size). In any event, a *partial effect due to regeneration during time T*, PE(T), would be added to those due to cell killing to get the total effect. PE(T) is positive or negative, respectively, as treatment time is lengthened or shortened.

To illustrate the application of the FDF method in comparison with the NSD method, we next rework Example 1 above and then proceed to a comparison of the methods using other examples.

*Solution to Example 1 (FDF method)*: A difference between the approaches is immediately apparent, since we must choose an $\alpha/\beta$ ratio to calculate the fractionation factor. Unfortunately these are not known for humans, and we must resort to the results of animal experimentation (Table 3.1), mindful of the comparisons between human and animal results presented in Section 3.5 (Table 3.7). This uncertainty, it is hoped, will have the salutary effect of convincing the user of the method to proceed with caution.

Suppose first that acute mucosal reactions are dose limiting, and that the overall times are the same in the 3- and 5-fractions/week schedules. From Table 3.1 the appropriate $\alpha/\beta$ is about 8 Gy, so that the TE for $30 \times 2$ Gy in $T$ days is

$$\begin{aligned} \text{TE} &= (8 + 2) \times 60 + \text{PE}(T) \\ &= 600 + \text{PE}(T) \end{aligned}$$

228  *Fractionation in Radiotherapy*

For the unknown number of fractions, $N$, then, we have

$$TE(30 \times 2\,Gy) = TE(N \times 3\,Gy)$$
$$600 + PE(T) = (8 + 3) \times N \times 3 + PE(T)$$

The PE($T$) cancels out so

$$600 = 33N$$
$$N = 18 \cdot 2$$

Rounding down to 18 fractions, we obtain the same answer as obtained by the NSD method, namely that $18 \times 3\,Gy$ in $T$ weeks is equivalent to $30 \times 2\,Gy$ in $T$ weeks (for acute mucosal tolerance).

This answer is not overly sensitive to the value of $\alpha/\beta$ chosen for mucosa. The results for other choices: $\alpha/\beta = 6\,Gy$ ($N = 17 \cdot 8$), $10\,Gy$ ($N = 18 \cdot 5$), $12\,Gy$ ($N = 18 \cdot 7$).

Suppose instead that *late-skin reactions* were dose limiting in a postoperative breast treatment of $30 \times 2\,Gy$. Here the $\alpha/\beta$ value is unknown, so we do the calculations for several choices. Proliferation will have no effect. First choose $\alpha/\beta = 3\,Gy$:

$$TE(30 \times 2\,Gy) = TE(N \times 3\,Gy)$$
$$(3 + 2) \times 60 = (3 + 3) \times N \times 3$$
$$300 = 18N$$
$$N = 16 \cdot 7$$

which (to be conservative) rounds down to 16. The results for other choices of $\alpha/\beta$ : $\alpha/\beta = 2\,Gy$ ($N = 16 \cdot 0$), $4\,Gy$ ($N = 17 \cdot 1$). We conclude that conservative management would dictate giving $16 \times 3\,Gy$, not $18 \times 3\,Gy$. This is corroborated by clinical experience (Montague 1968) as shown in Table 3.5.

**Example 2** (Hall 1978): It had been planned to give a course of 30 fractions of $2 \cdot 1\,Gy$ 5 times/week. After 12 fractions, it is decided to change to a dose of $2 \cdot 5\,Gy$ and treat only 3 times/week. How many more doses must be given?

*Solution (NSD method)*: The original planned course represents a TDF of 107; this is found in Table 14-5 (Hall 1978), in the column for 30 fractions, and on the line for $2 \cdot 1\,Gy$/fraction. The first 12 doses result in a TDF of 43, again found in Table 14-5, in the column for 12 fractions and on the line for $2 \cdot 1\,Gy$/fraction. The extra TDF required is $107 - 43$, i.e. 64. To achieve this at the rate of 3 fractions/week, Hall's Table 14-3 on the line for $2 \cdot 5\,Gy$/day shows that 15 fractions are required.

*Solution (FDF method):* If the dose is limited by the oral mucosa, the $\alpha/\beta$ is approximately 8 Gy. Therefore the total effect of $30 \times 2 \cdot 1$ Gy is TE $= (8 + 2 \cdot 1) \times 63 = 636 \cdot 3$. This is to be equated to two consecutive treatments, first with $12 \times 2 \cdot 1$ Gy and afterward with $N \times 2 \cdot 5$ Gy. The times are different in the two regimens (6 weeks versus 7·5 weeks), so:

$$636 \cdot 3 + \text{PE(6 weeks)} = (8 + 2 \cdot 1) \times 25 \cdot 2 + (8 + 2 \cdot 5) \times N \times 2 \cdot 5 + \text{PE(7·5 weeks)}$$
$$= 254 \cdot 52 + 26 \cdot 25N + \text{PE(7·5 weeks)}$$

The equations for adjustments in the fractionation without the effects of proliferation now read

$$636 \cdot 3 = 254 \cdot 52 + 26 \cdot 25N$$

which gives $N = 14 \cdot 54$, close to $N = 15$ obtained by the NSD method. Higher (or lower) values of $N$ result if $\alpha/\beta$ is a little bigger (or smaller) than 8 Gy. We next must compensate for the difference in the time: PE(7·5 weeks) − PE(6 weeks) = PE (1·5 weeks), i.e. we must compensate for an extra 1½ weeks' proliferation, and for this a dose equivalent of proliferation must be added in terms of extra treatments. For example, at 60 cGy/day about 6 Gy worth of proliferation must be accounted for, i.e. two extra treatments must be given. There are, unfortunately, no hard data for the dose equivalent of proliferation (cf. Section 4.2), as this varies between acutely responding tissues and tumours and may depend on time after start of treatment.

If treatment is limited by necrosis and edema of the laryngeal cartilage, no values of $\alpha/\beta$ are known but again we assume one in the range typical of late responses, i.e. 1−4 Gy. For $\alpha/\beta = 3$ Gy, for example, we calculate TE $= (3 + 2 \cdot 1) \times 63 = 321 \cdot 3$, so

$$321 \cdot 3 = (3 + 2 \cdot 1) \times 25 \cdot 2 + (3 + 2 \cdot 5) \times N \times 2 \cdot 5$$
$$= 128 \cdot 52 + 13 \cdot 75 \times N$$

which gives $N = 14 \cdot 0$, one treatment less than predicted by the NSD method. No special consideration is necessary for proliferation with late responses. Again, this result is corroborated by clinical experience (cf. Table 3.4).

**Example 3** (Hall 1978): A standard plan considered to result in normal tissue tolerance consists of 16 doses of 1·9 Gy, given as 5 fractions/week, followed by 10 doses of 2·8 Gy given as 3 fractions/week. What regimen would produce an equivalent effect given at the rate of 2 fractions/week throughout?

*Solution (NSD method)*: Referring to Hall's Table 14-5, 16 doses of 1·9 Gy results in a TDF of 49; referring to his Table 14-3, 10 doses of 2·8 Gy results in a TDF of 51. TDF factors are proportional to partial tolerances and are therefore additive. The total TDF is 49 + 51, i.e. 100.

For an equivalent treatment given at the rate of 2 fractions/week, any combination of number of fractions and dose/fraction may be chosen from his table 14-2, which results in TDF of 100; for example, 12 fractions of 4 Gy, or 17 fractions of 3·2 Gy.

*Solution (FDF method)*: For a tissue characterized by $\alpha/\beta = 10$ Gy, the total effect of the standard plan is TE = PE(7 weeks) + (10 + 1·9) × 30·4 + (10 + 2·8) × 28 = PE(7 weeks) + 720·16. In order that the times match, we would have to give 14 fractions in 7 weeks, 2 fractions/week. Therefore, it remains to determine the dose per fraction, $d$:

$$720 \cdot 16 = (10 + d) \times 14 \times d$$
$$= 140d + 14d^2$$

i.e. $14d^2 + 140d - 720.16 = 0$

This is a quadratic equation in the unknown dose per fraction, $d$. It will be recalled from algebra that these equations are of the form

$$ad^2 + bd + c = 0$$

and have the solutions

$$d = \frac{-b \pm \sqrt{b^2 - 4ac}}{2a}$$

One of these will be negative, and this will be rejected in favour of the positive solution

$$d = \frac{-b + \sqrt{b^2 - 4ac}}{2a}$$

The positive solution of the present quadratic is $d = 3 \cdot 74$ Gy. We conclude that $14 \times 3 \cdot 74$ Gy given twice weekly for 7 weeks would be equivalent, for an acute response characterized by $\alpha/\beta = 10$ Gy, to the standard plan.

**Example 4** (Hall 1978): As an experimental treatment for carcinomas of the bladder, it is proposed to give 10 doses of 2·7 Gy (5 fractions/week) followed by a 3-week rest period, before a further 10 doses of 2·7 Gy.

What daily dose given in 30 fractions would be expected to produce the same effect?

*Solution (NSD method)*: Ten doses of 2·7 Gy, 5 fractions/week, is seen from Hall's Table 14-5 to produce a TDF of 52.

By the time the second half of the treatment is started, the TDF of the first part of the protocol will have decayed with time. From Hall's Table 14-6, the decay factor is 0·89, corresponding to 11 days of treatment followed by 21 days of rest. The total TDF is therefore 52 × 0·89 + 52, i.e. 98.

The daily dose, given in 30 fractions (5 times/week), which results in this same TDF of 98, may be looked up directly in Hall's Table 14-5; the result is 1·99 Gy. A TDF of 99 would result from daily fractions of 2 Gy, while a TDF of 91 would result from 1·9 Gy daily; the 1·99 is obtained by interpolation between these figures.

*Solution (FDF method)*: Since the degree of stimulated proliferation during a rest period is likely to be widely variable among tissues, we do not feel that anything more than a guess can be made at its dose-equivalent. Calculations would proceed as above to find a schedule equivalent in cell killing, and then a more-or-less arbitrary dose would be subtracted to account for the missing rest period.

**Example 5**: In order to increase the size of individual doses used in conjunction with misonidazole, a radiotherapy centre replaced 5 times weekly treatment with 6 fractions/18 days. As a result, the dose to the spinal cord changed from 20 × 2·5 Gy/4 weeks to 6 × 5·8 Gy/18 days (Dische *et al.* 1981). Would these regimens be expected to be isoeffective for cord injury?

*Solution (NSD method)*: From the TDF Tables for 5 treatment days/week, TDF = 93, while for treatment twice weekly TDF = 88, so a lower incidence of myelopathy would be expected from the twice weekly treatments.

*Solution (FDF method)*: For this 5 times/week schedule, assuming $\alpha/\beta = 3$ Gy for the cord, TE = $(3 + 2·4) \times 48 = 259·2$. Proliferation can be neglected, and so the appropriate number $N$ of treatments in 5·8 Gy fractions is calculated from

$$259·2 = (3 + 5·8) \times N \times 5·8$$
$$= 51·04N$$

i.e. $N = 5·1$; in fractions of size 5·6 Gy, $N = 5·2$. Thus the FDF method indicates 5 (conservatively) doses of 5·8 Gy or 5 doses of 5·6 Gy. The FDF prediction for the fractional dose to be given in 6 treatments would

be calculated as:
$$259 \cdot 2 = (3+d) \times 6 \times d$$
$$= 18d + 6d^2,$$

a quadratic whose positive root is $d = 5 \cdot 2$ Gy. All of these indicate much more conservative treatment than prescribed by the NSD method.

The treatment with $6 \times 5 \cdot 8$ Gy resulted in 8 cases of radiation myelitis out of 70 treated (Dische et al. 1981), as opposed to 1 out of 22 with $2 \cdot 5$ Gy fractions. This patient received treatment equivalent to a TDF of $90 \cdot 9$, lower than the average.

**Example 6** (hyperfractionation with twice-a-day treatments separated by 4 or 8 hours): In a clinical trial of hyperfractionation by the EORTC, head-and-neck cancers were treated with 70 fractions of $1 \cdot 15$ Gy, two times/day, in 7 weeks (Horiot et al. 1985). Suppose that the repair half-time of the dose-limiting late-responding tissue is $1 \cdot 5$ hours. To what conventional (one treatment per day) schedule using 2 Gy fractions is this regimen equivalent for late effects, if $\alpha/\beta = 3$ Gy, for 4-h intervals? For 8-h intervals?

*Solution (FDF method)*: When there is a possibility of incomplete repair, the fractionation factor is changed from $\alpha/\beta + d$ to

$$\text{fractionation factor} = \alpha/\beta + d + d \times h_\text{M} \quad (6.5)$$
$$= \alpha/\beta + d(1 + h_\text{M}).$$

The *incomplete-repair factors* ($h_\text{M}$) are tabulated in Table 6.3 for different numbers of treatments per day ($M$), repair halftimes, and interfraction intervals. When the incomplete-repair factors are larger, repair is less complete, and so the fractionation factors increase. This will require a reduction in the dosage factor, i.e. in the total dose, to give the same total effect.

In the present case for 4-h intervals $h_\text{M} = 0 \cdot 1575$, so the total effect would be

$$\text{TE} = (\alpha/\beta + d + d \times h_\text{M}) \times D$$
$$= (3 + 1 \cdot 15 + 1 \cdot 15 \times 0 \cdot 1575) \times 80 \cdot 5$$
$$= 348 \cdot 65$$

This would be equivalent to $N \times 2$ Gy given conventionally, where N is determined from

$$348 \cdot 675 = (\alpha/\beta + 2) \times N \times 2$$
$$= 10N$$
$$N = 35 \text{ fractions.}$$

Table 6.3. Incomplete-repair factors $h_M$ for MFD treatment with $M$ treatments/day

| Repair halftime (h) | Interval (h) | | | | |
|---|---|---|---|---|---|
| | 3 | 4 | 5 | 6 | 8 |
| 0·5  | 0·0156 | 0·0039 | 0·0010 | 0·0002 | — |
|      | 0·0210 | 0·0052 | 0·0013 | 0·0003 | — |
| 0·75 | 0·0625 | 0·0248 | 0·0098 | 0·0039 | 0·0006 |
|      | 0·0859 | 0·0335 | 0·0132 | 0·0052 | 0·0008 |
| 1·0  | 0·1250 | 0·0625 | 0·0312 | 0·0156 | 0·0039 |
|      | 0·1771 | 0·0859 | 0·0423 | 0·0210 | 0·0052 |
| 1·25 | 0·1895 | 0·1088 | 0·0625 | 0·0359 | 0·0118 |
|      | 0·2766 | 0·1530 | 0·0859 | 0·0487 | 0·0159 |
| 1·5  | 0·2500 | 0·1575 | 0·0992 | 0·0625 | 0·0248 |
|      | 0·3750 | 0·2265 | 0·1388 | 0·0859 | 0·0335 |
| 2·0  | 0·3536 | 0·2500 | 0·1768 | 0·1250 | 0·0625 |
|      | 0·5547 | 0·3750 | 0·2565 | 0·1771 | 0·0859 |
| 2·5  | 0·4353 | 0·3299 | 0·2500 | 0·1895 | 0·1088 |
|      | 0·7067 | 0·5124 | 0·3750 | 0·2766 | 0·1530 |
| 3·0  | 0·5000 | 0·3969 | 0·3150 | 0·2500 | 0·1575 |
|      | 0·8333 | 0·6341 | 0·4861 | 0·3750 | 0·2265 |
| 4·0  | 0·5946 | 0·5000 | 0·4204 | 0·3536 | 0·2500 |
|      | 1·0285 | 0·8333 | 0·6784 | 0·5547 | 0·3750 |

$M$ = number of treatments/day
Upper ($M = 2$); Lower ($M = 3$)

Details on the form of the incomplete-repair factors can be found in the Appendix (Section 7.2).

With 8-h intervals $h_M = 0·0248$ so

$$\text{TE} = (3 + 1·15 + 1·15 \times 0·0248) \times 80·5$$
$$= 336·37$$

and this would be equivalent to less than 34 fractions of 2 Gy. Therefore the extra 4 hours would be equivalent to more than 2 Gy total spared dose. Since 35 × 2 Gy is expected to be close to tolerance, this spared dose could be important.

**Example 7** (combination of external beam and interstitial therapy): A total dose of 60 Gy in 1 week is planned for interstitial radium treatment of tongue cancer. After 3 days severe edema causes cessation of treatment by brachytherapy. The decision is made to complete treatment with external beam (2 Gy per fraction, 5 times/week) to achieve equivalence with a treatment of 30 × 2 Gy given conventionally 5 times/week. It is estimated that an average of 30 Gy has been delivered by the implant. How many 2 Gy treatments are required?

*Solution*: For continuous exposures the fractionation factor is changed

**Table 6.4. Continuous repair factors**

| Repair halftime (h) | Exposure time (h) | | | | | | Exposure time (days) | | | | | | |
|---|---|---|---|---|---|---|---|---|---|---|---|---|---|
| | 1 | 2 | 3 | 4 | 8 | 12 h | 1 | 1·5 | 2 | 2·5 | 3 | 3·5 | 4 |
| 0·5 | 0·6622 | 0·4774 | 0·3671 | 0·2959 | 0·1641 | 0·1130 | 0·0583 | 0·0393 | 0·0296 | 0·0238 | 0·0198 | 0·0170 | 0·0149 |
| 0·75 | 0·7517 | 0·5888 | 0·4774 | 0·3983 | 0·2339 | 0·1641 | 0·0861 | 0·0583 | 0·0441 | 0·0354 | 0·0296 | 0·0254 | 0·0223 |
| 1 | 0·8040 | 0·6622 | 0·5571 | 0·4774 | 0·2959 | 0·2115 | 0·1130 | 0·0769 | 0·0583 | 0·0469 | 0·0393 | 0·0338 | 0·0296 |
| 1·25 | 0·8382 | 0·7137 | 0·6165 | 0·5394 | 0·3504 | 0·2555 | 0·1390 | 0·0952 | 0·0723 | 0·0583 | 0·0488 | 0·0420 | 0·0369 |
| 1·5 | 0·8622 | 0·7517 | 0·6622 | 0·5888 | 0·3983 | 0·2959 | 0·1641 | 0·1130 | 0·0861 | 0·0695 | 0·0583 | 0·0502 | 0·0441 |
| 2 | 0·8938 | 0·8040 | 0·7276 | 0·6622 | 0·4774 | 0·3671 | 0·2115 | 0·1475 | 0·1130 | 0·0916 | 0·0769 | 0·0663 | 0·0583 |
| 2·5 | 0·9136 | 0·8382 | 0·7720 | 0·7137 | 0·5394 | 0·4269 | 0·2555 | 0·1803 | 0·1390 | 0·1130 | 0·0952 | 0·0822 | 0·0723 |
| 3 | 0·9272 | 0·8622 | 0·8040 | 0·7517 | 0·5888 | 0·4774 | 0·2959 | 0·2115 | 0·1641 | 0·1339 | 0·1130 | 0·0977 | 0·0861 |
| 4 | 0·9447 | 0·8938 | 0·8471 | 0·8040 | 0·6622 | 0·5571 | 0·3671 | 0·2693 | 0·2115 | 0·1739 | 0·1475 | 0·1280 | 0·1130 |

Details on the calculations of $g$ can be found in the Appendix (Section 7.3).

to

$$\text{fractionation factor} = \alpha/\beta + d \times g$$

where the *continuous repair factors* $g$ are set out in Table 6.4 for different exposure times and tissue-repair halftimes.

The partial effect for the continuous treatment is then

$$PE = (\alpha/\beta + d \times g) \times D \qquad (6.6)$$

where $D$ is the total dose given in $N = D/d$ continuous exposures, separated by times long compared with the repair halftime $T_{1/2}$. In the present case $N = 1$, so the total effect for $\alpha/\beta = 3$ Gy and $T_{1/2} = 1 \cdot 5$ h (typical late-effects values) and exposure time 72 h is

$$TE = (3 + 30 \times 0.0583) \times 30 + (3 + 2) \times N \times 2$$
$$= 142 \cdot 5 + 10 \times N$$

Since the desired total effect is $(3 + 2) \times 60 = 300$, we have

$$300 = 142 \cdot 5 + 10N, \text{ i.e.}$$

$$N = 15 \cdot 8 \text{ fractions.}$$

For acute mucositis we take $\alpha/\beta = 8$ Gy and $T_{1/2} = 0 \cdot 8$ h (cf. Tables 3.1 and 3.6). Then

$$TE = (8 + 2) \times 60$$
$$600 = (8 + 30 \times 0 \cdot 0316) \times 30 + (8 + 2) \times N \times 2$$
$$= 268 \cdot 4 + 20N$$
$$\text{i.e. } N = 16 \cdot 6 \text{ fractions.}$$

**Example 8** (palliation): A radiotherapy centre treats bladder carcinoma radically with 55 Gy/16 fractions/22 days. What dose should be used to treat with 8 fractions in 10 days, bearing in mind that the latter is to be used in a palliative situation? Further, what would be the dose using 4 fractions in 4 days?

*Solution*: From Table 3.1, the $\alpha/\beta$ value for late bladder damage is about 5 Gy. Therefore the total effect of the radical treatment is $TE = (5 + 3 \cdot 44) \times 55 = 464 \cdot 2$. For 8 fractions of dose per fraction $d$,

$$464 \cdot 2 = (5 + d) \times 8 \times d$$
$$= 40d + 8d^2$$
$$8d^2 + 40d - 464 \cdot 2 = 0$$

and the positive solution of this quadratic is $d = 5\cdot52$ Gy per fraction. Therefore the tolerance dose in 8-fractions should be $44\cdot2$ Gy/8 fractions/10 days. The palliation treatment used at Manchester is 35 Gy/8 fractions/10 days (Pointon 1985), which is seen to be about 9 Gy or 20% below tolerance. For treatment in 4 fractions,

$$464\cdot2 = (5 + d) \times 4 \times d$$
$$= 20d + 4d^2$$
$$4d^2 + 20d - 464\cdot2 = 0$$

and the positive solution is $d = 8\cdot56$ Gy per fraction. A 4-fraction treatment to full tolerance would be $34\cdot2$ Gy/4 fractions/4 days, and in palliative situations the dose would be reduced as above.

**Example 9** (total body irradiation with fractionated or fractionated-low-dose-rate radiation): A centre uses $6 \times 2$ Gy (10 cGy/min) in 3 days total-body irradiation prior to bone-marrow transplantation. The lung is considered the dose-limiting tissue. It is thought possible that a therapeutic gain might result by using low-dose-rate irradiation at each sitting. How much could the dose be boosted for equivalent lung damage by lowering the dose rate to 3 cGy/min?

*Solution*: The 10-cGy/min treatments each last 20 min = 1/3 h and by interpolation in Table 6.4 the appropriate $g$-factor is $0\cdot90$. We use $\alpha/\beta$ (lung) = $3\cdot2$ Gy from Table 3.1 and $T_{1/2}$ (lung) = $0\cdot72$ h from Table 3.6. From equation (6.6), therefore, the total effect of the 10-cGy/min fractionated treatments is

$$TE = (3\cdot2 + 2 \times 0\cdot90) \times 12$$
$$= 60$$

The 3-cGy/min treatments will each last $1\cdot11$ h, so by interpolation in Table 6.2 we find that $g = 0\cdot72$, and therefore for the unknown dose per fraction $d$ we have

$$60 = (3\cdot2 + 0\cdot72d) \times 6 \times d$$
$$= 19\cdot2d + 4\cdot32d^2$$
$$4\cdot32d^2 + 19\cdot2d - 60 = 0$$

and the positive root of the quadratic is $d = 2\cdot12$ Gy/fraction. Therefore the total dose can be increased from $12\cdot0$ Gy to $12\cdot7$ Gy without further injury to the lung by increasing the exposure time per treatment from 20 minutes to 1 hour.

**Example 10** (accelerated fractionation with three treatments per day separated by 4 or 6 hours): In a clinical trial of accelerated fractionation for head-and-neck tumours a cooperative group plans to give $3 \times 1\cdot 6$ Gy daily for 2 weeks (10 days), followed by a rest period to allow recuperation of the mucosa. This is to be followed by resumption of $3 \times 1\cdot 6$ Gy per day. How many additional $1\cdot 6$-Gy fractions may be given to yield late effects equivalent to those resulting from the comparison arm in the trial, $35 \times 2$ Gy/7 weeks, if 4-hour intervals are used? 6-hour intervals? Assume that for late effects $\alpha/\beta = 3$ Gy and the halftime for repair is $1\cdot 5$ h.

*Solution*: For the comparison arm TE $= (3 + 2) \times 70 = 350$. From Table 6.3 the incomplete repair factors are $0\cdot 2265$ for 4-h and $0\cdot 0859$ for 6-h fractionation intervals, assuming a repair time of $1\cdot 5$ h. The effect of proliferation can be neglected, so if $N$ is the number of $1\cdot 6$-Gy fractions given in the second course of therapy we have for 4-h intervals:

$$350 = (3 + 1\cdot 6 \times 0\cdot 2265) \times 48 + (3 + 1\cdot 6 \times 0\cdot 2265) \times N \times 1\cdot 6$$
$$= 161\cdot 4 + 5\cdot 38 \times N$$
$$N = 35 \text{ fractions}$$

and for 6-h intervals:

$$350 = (3 + 1\cdot 6 \times 0\cdot 0859) \times 48 + (3 + 1\cdot 6 \times 0\cdot 0859) \times N \times 1\cdot 6$$
$$= 150\cdot 6 + 5\cdot 02\, N$$
$$N = 39\cdot 7 \text{ fractions}$$

Therefore an extra $8$ Gy $= 5 \times 1\cdot 6$ Gy dose-equivalent of sparing would accrue from the use of 6-h as opposed to 4-h intervals.

## 6.11. The biological hazards of irradiation

**Whole-body syndromes**

There are three classical syndromes following whole-body exposure—the neurological, gastrointestinal, and bone marrow syndromes (Bond *et al.* 1965). These occur over different ranges of dose, and after different latency periods (cf. Section 1.3). The syndromes can lead to death, and the characteristic shape of the curve of latency period to death versus dose is shown for several animal species in Figure 6.24. The curve shape and approximate position is expected to be similar in man, but its exact position is unknown. Before discussing each of these syndromes, the prodromal phase will be considered.

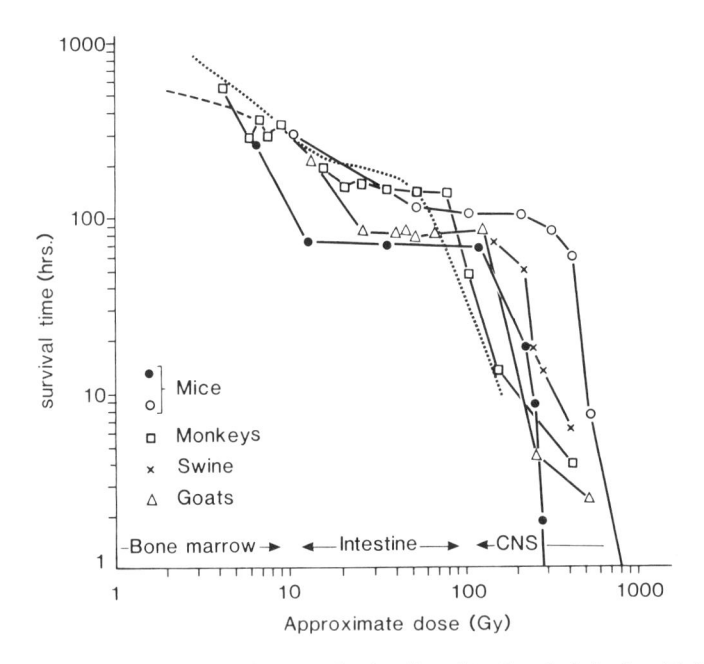

Figure 6.24. Survival times of various species irradiated to the whole body with increasing dose. The arrows denote the tissues primarily responsible for death. Redrawn from Bond et al. (1965).

The prodromal phase comprises the initial symptoms appearing in the first 48 hours following irradiation. The reaction is mediated through the response of the autonomic nervous system, and is expressed as gastrointestinal and neuromuscular symptoms such as nausea, vomiting, fatigue, apathy. The neural control mechanism for emesis is in the medulla oblongata in the brain, and irradiation of the head alone to high doses, or the abdomen alone to low doses, will produce the symptoms. The latency period is dose-dependent, and after high doses, all symptoms appear within 15 minutes. In man, acute doses to the abdomen to give the symptoms in 50% of radiotherapy patients following whole-body irradiations have been estimated to be approximately $0 \cdot 6$ Gy (anorexia), $1 \cdot 2$ Gy (nausea), and $1 \cdot 8$ Gy (vomiting). Low dose rates and fractionated doses are less effective in inducing prodromal responses, but quantitative relationships have not yet been established.

The neurological syndrome occurs after doses higher than about 100 Gy in most species, and the latent period is dose-dependent. The severe symptoms and signs of the prodromal phase lead directly into the neurological syndrome, characterized by transient periods of depressed or enhanced motor activity, resulting in total incapacitation and death.

This can occur in a few hours after very high doses of 1000 Gy. There is no known curative treatment for this syndrome.

The gastrointestinal syndrome occurs after doses between about 10 and 50 Gy in most species. The mean time to death is *independent* of dose, as expected for the response to high doses of a hierarchical tissue (cf. Section 1.3 and Figure 1.5), and it is 3·5 to 9 days depending on the species. The symptoms and signs follow those of the prodromal phase, and include diarrhoea, decreased intestinal absorption, and weight loss. The syndrome occurs as a result of denudation of the intestinal mucosa following sterilization of the clonogenic cells. Hence the latter are the target-cells for this syndrome. The effects of the lack of a fully functional mucosa are aggravated by a lack of leukocytes, and by haemorrhages and bacteraemia. The latent period is dependent on the turnover time of the epithelium and on the bacterial content of the gut. The incidence of death can be reduced by transfusion of balanced salt solutions and antibiotics.

Effects in the intestine are reduced by fractionation and by exposures at low dose rates, and there is a good correspondence between the sparing of the clonogenic cells and of the incidence of gastrointestinal failure (cf. Figure 2.6).

The bone-marrow syndrome occurs between 2 and 10 Gy, and is associated variously among species with granulocytopenia, thrombocytopenia, and lymphopenia. Granulocytopenia is usually considered to be the injury of prime importance. Anaemia occurs as a result of haemorrhages, and hence is associated with thrombocytopenia, but it does not correlate with time of death. The target-cells for this syndrome are the marrow precursor cells, particularly the granulocyte-macrophage precursors and the bone-marrow stem-cells. Death occurs mostly in the third week after irradiation, and for man this extends up to week 6. In cases where the injury is only just sufficient to produce the syndrome, death can be prevented by appropriate antibiotic treatment and transfusions of fluids and mature blood cells. After higher doses, transplantation of marrow (preferably isogeneic) is required to repopulate the sterilized endogenous marrow and regenerate the blood-cell populations.

When one syndrome is prevented, another may become apparent depending on the dose. A good example is total-body irradiation (TBI) and marrow transplantation in the treatment of leukaemia. In this case the lung is the dose-limiting tissue. Tolerance doses for interstitial pneumonitis in man are about 8 Gy (single dose) or about 12 Gy (6 fractions). When radiation-induced pneumonitis occurs, it does so usually between 1 and 7 months after irradiation. The likely target cells for pneumonitis are the type-2 alveolar cells and the endothelial cells (see Section 1.3). The above TBI doses result in various long-term complications, e.g. cataracts and infertility (reviewed by Deeg et al. 1984; Hendry 1987b).

### Effects on the embryo and the fetus

The effects of radiation on the embryo and the fetus are due primarily to cell killing. This can kill the embryo in the early stages of development, or can lead to subsequent malformations when the embryo is irradiated in the later stages of organogenesis. The sensitivity of the embryo concerning mortality is highest soon after implantation and during early organogenesis, and then it decreases at later developmental stages. LD50 values are about $1 \cdot 5$ Gy in rodents.

The sensitivity to induced malformation varies markedly with the type of defect (UNSCEAR 1986). For a given species there is a particular relationship between the type of malformation induced and the age at irradiation, which correlates with major phases of differentiation and organization of the relevant structure. Similar types of malformations are induced by irradiation of different species at comparative ages of development. There are examples of the incidence being linear or curvilinear with increasing dose. In man, the best documented effect is microencephaly, in severe cases accompanied by mental retardation.

### Carcinogenesis

Radiation acts both as an initiator and as a promoter of the expression of neoplasia. Cancer can arise from a single transformed cell, but the time course and probability of any transformed cell inducing the cancer depends on a large number of factors, including micro-environmental, hormonal and immunological influences.

The dose—incidence curve for many cancers including leukemia is bell-shaped. There is an increasing incidence with dose at low doses, which is considered to be curvilinear with no threshold dose. The incidence reaches a maximum and then declines after high doses. This is due to sterilization of the transformed cells after high doses. The maximum incidence and the dose at which this occurs vary among tumour types and species, depending on the relative sensitivities of the target cells to transformation and sterilization, and the relative effects of secondary influences referred to above (UNSCEAR 1977). With myeloid leukemia in mice, a maximum incidence of $20-40\%$ is induced by doses of 2 to 3 Gy. For lung tumours, there is an incidence of about $85\%$ after 15 Gy. In rats, the peak incidence for lung and skin tumours is reached after high doses of 25 to 30 Gy.

The incidence of tumours in most cases is decreased by the use of low dose rates, and is increased after high-LET radiations. RBE values approach values of 100 after very low doses.

In man, the mean latency period to diagnosis is about 10 years for leukemia and about 25 years for various solid tumours. The evidence concerning the risks of cancer induction come from five sources:

(a) occupational exposure, e.g. radiologists and miners;
(b) survivors of atomic bombs;
(c) radiotherapy of malignant conditions, e.g. cancer of the uterus following radium treatment of cervix cancer;
(d) radiotherapy of benign conditions, e.g. leukemia induction after spinal irradiation for ankylosing spondylitis,
(e) radiodiagnosis, e.g. liver cancer after thorotrast administration.

The risks per $10^5$ persons per cGy are higher for thyroid and breast cancer (100) than for lung cancer or leukemia (25 to 50), stomach, liver, and large intestine (10 to 15), and bone, oesophagus, small intestine, bladder, pancreas, rectum, and lymphatic tissue (2 to 5). The risks for malignancies arising as a consequence of irradiation of the fetus *in utero* (200−250) are higher than those following total-body irradiation of the adult at low doses (100). Leukemia accounts for about one fifth of all induced cancers.

## Life shortening

The life span of mice, rats, and dogs is reduced by about 5% per Gy for acute exposures (UNSCEAR 1982). There is little change in this figure for dose rates down to $0 \cdot 004$ Gy per minute, and little effect of fractionation. The cause of life shortening is primarily tumour induction, and there is no clear evidence for a contribution from acceleration of age-related somatic diseases. The amount of life shortening is usually higher in females due to the induction of tumours of the genital tract. As expected, there is less life shortening when animals are irradiated at increasing ages, but there also is less when animals are irradiated *in utero*.

In man, studies of the pioneer radiologists in America showed that cancer induction could not account for all of the life shortening, and there was probably a contribution from nonneoplastic conditions. However, in more extensive studies including the A-bomb survivors, an increased prevalence of cancer accounted for all of the effects.

## The biological basis of radiation protection

It is generally considered that there is no safe dose of radiation, and that all doses, however small, carry a probability of harm (ICRP 26,27, 1977). Harm can be somatic injury or hereditary effects, and an important distinction is made between *stochastic* and *nonstochastic* effects. As discussed in Section 6.7, stochastic effects are those for which the probability of occurrence, rather than the severity of the effect, is a function of dose and for which there is no threshold dose. Nonstochastic effects are those for which the severity of the effect varies with dose, and for which a threshold may occur (see Figure 6.17).

At the levels of low and chronic exposure involved in radiation protection, hereditary effects are regarded as stochastic. With uniform whole-body irradiation, the hereditary detriment is likely to be less than that due to somatic effects. Carcinogenesis is a stochastic effect and is regarded as the main somatic risk from irradiation at low doses and therefore the main problem in protection. Nonstochastic effects include cataracts of the lens, desquamation of the skin, haematological deficiencies, and impairment of fertility.

Occupational dose-equivalent limits are quoted in *sieverts* (Sv), which are doses in gray (Gy) multiplied by a quality factor which depends on the particular detriment concerned. When only part of the body is irradiated, the limit for some tissues may be greater than that allowed for uniform exposure. There are weighting factors that express the relative risks for different tissues concerning stochastic risks, e.g. malignancies and hereditary detriment. These factors are shown in Table 6.5.

For uniform whole-body exposure, the total risk of malignancy is taken to be at least three times the total hereditary risk. For nonuniform exposure, the sum of the products of the weighting factors and the respective dose-equivalent limits is the effective dose equivalent, and this must not exceed $0 \cdot 05$ Sv per year.

For nonstochastic harm, the annual limit is set at $0 \cdot 15$ Sv for the lens, $0 \cdot 5$ Sv for all other tissues, and $0 \cdot 05$ Sv for whole-body irradiation. The bases for these limits are occupational experience of continuous low level exposures and extrapolations from prolonged radiotherapy treatments (ICRP 41 1984; Field & Upton 1985).

Table 6.5. Relative risk for tissues

| Tissue | Weighting factor |
|---|---|
| Gonads | $0 \cdot 25$ |
| Breast | $0 \cdot 15$ |
| Red bone marrow | $0 \cdot 12$ |
| Lung | $0 \cdot 12$ |
| Thyroid | $0 \cdot 03$ |
| Bone surfaces | $0 \cdot 03$ |
| Remainder | $0 \cdot 30$ |
|  | $1 \cdot 00$ |

## 6.12. Further reading

**References for syllabus topics not covered**

*Cell biology*
Molecular Biology of the Cell, 1983, B. Albert, D. Bray, J. Lewis, M. Raff, K. Robert and J. D. Watson. (New York and London: Garland Publishing Inc.).

*Radiation chemistry*
The Chemical Basis of Radiation Biology, 1987, C. von Sonntag, (London: Taylor & Francis).

*Genetics and other aspects of oncology*
Introduction to the Cellular and Molecular Biology of Cancer, 1986, Eds. L. M. Franks and N. M. Teich (Oxford: Oxford University Press).

*Hyperthermia*
Hyperthermia and Cancer, 1982, G. M. Hahn (New York: Plenum Press).
Hyperthermic Oncology, Volume 2, 1985, Ed. J. Overgaard, (London: Taylor & Francis).

*Chemotherapy*
The Anticancer Drugs, 1979, W. B. Pratt and R. W. Ruddon (Oxford University Press).
Basic Principles of Cancer Chemotherapy, 1980, T. J. Priestman (Montedison Pharmaceuticals Ltd)

**Further reading on syllabus topics presented in this chapter**

*Cell kinetics*
An Introduction to Cell Population Kinetics, 1977, W. A. Aherne, R. S. Camplejohn and N. A. Wright, (London: Edward Arnold).
Cell Kinetics and Cancer Therapy, 1982, J. Denekamp (Springfield, USA: C. C. Thomas).
Growth Kinetics of Tumours, 1977, G. G. Steel (Oxford: Clarendon Press).
Stem Cells: Their Identification and Characterisation, 1983, Ed. C. S. Potten (Edinburgh: Churchill-Livingstone).

*Cell survival*
The Radiobiology of Cultured Mammalian Cells, 1967, M. M. Elkind and G. F. Whitmore. (New York: Gordon & Breach).
Cell Clones: Manual of Mammalian Cell Techniques, 1985, Eds. C. S. Potten and J. H. Hendry (Edinburgh: Churchill-Livingstone).

*High-LET radiation*
*Fast Neutrons in the Treatment of Cancer*, 1979, M. Catterall and D. K. Bewley, (London: Academic Press).
*Heavy Particle Radiotherapy*, 1980, M. R. Raju (New York: Academic Press).
*Nuclear Particles in Cancer Therapy*, 1981, J. F. Fowler. Medical Physics Handbooks No. 8 (Bristol: Adam Hilger).

*Tissue responses*
*Radiation Histopathology*, 2 vols., 1981, G. Casarett, (Boca Raton, Fla, USA: CRC Press).
*Cytotoxic Insult to Tissue: Effects on Cell Lineages*, 1983, Eds. C. S. Potten and J. H. Hendry (Edinburgh: Churchill-Livingstone).
*Radiation and Skin*, 1985, C. S. Potten (London: Taylor & Francis).

*Radiation hazards*
*Nuclear Radiation: Risks and Benefits*, 1983, E. E. Pochin (Oxford University Press).
International Commission on Radiological Protection, 1977, Publication 26, *Annals of the ICRP*, 1, No. 3, (Oxford: Pergamon Press).
International Commission on Radiological Protection, 1977, Publication 27, Problems in developing an index of harm, *Annals of the ICRP*, 1, No. 4, (Oxford: Pergamon Press).
International Commission on Radiological Protection, 1984, Publication 41, 'Non-stochastic effects of ionizing radiation', *Annals of the ICRP*, 14, No. 3, (Oxford: Pergamon Press).
United Nations Committee on the Effects of Atomic Radiation (UNSCEAR), 1977, 1982 and 1986 reports to the General Assembly, New York.


**General texts**

*Clinical Radiobiology*, 1977, W. B. Duncan and A. H. W. Nias (Edinburgh: Churchill-Livingstone).
*Radiobiology for the Radiologist*, 1978, E. J. Hall. (New York: Harper & Row).
*Biologic Aspects of Radiation Therapy*, in *Textbook of Radiotherapy*, 1980, Ed. G. H. Fletcher (Philadelphia: Lea and Febiger).
*Biological Effects of Radiation*, 1983, J. E. Coggle (London: Taylor & Francis).
*The Biological Basis of Radiotherapy*, 1983, Eds. G. G. Steel, G. E. Adams and M. J. Peckham (New York: Elsevier).

# Chapter 7
# Appendix

In this chapter we derive the various formulae necessary for an understanding of the time factor in terms of cellular repair processes. It is intended mainly for modellers and is written in a terse format. However, the general reader can find particular parts of interest to him by neglecting the formulae as necessary and picking out the main ideas.

## 7.1. The time factor in radiotherapy

*Time factor* is the term used to denote the dependence of the biological effect of a low-LET (see Section 6.2) irradiation on the time over which it is delivered. The time ($t$) of delivery of a dose may vary because the dose is split into numbers of small doses separated by variable intervals (fractionated) or because the dose is given in one shot but at variable dose rates (continuous).

In general, biologically isoeffective doses increase with increasing time, mainly because of cellular repair processes and regeneration through cellular division. In either case a population of cells that survives the earlier stages of a prolonged irradiation is rendered more likely to survive its latter stages because its constituent cells repair radiation-induced damage or because survivors increase their number by cell division. The probability of survival of the population is thereby enhanced, and injury to a tissue in which the population constitutes the renewing cells is correspondingly reduced.

The time factor was at first modelled as a simple power function of $t$ (Chapter 5), wherein isoeffective doses increased as $D = \text{constant} \times t^p$, $0 < p < 1$. In rapidly renewing tissues such as gut and skin, $p$ will be influenced by both repair and repopulation. In the late-responding tissues, where target-cell renewal is very slow, $p$ is by contrast almost exclusively determined by cellular repair processes, and can in fact be derived in terms of the basic parameters of cell survival and response to fractionated and continuous irradiations (Thames 1987a).

In the following we will be concerned exclusively with the time factor as determined by cellular repair processes and will neglect any influence of regeneration of survivors. Furthermore, we will assume constant values of the parameters during the irradiation and neglect changes that can occur because of progression in the division cycle (Section 6.6) during exposure.

## 7.2. Repair during fractionated exposures: the IR model

After irradiation mammalian cells retain their ability to divide and give birth to daughters that are also capable of division with a dose-dependent probability whose logarithm is approximately a second degree polynomial in dose (Figure 3.15, upper left). If a dose $x$ is given twice and sufficient time (of the order of several hours) is allowed between doses ($\Delta t$), the survival probability for the second dose is the same as that for the first dose: memory of the first dose is lost because of repair of some of the injury it induced (Figure 3.15, upper curve in lower right inset). If no time is allowed, survival is described by a continuation of the curve in the upper-left part of Figure 3.15, i.e. by response to a single dose $2x$. In intermediate cases, it is envisioned that an initial segment of the survival curve, equivalent to the dose $\theta x$ (where $\theta$ is a number between 0 and 1), is not repeated, and survival after the second dose is described by the heavy portion of the initial shoulder (Oliver 1964). The factor $\theta$ determines the rate at which repair proceeds, i.e. the repair kinetics. Oliver assumed an exponential form for $\theta$:

$$\theta = \exp(-\mu \Delta t) \tag{7.1}$$

Log survival after split dose (i.e. 2 doses) is given by

$$\ln \text{s.f. (2 doses of size } x\text{, interval } \Delta t) = \ln f(x) + \ln [f(x + \theta x)/f(\theta x)], \tag{7.2}$$

where

$$f(x) = \text{surviving fraction after dose } x.$$

If survival is adequately described by the linear-quadratic (LQ) model

$$f(x) = \exp(-\alpha x - \beta x^2) \tag{7.3}$$

then after a little algebra equation (7.2) becomes

$$\ln \text{s.f.} \text{ (2 doses of size } x, \text{ interval } \Delta t) = -2\alpha x - 2\beta x^2 - 2\beta x^2 \theta. \quad (7.4)$$

Thus, for long $\Delta t$, $\theta \simeq 0$ and $\ln \text{s.f.} = -2\alpha x - 2\beta x^2 = 2 \ln f(x)$, i.e. there is an equal response from each dose because of complete repair and recovery of all the initial segment of the survival curve (upper curve in lower inset, Figure 3.15). If there is no break between the dose ($\Delta t = 0$), then $\ln \text{s.f.} = -2\alpha x - 4\beta x^2 = \ln f(2x)$, i.e. the response to a single dose of size $2x$.

We now generalize equation (7.2) to $n$ fractions, under the assumption that cell proliferation is negligible. After a third dose $x$, given at the same interval $\Delta t$ after the second dose, the dose equivalent of incomplete repair is $\theta x + \theta^2 x$. The first term, $x \exp(-\mu \Delta t)$, represents unrepaired injury from the second dose. The second term, $\theta^2 x = x \exp -\mu(2\Delta t)$, represents unrepaired injury from the first dose, given $2\Delta t$ before the third dose. The response to the third dose follows the curve describing the response to the second dose, except that the initial segment equivalent to the dose ($\theta x + \theta^2 x$) is omitted.

These considerations suggest that the proper change in equation (7.2) to account for the third dose is

$$\ln \text{s.f.} \text{ (3 doses of size } x, \text{ interval } \Delta t) = \ln f(x) + \ln [f(x + \theta x)/f(\theta x)]$$
$$+ \ln [f(x + \theta x + \theta^2 x)/f(\theta x + \theta^2 x)].$$

Let $s_n(x,\theta) = \text{s.f.}$ ($n$ doses of size $x$, interval $\Delta t$).

Then the generalization to $n$ doses is

$$\ln s_n(x,\theta) = \ln f(x) + \ln [f(x + \theta x)/f(\theta x)]$$
$$+ \ln [f(x + \theta x + \theta^2 x)/f(\theta x + \theta^2 x)] + \cdots$$
$$+ \ln [f(x + \theta x + \cdots \theta^{n-1} x)/f(\theta x + \theta^2 x + \cdots + \theta^{n-1} x)]. \quad (7.5)$$

In connection with equation (7.5), note that if $\Delta t$ is large and thus $\theta = 0$, then $f(0) = 1$ and $s_n(x,0) = f(x)^n$, i.e. complete repair during interfraction intervals lead to equal decrements in survival. On the other hand, if $\Delta t = 0$ then $\theta = 1$, and

$$s_n(x, 1) = f(x) \cdot [f(x + x)/f(x)] \cdot [f(x + x + x)/f(x + x)] \ldots = f(nx),$$

i.e. the response to a single dose of size $nx$.

A model linear in its parameters (the LQ model) is required in order to go further with the calculations. From equation (7.3) we have $\ln f(x) = -\alpha x - \beta x^2$, $\ln f(x + \theta x) = -\alpha(x + \theta x) - \beta(x + \theta x)^2$, etc. Substituting into equation (7.5), we find

$$\ln s_n(x,\theta) = \sum_{k=0}^{n-1} \left\{ \ln f\left(x\sum_{i=0}^{k} \theta^i\right) - \ln f\left(x\sum_{i=1}^{k} \theta^i\right) \right\}$$

$$= \sum_{k=0}^{n-1} \left\{ -\alpha x\left(1 + \sum_{i=1}^{k} \theta^i\right) - \beta x^2\left(1 + \sum_{i=1}^{k} \theta^i\right)^2 \right. \quad (7.6)$$

$$\left. + \alpha x \sum_{i=1}^{k} \theta^i + \beta x^2 \left(\sum_{i=1}^{k} \theta^i\right)^2 \right\}$$

$$= n(-\alpha x - \beta x^2) - 2\beta x^2 \sum_{k=0}^{n-1}\sum_{i=1}^{k} \theta^i.$$

When the summations of equation (7.6) are carried out, the result is

$$\left.\begin{array}{l}\ln s_n(x,\theta) = n \ln f(x) - n\beta x^2 h_n(\theta), \\ h_n(\theta) = (2/n)[\theta/(1-\theta)][n - (1-\theta^n)/(1-\theta)]\end{array}\right\} \quad (7.7)$$

Equations (7.6) and (7.7), mathematical representations of the incomplete-repair (IR) model for fractionated doses, provided expressions for log survival after $n$ doses of size $x$ with intervals $\Delta t$ between fractions. The following points may be made:

(a) Incomplete repair affects only the $\beta$-component of killing, and not the $\alpha$-component.
(b) The limiting behaviour of the function $h_n(\theta)$ in equation (7.7) is given by $h_n(0) = 0$ and $h_n(1) = n - 1$. Therefore $\ln s_n(x, 0) = n \ln f(x)$ (complete repair) and $\ln s_n(x, 1) = \ln f(nx)$.

Tests of equation (7.7) may be found in Thames (1985) and in Figure 3.17.

## 7.3. Repair during continuous, low-dose-rate exposures

An IR model for survival response after continuous exposures (with the assumptions of negligible cell proliferation and unchanging radiosensitivity) may be derived from equation (7.7) in a limiting process whereby $x$ and $\Delta t$ are allowed to tend toward zero as $n \to \infty$, but such that the total dose $D = nx$ and overall time $t = (n-1)\Delta t$ remain constant. Put otherwise, equation (7.7) may be thought of as an approximation to the effect of continuous irradiation at dose rate $v$, so that total dose

$$D = vt$$
$$= \text{dose rate} \times \text{exposure time}$$

# Appendix

is given in a sequence of $n$ small doses of size $x$, separated by intervals $\Delta t$. Therefore, after $n$ doses of size $x = v\Delta t = vt/n$ (we replace $n-1$ by $n$, as the latter is assumed very large compared with 1), the log surviving fraction is given by equation (7.7).

We now seek the limit of $\ln s_n$ as $\Delta t \to 0 (n \to \infty)$. For the first term we have

$$\lim_{n \to \infty} n \ln f(x) = \lim_{n \to \infty} n(-\alpha(vt/n) - \beta(vt/n)^2)$$
$$= -\alpha vt$$

This is the limiting response obtained when the dose rate is so low that survival is exponential. From the second term of equation (7.7) we have

$$\lim_{\Delta t \to 0} x^2[\theta/(1-\theta)][n - (1-\theta^n)/(1-\theta)]$$
$$= \lim_{\Delta t \to 0} (v\,\Delta t)^2 [\exp(-\mu\,\Delta t)/(1 - \exp(-\mu\,\Delta t))]$$
$$\times [t/\Delta t - (1-\exp(-\mu\,\Delta t))^{t/\Delta t}/(1 - \exp(-\mu\,\Delta t))],$$
$$= (vt)^2(\mu t - 1 + \exp(-\mu t)/(\mu t)^2$$

Therefore, if we designate the limit of $s_n$ by $S(vt,\mu)$:

$$S(vt,\mu) = \lim_{n \to \infty} s(vt/n, \exp(-\mu\,\Delta t))$$
$$= \text{s.f. (continuous dose } vt \text{ delivered at (low) dose rate } v \text{ for time } t, \text{ with repair constant } \mu)$$

then

$$\left.\begin{array}{l}\ln S(vt,\mu) = -\alpha(vt) - \beta\,(vt)^2\,g(\mu t),\\ g(\mu t) = 2[\mu t - 1 + \exp(-\mu t)]/(\mu t)^2\end{array}\right\}. \quad (7.8)$$

The following points may be raised in connection with equation (7.8), which is equivalent to the 'accumulation' model of Roesch (1978):

(a) Dose rate affects only the $\beta$-component (through the function $g$). At ever smaller dose rates the survival curve tends toward the exponential with a slope identical to the initial slope of the acute-dose survival curve.
(b) The function $g$ has the value $g(0) = 1$ for very short exposure times and tends gradually toward zero (concave side up) as $t$ increases.
(c) The emphasis above on the adjective 'low' to describe the dose rate $v$ derives from averaging many ($n$) small, acute exposures over the time $t$. When the limit is taken, the dose rate is 'low' during any finite time interval.

## 7.4. Tissue response to fractionated or continuous irradiation

We suppose that a particular response in a tissue (paralysis following irradiation of the cord, death from pneumonitis following exposure of the lungs, etc.) corresponds to precisely one level of depletion of a critical target-cell population whose survival is described by the IR model, equations (7.7) and (7.8) above. Further, cellular proliferation is assumed to have a negligible effect. Thus, let the positive number $E$ denote the negative of log surviving fraction of target cells in a tissue at this critical level:

$$E = -\ln \text{ s.f. (target cells)}$$

From equations (7.7) and (7.8) we have

$$E = n(\alpha x + \beta x^2) + n\beta x^2 h_n(\theta) \quad (7.9)$$
(fractionated exposure)

$$E = \alpha(vt) + \beta(vt)^2 g(\mu t)$$
(continuous growth)

The experimental data that may be used to test the isoeffect models of equation (7.9) are usually in the form of isoeffect doses (e.g. for 50% responders from a test population) determined under different fractionation or exposure conditions, i.e. different doses per fraction $x$ or exposure time $t$ (or equivalently, dose rate $v$). Since different tissues, with vastly different target-cell numbers or levels of depletion required to elicit response, may have very nearly the same fractionation response, it is necessary that the number $E$ (indeterminate in isoeffect experiments) be absorbed into the parameters $\alpha$ and $\beta$. For example, after division we may write

$$\left.\begin{array}{l}1 = n[(\alpha/E)x + (\beta/E)x^2] + n(\beta/E)x^2 h_n\theta \\ \text{(fractionated exposure)} \\ 1 = (\alpha/E)vt + (\beta/E)(vt)^2 g(\mu t) \\ \text{(continuous exposure)}\end{array}\right\} \quad (7.10)$$

More convenient representations for fitting data, similar to those suggested by Douglas & Fowler (1976), are obtained by dividing equation (7.10) by total dose $D$ ($nx$ or $vt$):

$$\begin{array}{l}1/D = (\alpha/E) + (\beta/E)x[1 + h_n(\theta)], \\ 1/D = (\alpha/E) + (\beta/E)Dg(\mu t)\end{array} \quad (7.11)$$

These we label 'reciprocal-dose' representations. When interfraction intervals are long and repair is complete between doses, $h_n = 0$ and

$$1/D = \alpha/E + (\beta/E)x \tag{7.12}$$

Incomplete repair will result in a divergence from linearity of reciprocal-dose graphs, i.e. in downward curvature of the reciprocal-dose graph. When the dose per fraction is large, however, as in the 1- and 2-fraction points, the same curvature would result if the true survival function were exponential at high doses (Taylor & Withers 1985).

## 7.5. The LPL model

The hypotheses on which the LPL (lethal, potentially lethal) model is based are as follows (Curtis 1982, 1986):

(1) Long-lived (minutes), spatially separated lesions (B-lesions in Figure 7.1) in the amount $\eta_{AB}$ per unit dose are created in cell nuclei by (low-LET) radiation. These lesions are repaired by a first-order enzymatic process, but may interact to produce irreparable lesions (C-lesions), one of which is sufficient to result in loss of cell-reproductive capacity; thus, the rate of the repair process will depend on the first power of the number of lesions, while their interaction and fixation will proceed at a rate dependent on its second power. The latter process may

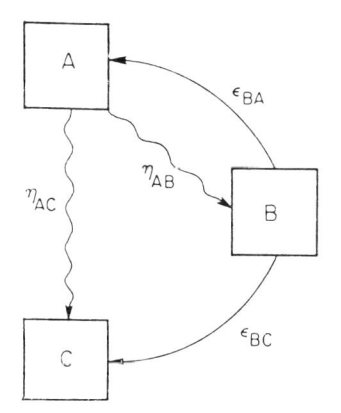

Figure 7.1. Hypothetical model of induction and repair of potentially lethal (B) and lethal, irreparable lesions (C) by radiation (from Pohlit & Heyder 1981). The numbers of B and C lesions are linearly related to dose; B lesions are repaired by a first-order process to the undamaged state (A), or are fixed by a second-order process to the irreparable state (C). (Reproduced with permission of Academic Press Inc. and the authors.)

also be interpreted as 'misrepair' (Tobias et al. 1980). Its probability depends on the overall concentration of lesions, not on their initial proximity.
(2) The lesions can interact with each other on a very short time scale (one second or less) to create an irreparable lesion, if they are created simultaneously and very close to each other (e.g. by a single charged particle, see Section 6.1). This is considered a C-lesion, created directly as a result of radiation, as shown in Figure 7.1 in the amount $\eta_{AC}$ per unit dose.
(3) $\eta_{AB}$ and $\eta_{AC}$ are independent of dose.

The part of the model having to do with repair, of most interest for our purposes, is as follows. Let $N_B(t)$ = mean number of repairable lesions per cell at time $t$, and $N_C(t)$ = mean number of irreparable lesions per cell at time $t$ (Figure 7.1). The differential equations describing the model are

$$dN_B/dt = -\varepsilon_{BA}N_B - \varepsilon_{BC}N_B^2; \; N_B(0) = \eta_{AB}x, \\ dN_C/dt = \varepsilon_{BC}N_B^2; \; N_C(0) = \eta_{AC}x, \quad (7.13)$$

whose solution is given by

$$N_B = \eta_{AB}x \exp(-\varepsilon_{BA}t)/[1 + (\eta_{AB}x/\varepsilon)(1 - \exp(-\varepsilon_{BA}t)], \\ N_C = \eta_{AB}x(1 + \eta_{AB}x/\varepsilon)(1 - \exp(-\varepsilon_{BA}t))/ \\ [1 + (\eta_{AB}x/\varepsilon)(1 - \exp(-\varepsilon_{BA}t))] \\ -\ln[1 + (\eta_{AB}x/\varepsilon)(1 - \exp(-\varepsilon_{BA}t))] + \eta_{AC}x. \quad (7.14)$$

In equation (7.14) $x$ is the radiation dose and

$$\varepsilon = \varepsilon_{BA}/\varepsilon_{BC}$$

To calculate survival the following assumptions are necessary: (1) all lesions are lethal, some repairable (B) and some irreparable (C); (2) all B-lesions become irreparable if the repair process is halted by some experimental treatment (fixation of damage); and (3) the distribution of lesions per cell is random (Poisson).

Therefore the surviving fractions at time $t$, $f(x, t)$, is given by

$$f(x, t) = \exp(-N_B - N_C)$$

which upon combining with equation (7.14) and substituting, becomes

$$f(x, t) = \exp(-(\eta_{AC} + \eta_{AB})x)[1 + (\eta_{AB}x/\varepsilon)(1 - \exp(-\varepsilon_{BA}t))]^\varepsilon. \quad (7.15)$$

Several remarks may be made in connection with the foregoing:
(1) The initial condition in equation (7.13) includes all the lesions of types

B and C induced by radiation alone; thus this is a high-dose-rate setting, in which induction of lesions by the radiation dose $x$ is essentially instantaneous in comparison with repair processes.

(2) Low-dose approximation of equation (7.15): when terms of order $(\eta_{AB}x)^3/\varepsilon^2$ may be neglected, i.e. at 'low' doses, the logarithm may be expanded in a Taylor series to give log survival:

$$\ln f(x,t) = -(\eta_{AC} + \eta_{AB}\exp(-\varepsilon_{BA}t))x - (\eta_{AB}^2/2\varepsilon)(1 - \exp(-\varepsilon_{BA}t))^2 x^2 \tag{7.16}$$

For long repair times after the dose $x$, equation (7.16) becomes

$$\ln f(x) = -\eta_{AC}x - (\eta_{AB}^2/2\varepsilon)x^2 \tag{7.17}$$

which is the LQ model equation (7.3), with

$$\left.\begin{array}{l}\alpha = \eta_{ac} \\ \beta = \eta_{AB}^2/2\varepsilon\end{array}\right\} \tag{7.18}$$

When this same low-dose restriction holds, the LPL model can be generalized to $n$ fractions, and shown to be equivalent to the IR model, equation (7.7) (Thames 1985). Similarly, when the dose rate $v$ is low enough that

$$2\eta_{AB}v/(\varepsilon\varepsilon_{BA}) \ll 1 \tag{7.19}$$

the LPL model can be generalized to continuous exposures; again it is equivalent to the corresponding IR model, equation (7.8) (Thames 1985).

As a result of the equivalence of the generalized LPL repair model and the IR model, explicit radiobiological assumptions on which the former rests may be used to interpret the latter. It is the repair of 'sublethal' damage (cf. Sections 3.1 and 6.4) that is accounted for in the IR model, and its application requires the assumption that sufficient time has been allowed after fractionated or continuous radiation exposures for all post-treatment ('potentially lethal') repair to be complete (Sections 3.2 and 6.4). The generalized LPL repair model accounts for both types of repair, although it makes no distinction between repair categories given differing operational definitions in experimental studies.

In the IR and generalized LPL models, repair kinetics is first-order regardless of dose and cannot be saturated. The shouldered survival curve results from hypotheses about one- and two-track actions in the IR model, since it assumes the LQ survival model holds, while it results from the interaction of radiation-induced lesions in the LPL model. Interestingly, it is not necessary to assume saturation of repair or depletion of critical factors to obtain the shouldered curve. The shoulder arises rather from the damage-fixation process, i.e. from the conversion of repairable lesions to irreparable lesions (cf. Figure 7.1). All these lesions are 'potentially' lethal, however, and can be fixed, e.g. by replating plateau-phase cells in fresh medium and causing their entry into the cell cycle, in which there are defined 'fixation points' (Iliakis 1980).

## 7.6. The time factor: slopes of isoeffect graphs

Assuming that the effect level $E$ is constant, equation (7.9) can be differentiated implicitly with respect to the number of fractions, $n$. We assume that repair is complete between fractions ($h_n = 0$) and recall that $x = D/n$. Thus,

$$0 = \alpha \, \partial D/\partial n + 2\beta x \, \partial D/\partial n - \beta x^2$$

which simplifies to

$$\frac{\partial \ln D}{\partial \ln n} = \frac{x}{\alpha/\beta + 2x} \qquad (7.20)$$

This is the so-called *number-of-fractions exponent* (exponent $0 \cdot 24$ in the Ellis (1967) NSD formula) that accounts for repair effects in fractionated treatments. It is called an exponent because it represents the repair component of the exponent $p$, i.e. the time factor (Section 7.1). Its values for various tissues and for changing dose per fraction $x$ are considered in Section 2.2 (see Table 2.5).

Similar calculations lead to the *fraction-size exponent* (slope of the graph of isoeffect dose versus (decreasing) dose per fraction):

$$\frac{\partial \ln D}{\partial(-\ln x)} = \frac{x}{\alpha/\beta + x} \qquad (7.21)$$

and this is the slope of the graphs presented on the cover of this book and in Figure 3.12. From these figures it can be seen that these slopes are greater for late effects (solid lines) than for early effects (dashed lines), which for a given dose per fraction $x$ leads from equation (7.21) to the inequality

$$(\alpha/\beta)_{\text{late}} < (\alpha/\beta)_{\text{early}} \qquad (7.22)$$

Finally, the time factor for continuous exposures has traditionally been expressed as a linear relationship between log isoeffect dose and log exposure time. We will call the slope of this representation the *exposure-time coefficient*. It may be calculated by differentiation of equation (7.9) for continuous exposures, and the result is

$$\frac{\partial \ln D}{\partial \ln t} = -\frac{(\mu t)Dg'(\mu t)}{\alpha/\beta + 2Dg(\mu t)} \qquad (7.23)$$

In equation (7.23) $\mu$ is the first-order repair rate constant, the prime denotes differentiation with respect to $\mu t$, and $g(\mu t)$ is given by equation (7.8). Application of equation (7.23) to the analysis of experimental and clinical data may be found in Section (2.3) and Table 2.6.

## 7.7. The time factor for arbitrary target-cell survival curves

The development in Section 7.6 and equations (7.20–7.23) were based on the assumption of the LQ model for target-cell survival. Suppose instead that survival is described by the function $f(x)$ where $x = $ dose, and that log survival, $\ln f$, has the concave-down shape shown in Figure 3.10. We assume that $\ln f$ satisfies: (1) $\partial \ln f(x)/\partial x < 0$ for $x > 0$, and (2) $\partial^2 \ln f(x)/\partial x^2 < 0$ for $x > 0$, but $f$ is otherwise arbitrary. For example, $f$ might satisfy an asymptotic condition like

$$\lim_{x \to \infty} d \ln f/dx = \text{constant},$$

as with the two-component model equation (6.3). We now derive expressions for the slopes of isoeffect graphs for tissues whose target-cell survival is described by $\ln f$.

Under the usual assumptions (equal effect per fraction, negligible proliferation, etc.), after $n$ doses of size $x$ that are sufficient for log cell kill $-E$ we have

$$E = -n \ln f(x) \qquad (7.24)$$

We differentiate equation (7.24) implicitly with respect to $n$, and recalling that $n = D/x$ we obtain

$$0 = -(\partial D/\partial n)(1/x)(\ln f) + (D/x^2)\ln f - (D/x) \, d \ln f/dx$$

which after some manipulation leads to

$$\partial \ln D/\partial \ln n = 1 - [\ln f/x]/[d \ln f/dx] \qquad (7.25)$$

This is the number-of-fractions exponent (cf. equation 7.20), and by reference to Figure 3.10 it will be seen that

$$\partial \ln D / \partial \ln n = 1 - (\text{slope of chord})/(\text{slope of tangent})$$
$$= 1 - D_0(\text{tangent})/D_0(\text{chord}) \quad (7.26)$$

The slope of the chord, $\ln f/x$, describes the fractionation response to repeated doses of size $x$, whereas the slope of the tangent, $d \ln f/dx$ (dashed line in Figure 3.10), describes the steepness of the response to a single dose of size $x$. Similarly,

$$\partial \ln D/\partial(-\ln x) = [d \ln f/dx]/[\ln f/x] - 1$$
$$= (\text{slope of tangent})/(\text{slope of chord}) - 1 \quad (7.27)$$
$$= D_0(\text{chord})/D_0(\text{tangent}) - 1,$$

i.e. the fraction-size exponent (cf. equation 7.21) is also related simply to the slopes of the tangent and chord as shown in Figure 3.10.

From equations 7.26–7.27 we arrive at an interesting relationship between the fraction-size exponent and the number-of-fractions exponent:

Fraction-size exp. = number-of-fractions exp./
$$(1 - \text{number-of-fractions exp.}) \quad (7.28)$$

If experimental conditions permit realization of the assumptions on which these calculations are based, then fulfillment of equation (7.28) constitutes a test of the target-cell hypothesis (Chapter 2).

# Glossary

$\alpha/\beta$ ratio — The ratio of the parameters $\alpha$ and $\beta$ in the equation describing the shape of the survival curve or the isoeffect plot (the higher the ratio the less is the curvature in the survival curve and the less steep is the isoeffect plot, i.e. the fractionation sensitivity is low).

Accelerated fractionation — Reduction in the overall time without a significant change in dose per fraction or total dose.

Angiogenesis — Production of new blood vessels, mediated through tumour-angiogenesis factor (TAF).

Apoptosis — Mode of cell death characterized by nuclear fragmentation, cell lysis, and phagocytosis of dense chromatin bodies by neighbouring cells.

Avalanche — Accelerating rate of cell proliferation induced by cell death.

Bone-marrow syndrome — The signs of haematopoietic failure as a result of irradiation (sterilization) of the bone marrow.

Cell-cycle time — The time between one mitosis and the next.

Cell loss factor ($\phi$) — The proportional loss of extra cells added by division. When all new cells are lost, the steady state is characterized by $\phi = 1 \cdot 0$. When half the new cells produced by division are lost, $\phi = 0 \cdot 5 = 1 - T_{pot}/T_{vol}$.

Chronic hypoxia — Persistent low oxygen concentrations such as exist on the periphery of tumour cords.

Clonogen — Abbreviation of clonogenic cell, capable of producing a clone of genetically identical daughter cells.

Colony-forming cells — Cells capable of repeated division and forming a colony comprising usually more than 50 cells.

| | |
|---|---|
| Compton effect | Absorption and scattering of photons by an atom, and ejection of an electron. |
| Conditional renewing (flexible) tissues | Tissues composed of cell populations capable of both division and function. |
| Continuous-repair factor ($g$) | Factor multiplied by the dose per fraction ($d$) to give the fractionation factor $= \alpha/\beta + d \times g$. |
| CRE | Cumulative radiation effect. At the tolerance level of effect, CRE = the nominal standard dose (NSD) in the Ellis formula. |
| $D_0$ | Dose which gives on average one lethal event per cell (mean lethal dose); dose which reduces survival to $e^{-1}$ (0·37 or 37%) of its previous value on the exponential portion of the survival curve. |
| Direct action | Ionization or excitation of a molecule by direct interaction with radiation. |
| Dosage factor | The product of the number of fractions and the dose per fraction, i.e. the total dose. |
| Dose-modifying factor (DMF) | Equal ratio of biologically equivalent doses for all levels of effect. |
| Doubling time | Time for a cell population to double its size. |
| Elastic scattering | Collision of particles with atoms or nuclei where kinetic energy of the incident particle equals kinetic energy of the recoil particles. |
| Elkind repair | Recovery of the shoulder on a survival curve when irradiation follows several hours after priming dose. |
| Exposure-time exponent | The power to which the overall time ($T$) is raised to calculate the increase in isoeffect dose ($D$) with increasing exposure time. |
| Extrapolated total dose (ETD) | Maximum isoeffect dose when the dose rate is very low, or when the number of fractions is very large using high dose rates. |
| Extrapolation number | Point of extrapolation of the exponential portion of a multi-target survival curve on the $y$-axis. |
| Field-size effect | The dependence of the effect on the size of the irradiated area. |
| Flexible tissues (conditional renewing) | Cell populations capable of both division and function. |

| | |
|---|---|
| Flexure dose (general definition) | Low-dose limit for effective fractionation; no detectable increase in isoeffect dose results when the fraction size is smaller than the flexure dose. |
| Flow cytometry | Technique for determination of cell kinetics parameters by measuring the change in DNA content of cells in different stages of the cell cycle. |
| Fractionation factor | The sum of the $\alpha/\beta$ ratio and the dose per fraction, i.e. the total dose. |
| Fractionation sensitivity | Rate of increase in total dose for isoeffect when the number of fractions is increased (dose per fraction decreased). High sensitivity = high rate of increase in total dose. |
| Free radical | A chemical species containing an unpaired electron. |
| Gastrointestinal syndrome | The signs and symptoms of intestinal failure. |
| GM−CFC | Colony-forming cells forming granulocytes and macrophages in culture. |
| gray (Gy) | Unit of absorbed dose. 1 Gy = 1 joule per kg (=100 rad). |
| Growth delay | Extra time required for an irradiated versus an un-irradiated tumour to reach a given size. |
| Growth fraction | The proportion of cells in cycle in a population. |
| Hierarchical tissues | Cell populations comprising a lineage of stem cells, proliferative cells, and mature cells. The mature cells do not divide. |
| Hyperfractionation | Increase in number of fractions and reduction in dose per fraction in the same overall time. |
| Hypofractionation | A reduction in the number of fractions, keeping the overall time similar. |
| Incomplete-repair factor ($h_M$) | Correction to the dose per fraction ($d$) to give the fractionation factor = $\alpha/\beta + d(1 + h_M)$; $M$ = number of treatments per day. |
| Indirect action | Transfer of energy to biological molecules through intermediary free radicals. |
| Interphase death | Cell death in the absence of mitosis. |
| Isoeffect plots | Doses for equal effect (e.g. ED50) plotted against dose per fraction or dose rate. |
| LD50/30 | Dose to produce lethality in 50% of subjects by 30 days. |

| | |
|---|---|
| Labelling index | Proportion or percentage of cells in S phase at any given time, determined using autoradiography. |
| Latency interval | Time between irradiation and expression of injury. |
| Linear energy transfer (LET) | The rate of energy loss along the track of an ionizing particle, imparted by charged particles of specified energy. Usually expressed in keV/$\mu$m. |
| Linear–quadratic (LQ) model | Model in which the effect ($E$) is a linear–quadratic function of dose ($d$) e.g. $E = \alpha d + \beta d^2$. |
| Log-phase cultures | Cell cultures increasing in size by the same proportion in equal intervals of time, i.e. those growing exponentially. |
| Mitotic death | Cell death caused by failure to complete mitosis correctly and produce two viable daughter cells. |
| Mitotic delay | Time delay induced in the $G_2$ phase prior to mitosis. |
| Mitotic index | Proportion or percentage of cells in mitosis at any given time. |
| Multi-target model | Model which assumes the presence of many targets in a cell, all of which require inactivation to kill the cell. |
| Neurological syndrome | Signs and symptoms of injury in the central nervous system leading to CNS failure within 48 hours. |
| Nonstochastic effect | An effect where the severity increases with increasing dose after a threshold region. |
| NSD | Nominal standard dose in the Ellis formula. |
| Number-of-fractions exponent | The power to which the number of fractions ($N$) is raised in power-law models, e.g. $N^{0.24}$. |
| Oxygen enhancement ratio (OER) | The ratio of dose given under anoxic conditions to the dose resulting in the same effect when given under oxic conditions. |
| Pair production | Absorption of photons with energies in excess of $1 \cdot 02$ MeV, conversion into an electron and a positron, and annihilation of these two to produce two photons each with an energy of $0 \cdot 51$ MeV. |
| Partial tolerance (PT) | A fraction ($n/N$) of the NSD, given in $n$ fractions out of a total of $N$ fractions resulting in tolerance. |
| Photoelectric effect | Absorption of photons by an atom, ionization of the atom, and emission of lower-energy photons. |
| Plateau-phase cultures | Cell cultures grown to confluency so that proliferation is markedly reduced. |

| | |
|---|---|
| Plating efficiency | The proportion or percentage of plated cells that forms colonies. |
| Poisson distribution | Distribution applicable when the probability of an event happening is small but the number of observations is large. The distribution of probabilities runs from zero to infinity, and an important characteristic of the distribution is that the mean equals the variance. |
| Potential doubling time ($T_{pot}$) | The volume-doubling time that would be measured in the absence of cell loss. |
| Potentially lethal damage | Injury which can be repaired in the radiation-free interval between irradiation and mitosis, and is lethal if not repaired. |
| Prodromal phase | The signs and symptoms in the first 48 hours following irradiation. |
| Quasi-threshold dose ($D_q$) | Point of extrapolation of the exponential portion of a multi-target survival curve on the $x$-axis. $D_q = D_0 \ln N$. |
| Radioresponsiveness | Rate of response of a tissue to irradiation. |
| Recoil proton | Proton emitted from the nucleus following collisions with heavy particles. |
| Redistribution | Change in the distribution of cells among the various phases of the cell cycle. |
| Relative biological effectiveness (RBE) | Ratio of doses of a reference radiation quality and the test radiation type that produce equal effect. |
| Reproductive integrity | Ability of cells to divide many times. |
| Self-renewal probability | Probability of self-renewal rather than differentiation at each division. |
| sievert (Sv) | Dose-equivalent in radiation protection. Doses in Gy are multiplied by a quality factor which depends on the particular detriment, to obtain sieverts. |
| Slow repair | Long-term recovery which takes place on a time scale of weeks to months, often associated with long-term intracellular repair. |
| Spheroid | Spherical colony of cells, usually tumour cells grown *in vitro*. |

| | |
|---|---|
| Split-dose recovery | Increase in survival when a dose is split into two equal fractions separated by various intervals of time, or the corresponding increase in total dose required for iso-survival. |
| Stem cells | Cells capable of self-renewal and of differentiation to produce all the various types of cells in a lineage. |
| Stochastic effect | An effect where the incidence, but not the severity, increases with increasing dose. |
| Sublethal damage | Nonlethal injury that can be repaired or accumulate with further dose to become lethal. |
| Target cell (general definition) | A (renewing) cell whose death contributes to a reduction in tissue function. |
| TDF | Time, dose and fractionation factors used with the Ellis formula. |
| Tissue-rescuing unit (TRU) | Unit of tissue capable of rescuing a tissue from failure. |
| Transient hypoxia | Low oxygen concentrations associated with the rapid closing and opening of blood vessels. |
| Transit cells | Maturing proliferative cells that amplify cell production in a hierarchical tissue. |
| Tumour bed effect (TBE) | Slower rate of tumour growth after irradiation due to stromal injury in the irradiated 'bed'. |
| Tumour cord | Sleeve of viable tumour growing around a capillary. |
| Volume-doubling time ($T_{vol}$) | Time for a tumour to double in size. |

# Bibliography

Abbatucci, J. S., de Lozier, T., Quint, R., Roussel, A. and Brune, D., 1978, Radiation myelopathy of the cervical spinal cord. Time, Dose and Volume factors. *International Journal of Radiation Oncology, Biology, Physics*, 4, 239–248.
Aherne, W. A., Camplejohn, R. S. and Wright, N. A., 1977, *An Introduction to Cell Population Kinetics* (London: Edward Arnold Ltd).
Ainsworth, E. J. and Leong, G. F., 1966, Recovery from radiation injury in dogs as evaluated by the split-dose technique. *Radiation Research*, 29, 131–42.
Albers-Schönberg, G., 1903, Röntgenstrahlenwirkung an den Hoden. *Münchener Medizinische Wochenschrift*, No. 43.
Alper, T., 1979, *Cellular Radiobiology* (Cambridge: The University Press), p. 320.
Alper, T., 1980, Survival curve models. *Radiation Biology in Cancer Research*, edited by R. E. Meyn and H. R. Withers (New York: Raven Press), pp. 3–18.
Alper, T., 1984, Implications of repair models for LET effects and other radiobiological phenomena. *British Journal of Cancer*, 49, Suppl. VI, 137–43.
Andrews, J. R. and Moody, J. M. 1956, The dose–time relationship in radiotherapy. *American Journal of Roentgenology*, 75, 590–6.
Andrews, J. R., 1965, Dose–time relationships in cancer radiotherapy, a clinical radiobiology study of extremes of dose and time. *American Journal of Roentgenology*, 93, 56–74.
Andrews, J. R., 1978. Models of human cancer radiotherapy. In *The Radiobiology of Human Cancer Radiotherapy*, (Baltimore: University Park Press), pp. 379–94.
Ang, K. Kian, Xu, F-X, van Uytsel, Luc and van der Schueren, Emmanuel, 1985a, Repopulation kinetics in irradiated mouse lip mucosa: the relative importance of treatment protraction and time distribution of irradiations. *Radiation Research*, 101, 162–9.
Ang, K. K., van der Kogel, A. and van der Schueren, E., 1985b, Lack of evidence for increased tolerance of rat spinal cord with decreasing fraction doses below 2 Gy. *International Journal of Radiation Oncology Biology Physics*, 11, 105–10.
Ang, K. K., Xu, F-X., Landuyt, W. and van der Schueren, E., 1985c, The kinetics and capacity of repair of sublethal damage in mouse lip mucosa during fractionated irradiations. *International Journal of Radiation Oncology, Biology, Physics*, 11, 1977–83.
Ang, K. K., Landuyt, W., Xu, F-X., Vanuytsel, L. and van der Schueren, E., 1987a. The effect of small radiation doses per fraction on mouse lip mucosa assessed using the concept of partial tolerance. *Radiotherapy and Oncology*, 8, 79–86.
Ang, K. K., Thames, H. D., van der Kogel, A. J. and van der Schueren, E., 1987b, Is there an influence of fraction size on repair kinetics in the spinal cord? *International Journal of Radiation Oncology Biology Physics*, 13, (in press).
Arcangeli, G., Friedman M. and Paoluzi, R., 1974, A quantitative study of late radiation effect on normal skin and subcutaneous tissues in human beings. *British Journal of Radiology*, 47, 44–50.

Arcangeli, G., Nervi, C., Cividalli, A., Mauro, F. and Pardini, M. D., 1984, Clinical implication of the radiobiological data in multiple fractions per day (MFD) radiotherapy. Proceedings of Varian's Fourth European Clinac Users Meeting, Varian, Zug, Switzerland, pp. 36—43.

Atkins, H. L., 1964, Massive dose techniques in radiation therapy of inoperable carcinoma of the breast. *American Journal of Roentgenology*, **91**, 80—9.

Bäckstrom, A., Jakobsson, P. A., Littbrand, B. and Wersall, I., 1973, Fractionation scheme with low individual doses in irradiation of carcinoma of the mouth. *Acta Radiologica*, **12**, 401—6.

Baclesse, F., 1949, Carcinoma of the Larynx. *British Journal of Radiology*, Supplement 3, pp. 1—63.

Barendsen, G. W., 1982, Dose fractionation, dose rate and iso-effect relationships for normal tissue responses. *International Journal of Radiation Oncology Biology Physics*, **8**, 1981—99.

Barendsen, G. W. and Broerse, J. J., 1969, Experimental radiotherapy of a rat rhabdomyosarcoma with 15 MeV neutrons and 300 kV X-rays. I. Effect of single exposures. *European Journal of Cancer*, **5**, 373—91.

Barendsen, G. W. and Broerse, J. J., 1970, Experimental radiotherapy of rat rhabdomyosarcoma with 15 MeV neutrons and 300 kV X-rays. II. Effects of fractionated treatments applied five times a week for several weeks. *European Journal of Cancer*, **6**, 89—109.

Barendsen, G. W., Roelse, H., Hermens, A. F., Madhuizen, H. T., van Peperzeel, H. A. and Rutgers, D. G., 1973, Clonogenic capacity of proliferative and non-proliferative cells of a transplantable rat rhabdomyosarcoma in relation to its radiosensitivity. *Journal of the National Cancer Institute*, **51**, 1521—7.

Barker, J. L., Montague, E. D. and Peters, L. J., 1980, Clinical experience with irradiation of inflammatory carcinoma of the breast with and without elective chemotherapy. *Cancer*, **45**, 625—9.

Baserga, R., 1986, Molecular biology of the cell cycle. *International Journal of Radiation Biology*, **49**, 219—26.

Bates, T. D. 1975, A prospective clinical trial of post-operative radiotherapy delivered in three fractions per week versus two fractions per week in breast carcinoma. *Clinical Radiology*, **26**, 297—304.

Bates, T. D. and Peters, L. J., 1975, Danger of the clinical use of the NSD formula for small fraction numbers. *British Journal of Radiology*, **48**, 773.

Battermann, J. J., Breur, K., Hart, G. A. M. and Peperzeel, H. A. Van, 1981, Observations on pulmonary metastases in patients after single doses and multiple fractions of fast neutrons and cobalt-60 gamma rays. *European Journal of Cancer*, **17**, 539—548.

Baverstock, K. F., Papworth, D. G. and Townsend, K. M., 1985, Man's sensitivity to bone marrow failure following whole-body exposure to low LET ionizing radiation: inferences to be drawn from animal experiments. *International Journal of Radiation Biology*, **47**, 397—411.

Becker, A. J., McCulloch, E. A., Siminovitch, L. and Till, J. E., 1965, The effect of differing demands for blood cell production in DNA synthesis by haemopoietic colony-forming cells of mice. *Blood*, **26**, 296—308.

Bedford, J. S., Mitchell, J. B. and Fox, M. H., 1980, Variations in responses of several mammalian cell lines to low dose-rate irradiation. In *Radiation Biology in Cancer Research*, edited by R. E. Meyn and H. R. Withers (New York: Raven Press), pp. 251—62.

Beer, J. Z., 1979, Heritable lesions affecting proliferation of irradiated mammalian cells. In *Advances in Radiation Biology*, 8, edited by J. T. Lett and H. Adler (New York: Academic Press), pp. 363—417.

Benjamin, A., Reuss, A., Sluka, A. and Schwarz, G., 1906, Einwirkung auf das Blut. *Wiener Klinische Wochenschrift*, no. 26.

Bennett, M. R., 1978, The treatment of Stage III squamous carcinoma of the cervix in air and hyperbaric oxygen. *British Journal of Radiology*, **51**, 68 (abstract).

Bergonié, J. and Tribondeau, L., 1906, *Comptes Rendus de l'Académie des Sciences*, **143**, 983 (1959, Translation of original article: Interpretation of some results of

radiotherapy and an attempt at determining a logical technique of treatment. *Radiation Research*, 11, 587−94).
Berry, R. J., Wiernik, G., Patterson, R. J. S. and Hopewell, J. W., 1974, Excess late subcutaneous fibrosis after irradiation of pigskin consequent upon the application of the NSD formula. *British Journal of Radiology*, 47, 277−81.
Bertalanffy, F. D. and Leblond, C. P., 1953, The continuous renewal of the two types of alveolar cells in the lungs of the rat. *Anatomical Record*, 115, 515.
Blackett, N. M., Roylance, P. J. and Adams, K., 1964, Studies of the capacity of bone-marrow cells to restore erythropoiesis in heavily irradiated rats. *British Journal of Haematology*, 10, 453−467.
Blackett, N. M., 1968, Investigation of bone-marrow stem cell proliferation in normal, anemic, and irradiated rats, using methotrexate and tritiated thymidine. *Journal of the National Cancer Institute*, 41, 909−18.
Bogaert, W. van den, van der Schueren, E., Tongelen, C. V., Horiot, J. C., Chaplain, G., Arcangeli, G., Gonzalez, D. and Svoboda, V., 1985, Late results of multiple fractions per day (MFD) with misonidazole in advanced cancer of the head and neck. A pilot study of the EORTC radiotherapy group, *Radiotherapy and Oncology*, 3, 139−44.
Bond, V. P., Fliedner, T. M. and Archambeau, J. O., 1965, *Mammalian Radiation Lethality: A Disturbance in Cellular Kinetics* (New York: Academic Press).
Borak, J., 1937, Spätergebnisse der fraktionierten Langbestrahlungsmethode. *Strahlentherapie*, 58, 585−94.
Braby, L. A. and Roesch, W. C., 1978, Testing of dose-rate models with *Chlamydomonas reinhardi*. *Radiation Research*, 76, 259−70.
Braun, R. and Holthusen, H., 1929, Einfluss der Quantengrösse auf die biologische Wirkung verschiedener Röntgenstrahlenqualitäten. *Strahlentherapie*, 34, 707−34.
Breiter, N. and Trott, K. R., 1986. Chronic radiation damage in the rectum of the rat after protracted fractionated irradiation. *Radiotherapy and Oncology*, 7, 155−64.
Brenk, H. A. S. van den, 1971, Radiation effects on the pulmonary system. In *Pathology of Irradiation*, edited by C. C. Berdjis (Baltimore: Williams and Wilkins), pp. 569−91.
Broerse, J. J., 1969, Dose mortality studies for mice irradiated with X-rays, gamma rays, and 15 MeV neutrons. *International Journal of Radiation Biology*, 15, 115−24.
Broerse, J. J. and Barendsen, G. W., 1969, Recovery of cultured cells after fast-neutron irradiation. *International Journal of Radiation Biology*, 15, 335−9.
Brown, J. M., 1970, The effect of acute X-irradiation on the cell proliferation kinetics of induced carcinomas and their normal counterpart. *Radiation Research*, 43, 627−53.
Brown, J. M., 1985, Sensitizers and protectors in radiotherapy. *Cancer*, 55, (Suppl.), 2222−8.
Brown, J. M. and Berry, R. J., 1969, Effects of X-irradiation on the cell population kinetics in a model tumour and normal tissue system: implications for the treatment of human malignancies. *British Journal of Radiology*, 42, 372−7.
Brown, J. M. and Probert, J. C., 1975, Early and late radiation changes following a second course of irradiation. *Radiology*, 115, 711−16.
Broxmeyer, H. E., Galbraith, P. R. and Baker, F. L., 1976, Relationship of colony-stimulating activity to apparent kill of human colony forming cells by irradiation and hydroxyurea. *Blood*, 47, 403−11.
Burrows, E. H., 1986, *Pioneers and Early Years: A History of British Radiology* (London: Colophon Limited).
Byhardt, R. W., Greenberg, M. and Cox, J. D., 1977, Local control of squamous carcinoma of oral cavity and oropharynx with 3 versus 5 treatment fractions per week. *International Journal of Radiation Oncology Biology Physics*, 2, 415−20.
Cairns, J. 1975, Mutation selection and the natural history of cancer. *Nature*, 255, 197−200.
Caldwell, W. L., 1975, Time-dose factors in fatal post-irradiation nephritis. *Cell Survival after Low Doses of Radiation*, edited by T. Alper (Bristol: J. Wright), pp. 328−32.
Calkins, J., 1971, A method of analysis of radiation response based on enzyme kinetics. *Radiation Research*, 45, 50−62.
Casarett, G. W., 1964, Similarities and contrasts between radiation and time pathology.

*Advances in Gerontological Research*, edited by B. Strehler (New York: Academic Press), pp. 109—63.
Casarett, G. W., 1981, *Radiation Histopathology*, 2 Vols. (Boca Raton, Florida : CRC Press).
Chaoul, H., 1932, Über den Einfluss der Verdünnung und Fraktionierung der R-dosis auf die Hautreaktion. *Fortschritte Röntgenstrahlen*, 46, 83—5.
Chen, F. D., 1986, *A cellular analysis of residual injury in skin*. Ph.D. Thesis, University of Manchester (U.K.).
Chen, F. D. and Hendry, J. H., 1986a, The radiosensitivity of microcolony- and macrocolony-forming cells in mouse tail epidermis. *British Journal of Radiology*, 59, 389—95.
Chen, F. D. and Hendry, J. H., 1986b, Effects of field size on the incidence of skin healing and the survival of epidermal colony-forming cells after irradiation. *British Journal of Cancer*, 53 *(Supplement VII)*, 73—4.
Chen, K. Y. and Withers, H. R., 1972, Survival characteristics of stem cells of gastric mucosa in C3H mice subjected to localized gamma irradiation. *International Journal of Radiation Biology*, 21, 521—34.
Chervenick, P. A. and Boggs, D. R., 1971, Patterns of proliferation and differentiation of hematopoietic stem cells after compartment depletion. *Blood*, 37, 568—80.
Choi, C. H. and Suit, H. D., 1975, Evaluation of rapid radiation treatment schedules utilizing two treatment sessions per day. *Radiology*, 116, 703—707.
Choi, K. N., Withers, H. R. and Rotman, M., 1985, Metastatic melanoma in brain: rapid treatment of large dose fractions. *Cancer*, 56, 10—15.
Christie Hospital and Holt Radium Institute, Manchester, 1939, Five year statistical report on the results of radium therapy for the years 1932—1933. (Stockport: R. Berry and Co. Ltd,).
Chwalinski, S. and Potten, C. S., 1986, Radiation-induced mitotic delay: duration, dose and cell position dependence in the crypts of the small intestine in the mouse. *International Journal of Radiation Biology*, 49, 809—19.
Coggle, J. E., 1987, Proliferation of type II pneumonocytes after X-irradiation. *International Journal of Radiation Biology*, 57, 393—9.
Cohen, L., 1949a, Clinical radiation dosage, Pt.I, *British Journal of Radiology*, 22, 160—3.
Cohen, L., 1949b, Clinical radiation dosage, Pt. II, *British Journal of Radiology*, 22, 706—13.
Cohen, L., 1952, Radiotherapy in breast cancer. 1. The dose—time relationship: theoretical considerations. *British Journal of Radiology*, 25, 636—42.
Cohen, L., 1960, The statistical prognosis in radiation therapy: a study of optimal dosage in relation to physical and biological parameters for epidermoid cancer. *American Journal of Roentgenology*, 84, 741—9.
Cohen, L., 1966, Radiation response and recovery: radiobiological principles and their relation to clinical practice. In *The Biological Basis of Radiation Therapy*, edited by E. E. Schwartz (London: Pitman), pp. 208—348.
Cohen, L., 1983, *Biophysical Models in Radiation Oncology*. (Boca Raton, Florida: CRC Press).
Cohen, L. and Kerrich, J. E., 1951, Estimation of biological dosage factors in clinical radiotherapy. *British Journal of Cancer*, 5, 180—94.
Cohen, L. and Scott, M. J., 1968, Fractionation procedures in radiation therapy: a computerized approach to evaluation. *British Journal of Radiology*, 41, 529—33.
Cole, M. P. and Hunter, R. D., 1985, Female genital tract. In *The Radiotherapy of Malignant Disease*, edited by E. C. Easson and R. C. S. Pointon (Berlin, Heidelberg, New York, Tokyo: Springer-Verlag) pp. 281—309.
Coultas, P. G., 1984, Type II cell turnover after lung irradiation. *British Journal of Radiology*, 57, 440 (Abstract).
Coutard, H., 1929, Die Röntgenbehandlung der epithelialen Krebse der Tonsillengegend. *Strahlentherapie*, 33, 249—52.
Coutard, H., 1932, Roentgentherapy of epitheliomas of the tonsillar region, hypopharynx, and larynx from 1920 to 1926. *American Journal of Roentgenology*, 28, 313—31 and 343—8.

Coutard, H., 1934, Principles of X-ray therapy of malignant disease. *Lancet*, 2, 1–8.
Coutard, H., 1937, Röntgentherapie der Karzinome. *Strahlentherapie*, 58, 561–4.
Cowell, M. A. C., 1937, 14th Annual Report, British Empire Cancer Campaign, 97–130.
Cowell, M. A. C., 1938, 15th Annual Report, British Empire Cancer Campaign, 162–72.
Cox, R. and Masson, W. K., 1974, Changes in radiosensitivity during the *in vitro* growth of diploid human fibroblasts. *International Journal of Radiation Biology*, 26, 193–6.
Cox, J. D., Byhardt, R. W., Komaki, R. and Greenberg, M., 1980, Reduced fractionation and the potential of hypoxic cell sensitizers in irradiation of malignant epithelial tumours. *International Journal of Radiation Oncology Biology Physics*, 6, 37–40.
Croizat, H., Frindel, E. and Tubiana, M., 1979, Long-term radiation effects on the bone marrow stem cells of C3H mice. *International Journal of Radiation Biology*, 36, 91–9.
Curtis, H. J., 1967, Biological mechanisms of delayed radiation damage in mammals. *Current Topics in Radiation Research*, 3, edited by M. Ebert and A. Howard (Amsterdam: North Holland), pp. 139–74.
Curtis, S. B., 1982, Ideas on the unification of radiobiological theories. *Lawrence Berkeley Laboratory Report*, 13159.
Curtis, S. B., 1986, Lethal and potentially lethal lesions induced by radiation – a unified repair model. *Radiation Research*, 106, 252–71.
Dale, R. G., Trott, K. R. and Huczkowski, J., 1987, Dose rate dependence of recovery kinetics as deduced from a linear-quadratic analysis of the effects of fractionated irradiations at varying dose rates. *British Journal of Radiology* (in press).
Davis, L. W., Moss, W., Leibel, S., Newall, J., Sagerman, R., Sunthaligam, N. and Wassermann, T., 1985, Essentials and guidelines for radiation oncology residency training programs. *International Journal of Radiation Oncology Biology Physics*, 11, 1009–16.
Deeg, H. J., Storb, R. and Thomas, E. D., 1984, Bone marrow transplantation: A review of delayed complications. *British Journal of Haematology*, 57, 185–208.
Denekamp, J., Ball, M. M. and Fowler, J. F., 1969, Recovery and repopulation in mouse skin as a function of time after X-irradiation. *Radiation Research*, 30, 361–70.
Denekamp, J., 1970, The cellular proliferation kinetics of animal tumors. *Cancer Research*, 30, 393–400.
Denekamp, J., 1972, The relationship between the 'cell loss factor' and the immediate response to radiation in animal tumours. *European Journal of Cancer*, 8, 335–40.
Denekamp, J., 1973, Changes in the rate of repopulation during multifraction irradiation of mouse skin. *British Journal of Radiology*, 46, 381–7.
Denekamp, J., 1975, Changes in the rate of proliferation in normal tissues after irradiation. In *Radiation Research: Biomedical, Chemical and Physical Perspectives*, edited by O. F. Nygaard, H. I. Adler and W. K. Sinclair (New York: Academic Press), pp. 810–25.
Denekamp, J., 1977, Tumour regression as a guide to prognosis: a study with experimental animals. *British Journal of Radiology*, 50, 271–9.
Denekamp, J., 1986, Cell kinetics and radiation biology. *International Journal of Radiation Biology*, 59, 357–80.
Denekamp, J. and Fowler, J. F., 1977, Cell proliferation kinetics and radiation therapy. *Cancer*, 6, edited by F. F. Becker (New York and London: Plenum), pp. 101–37.
Denekamp, J. and Thomlinson, R. H., 1971, The cell proliferation kinetics of four experimental tumours after acute X-irradiation. *Cancer Research*, 31, 1279–84.
Denekamp, J., Stewart, F. A. and Douglas, B. G., 1976, Changes in the proliferation rate of mouse epidermis after irradiation: continuous labelling studies. *Cell and Tissue Kinetics*, 9, 19–29.
Deschavannes, P. J., Fertil, B. and Malaise, E., 1980a, Radiosensitivity and repair of radiation damage in human HF19 fibroblasts. *International Journal of Radiation Biology*, 38, 167–77.
Deschavannes, P. J., Guichard, M. and Malaise, E. P., 1980b, Radiosensitivity of mouse kidney cells determined with an *in vitro* colony method. *International Journal of Radiation Oncology Biology Physics*, 6, 1551–8.
Devik, F., 1962, Studies on the duration of DNA-synthesis and mitosis in irradiated and regenerating epidermis cells in mice, by means of tritium-labelled thymidine. *International Journal of Radiation Biology*, 5, 59–66.

Dische, S., Martin, W. M. C. and Anderson, P., 1981, Radiation myelopathy in patients treated for carcinoma of bronchus using a six fraction regime of radiotherapy. *British Journal of Radiology*, **54**, 29–35.

Douglas, B. G., 1982a, Implications of the quadratic cell survival curve and human skin radiation 'tolerance doses' on fractionation and superfractionation dose selection. *International Journal of Radiation Oncology Biology Physics*, **8**, 1135–42.

Douglas, B. G., 1982b, Superfractionation: its rationale and anticipated benefits. *International Journal of Radiation Oncology Biology Physics*, **8**, 1143–53.

Douglas, B. G. and Worth, A., 1982, Superfractionation in glioblastoma multiforme: Results of a phase II study. *International Journal of Radiation Oncology Biology Physics*, **8**, 1787–94.

Douglas, B. G. and Fowler, J. F., 1976, The effect of multiple small doses of X-rays on skin reactions in the mouse and a basic interpretation. *Radiation Research*, **66**, 401–26.

Down, J. D. and Steel, G. G., 1983, The expression of early and late damage after thoracic irradiations: A comparison between CBA and C57BL mice. *Radiation Research*, **96**, 603–10.

Down, J. D., Easton, D. F. and Steel, G. G., 1986, Repair in mouse lung during low dose-rate irradiation. *Radiotherapy Oncology*, **6**, 29–42.

Dritschillo, A., Bruckman, T. E., Cassady, J. R. and Belli, J. A., 1981, Tolerance of brain to multiple courses of radiation therapy. 1. Clinical experiences. *British Journal of Radiology*, **54**, 782–6.

Duffy, J., Arnesen, A. N. and Edward, L. V., 1934. The rate of recuperation of human skin following irradiation. *Radiology*, **23**, 486–90.

DuSault, L. A., 1956, Time–dose relationships. *Radiology*, **75**, 597–606.

Duthie, M. B. and Gupta, N. K., 1985, Head and neck. In *The Radiotherapy of Malignant Disease*, edited by E. C. Easson and R. C. S. Pointon (Berlin, Heidelberg, New York, Tokyo: Springer-Verlag), pp. 154–213.

Dutreix, J. and Sahatchiev, A., 1975, Clinical radiobiology of low dose-rate radiotherapy. *British Journal of Radiology*, **48**, 846–50.

Dutreix, J., Wambersie, A. and Bounik, C., 1973, Cellular recovery in human skin reactions. Application to dose, fraction number, overall time relationship in radiotherapy. *European Journal of Cancer*, **9**, 159–67.

Dyke, J. van, Keane, T. J., Kans, et al., 1981, Radiation pneumonitis following large single dose irradiation. A re-evaluation based on absolute dose to lung. *International Journal of Radiation Oncology Biology Physics*, **1**, 461–7.

Eder, J. M., 1922, Das Jubiläum einer Wiener Entdeckung. *Neue Freie Presse* (7 Jan 1922).

Edsmyr, F., Andersson, L., Espoti, P. L., Littbrand, B. and Nilsson, B., 1985, Irradiation therapy with multiple small fractions per day in urinary bladder cancer. *Radiotherapy and Oncology*, **4**, 197–203.

El-Mofty, S. K. and Kahn, A. J., 1981, Early membrane injury in lethally irradiated salivary gland cells. *International Journal of Radiation Biology*, **39**, 55–62.

Elkind, M. M., 1960, Cellular aspects of tumour therapy. *Radiology*, **74**, 529–41.

Elkind, M. M., 1976, Fractionated dose radiotherapy and its relationship to survival curve shape. *Cancer Treatment Review*, **3**, 1–15.

Elkind, M. M., 1977, The initial part of the survival curve. Implications for low-dose, low-dose-rate responses. *Radiation Research*, **71**, 9–23.

Elkind, M. M. and Sutton, H., 1959, X-ray damage and recovery in mammalian cells in culture. *Nature*, **184**, 1293–5.

Elkind, M. M. and Sutton, H., 1960, Radiation response of mammalian cells grown in culture. I. Repair of X-ray damage in surviving Chinese hamster ovary cells. *Radiation Research*, **13**, 556–93.

Elkind, M. M. and Whitmore, G. F., 1967, *The Radiobiology of Cultured Mammalian Cells*, (New York: Gordon & Breach).

Elkind, M. M., Han, A. and Volz, K. W., 1963, Radiation response of mammalian cells grown in culture. IV. Dose dependence of division delay and postirradiation growth of surviving and nonsurviving Chinese hamster ovary cells. *Journal of the National Cancer Institute*, **30**, 705–21.

Elkind, M. M., Sutton-Gilbert, H., Moses, W. B., Alescio, T. and Swain, R. W., 1965,

Radiation response of mammalian cells grown in culture. *Radiation Research*, **25**, 359–76.
Ellis, F., 1942, Tolerance dosage in radiotherapy with 200 kV X-rays. *British Journal of Radiology*, **15**, 348–50.
Ellis, F., 1963, Fractionation and dose-rate. *British Journal of Radiology*, **36**, 153–62.
Ellis, F., 1967, Fractionation in radiotherapy. In *Modern Trends in Radiotherapy*, Vol. 1, edited by Deeley and Wood (London: Butterworths), pp. 34–51.
Ellis, F., 1968a, Time, fractionation and dose-rate in radiotherapy. *Frontiers of Radiation Therapy Oncology*, **3**, 131–40.
Ellis, F., 1968b, The relationship of biological effect to dose-time-fractionation factors in radiotherapy. In *Current Topics in Radiation Research*, Vol. 4, edited by M. Ebert and A. Howard (Amsterdam: North Holland Publishing Co.), pp. 359–97.
Ellis, F., 1969, Dose time and fractionation; a clinical hypothesis. *Clinical Radiology*, **20**, 1–7.
Emery, E. W., Denekamp, J., Ball, M. M. and Field, S. B., 1970, Survival of mouse skin epithelial cells following single and divided doses of X-rays. *Radiation Research*, **41**, 450–66.
Essen, C. F., von, 1960, Roentgen therapy of skin and lip carcinoma: factors influencing success and failure. *American Journal of Roentgenology*, **83**, 556–72.
Etoh, H., Taguchi, Y. H. and Tabachnick, J., 1975, Movement of beta-irradiated epidermal basal cells to the spinous-granular layers in the absence of cell division. *Journal of Investigative Dermatology*, **64**, 431–5.
Fajardo, L. F. and Stewart, J. R., 1971, Capillary injury preceding radiation-induced myocardial fibrosis. *Radiology*, **101**, 425–33.
Field, S. B., Hornsey, S. and Kutsutani, Y., 1976, Effects of fractionated irradiation on mouse lung and a phenomenon of slow repair. *British Journal of Radiology*, **49**, 700–7.
Field, S. B. and Upton, A. C., 1985, Non-stochastic effects: compatibility with present ICRP recommendations. *International Journal of Radiation Biology*, **48**, 81–94.
Fisher, D. R., 1985, *Studies on residual damage in irradiated liver*, Ph.D. Thesis, University of Manchester, UK.
Fisher, D. R. and Hendry, J. H., 1986. Response of clonogenic hepatocytes to fractionated irradiation. *British Journal of Cancer*, **53**, (Suppl. VII), 298–9.
Fisher, D. R. and Hendry, J. H., 1987, Dose fractionation and hepatocyte clonogens: $\alpha/\beta \simeq 1-2$ Gy, and decreases with increasing delay before assay. *Radiation Research* (submitted).
Fisher, D. R., Hendry, J. H. and Scott, D., 1987, Long-term repair *in vivo* of colony-forming ability and chromosomal injury in X-irradiated mouse hepatocytes. *Radiation Research* (submitted).
Fletcher, G. H., 1980, *Textbook of Radiotherapy*, 3rd edition. (Philadelphia: Lea & Febiger), pp. 202–3.
Fletcher, G. H. and Barkley, H. T., 1974, Present status of the time factor in clinical radiotherapy. I. The historical background of the recovery experiments. *Journal de Radiologie et de l'Électrologie*, **55**, 443–51.
Fletcher, G. H., Barkley, H. T. and Shukovsky, L. J., 1974, Present status of the time factor in clinical radiotherapy. II. The nominal standard dose formula. *Journal de Radiologie et de l'Électrologie*, **55**, 745–51.
Fletcher, G. H. and Shukovsky, L. J., 1975, The interplay of radiocurability and tolerance in the irradiation of human cancers. *Journal de Radiologie et de l'Électrologie*, **56**, 383–400.
Fliedner, T. M., Nothdurft, W. and Heit, H., 1984, Biological factors affecting the occurrence of radiation syndromes. In *Response of Different Species to Total Body Irradiations*, edited by J. J. Broerse and T. J. MacVittie, (Dordrecht, The Netherlands: Martinus Nijhoff Publishers), pp. 209–19.
Forssell, G., Berven, E., Reuterwall, O. and Sievert, R., 1939, King Gustav V's Stockholm Jubilee Clinic for Radiotherapy and Research in Cancer. *Acta Radiologica, Suppl.* **38**, 5–80.
Fowler, J. F., 1971, Experimental animal results relating to time–dose relationships in radiotherapy and the 'ret' concept. *British Journal of Radiology*, **44**, 81–90.

Fowler, J. F., 1983, Dose—response curves for organ function or cell survival. *British Journal of Radiology*, 56, 497—500.
Fowler, J. F., 1984a, Review: Total doses in fractionated radiotherapy—implications of new radiobiological data. *International Journal of Radiation Biology*, 46, 103—20.
Fowler, J. F., 1984b, What next in fractionated radiotherapy? *British Journal of Cancer*, 49, Suppl. VI, 285—300.
Fowler, J. F., 1985, Chemical modifiers of radiosensitivity. Theory and reality. *International Journal of Radiation Oncology, Biology, and Physics*, 11, 665—74.
Fowler, J. F., 1986, Fading times required for apparently complete repair in irradiated tissues. *International Journal of Radiation Biology*, 50, 601—7.
Fowler, J. F. and Stern, B. E., 1960, Dose-rate effects: some theoretical and practical considerations. *British Journal of Radiology*, 33, 389—95.
Fowler, J. F. and Stern, B. E., 1963, Dose—time relationships in radiotherapy and the validity of cell survival curve models. *British Journal of Radiology*, 36, 163—72.
Fowler, J. F., Denekamp, J., Delapeyre, C., Harris, S. and Sheldon, P., 1974, Skin reactions in mice after multifraction X-irradiation. *International Journal of Radiation Biology*, 25, 213—23.
Fowler, J. F., Joiner, M. C. and Williams, M. V., 1983, Low doses per fraction in radiotherapy: a definition for flexure dose. *British Journal of Radiology*, 56, 599—602.
Fowler, J. F., Morgan, M. A., Silvester, J. A., Bewley, D. K. and Turner, B. A., 1963, Experiments with fractionated X-ray treatment of the skin of pigs. I. Fractionation up to 28 days. *British Journal of Radiology*, 36, 188—96.
Frankfurt, O. S., 1967, Cell proliferation and differentiation in the squamous epithelium of the forestomach of the mouse. *Experimental Cell Research*, 46, 603—6.
Freund, L., 1897a, Ein mit Röntgen-Strahlen behandelter Fall von Naevus pigmentosus piliferus. *Wiener Medizinische Wochenschrift*, 47 (Number 10), 428—34.
Freund, L., 1897b, Nachtrag zu den Artikel 'Ein mit Röntgen-Strahlen behandelter Fall von Naevus pigmentosus pilferus'. *Wiener Medizinische Wochenschrift*, 47, (Number 19), 856—60.
Freund, L., 1927, Zur Geschichte der 'Schwachbestrahlung'. *Strahlentherapie*, 25, 593—6.
Freund, L., 1937, 40 Jahre österreichische Forschungsarbeit auf dem Gebiete der medizinischen Röntgenologie. *Strahlentherapie*, 58, 499—522.
Freund, L., 1948, Ein Beitrag zur Geschichte der Entstehung der Röntgentherapie. *Neuburger-Festschrift* (Vienna), pp. 144—51.
Fu, K. K., Newman, H. and Phillips, T. L., 1975, Treatment of locally recurrent carcinoma of the nasopharynx. *Radiology*, 117, 425—31.
Geraci, J. P., Jackson, K. L., Christensen, C. M., Parker, R. G., Fox, M. S. and Thrower, P. D., 1974, The relative biological effectiveness of cyclotron fast neutrons for early and late damage to the small intestine of the mouse. *European Journal of Cancer*, 10, 99—102.
Geraci, J. P., Jackson, K. L., Christensen, C. M., Thrower, P. D. and Weyor, B. S., 1977, Acute and late damage in the mouse intestine following multiple fractionation of neutrons or X-rays. *International Journal of Radiation Oncology Biology Physics*, 2, 693—6.
Gilbert, C. W., 1969, The relationship between the mortality of whole animals and the survival curve for single cells. *International Journal of Radiation Biology*, 16, 287—90.
Gilbert, C. W., Hendry, J. H. and Major, D., 1980, The approximation in the formulation for survival $S = \exp - (\alpha D + \beta D^2)$. *International Journal of Radiation Biology*, 37, 469—71.
Glasser, O., 1937, Roentgentherapie mit Ultraspannungen in Nordamerika. *Strahlentherapie*, 60, 557—74.
Glasser, O., 1959, *Wilhelm Conrad Röntgen und die Geschichte der Röntgenstrahlen* (2nd edition). (Berlin—Göttingen—Heidelberg: Springer-Verlag), pp. 328—67.
Glocker, R., Hayer, Langendorff, H. and U. Reuss, I., 1931, Gesetzmässigkeit der Zeitfaktorwirkung bei Röntgenbestrahlung. *Strahlentherapie*, 42, 148—59.
Gonzales-Gonzales, D., Breur, K. and van den Schueren, E., 1980, Preliminary results in advanced head and neck cancer with radiotherapy by multiple fractions a day. *Clinical Radiology*, 31, 417—21.

Goitein, M., 1976, Review of parameters characterising response of normal connective tissue to radiation. *Clinical Radiology*, **27**, 389—404.

Goodhead, D. T., 1980 Models of radiation inactivation and mutagenesis. In *Radiation Biology in Cancer Research*, edited by R. E. Meyn and H. R. Withers (New York: Raven Press), pp. 231—47.

Gould, M. N. and Clifton, K. H., 1977, The survival of mammary cells following irradiation *in vivo*: a directly generated single-dose-survival curve. *Radiation Research*, **72**, 343—52.

Gould, M. N. and Clifton, K. H., 1979, Evidence for a unique *in situ* component of the repair of radiation damage. *Radiation Research*, **77**, 149—55.

Gragg, R. L., Humphrey, R. M., Thames, H. D. and Meyn, R. E., 1978, The response of Chinese hamster ovary cells to fast-neutron radiotherapy beams. III. Variations in relative biological effectiveness with position in the cell cycle. *Radiation Research*, **76**, 283—91.

Gray, A. J., 1986, Treatment of advanced head and neck cancer with accelerated fractionation. *International Journal of Radiation Oncology Biology Physics*, **12**, 9—12.

Gray, J. W., Dobbeare, F., Pallaricini, M. G., Beisker, W. and Waldman, F., 1986, Cell cycle analysis using flow cytometry. *International Journal of Radiation Biology*, **49**, 237—55.

Gray, L. H. and Scholes, M. E., 1951, The effect of ionizing radiations on the broad bean root — Part VIII. *British Journal of Radiology*, **24**, 285—91.

Green, N. and Melbye, R. W., 1982, Lung cancer: retreatment of local recurrence after definitive irradiation. *Cancer*, **49**, 865—68.

Griem, M. L., Dimitrievich, G. S. and Lee, R. M., 1979, The effect of X-irradiation and adriamycin on proliferating and nonproliferating hair coat of the mouse. *International Journal of Radiation Oncology Biology Physics*, **5**, 1261—4.

Griffin, C. S. and Hornsey, S., 1986, The effect of neutron dose rate on jejunal crypt survival. *International Journal Radiation Biology*, **49**, 589—95.

Guzman, E. and Lajtha, L. G., 1970, Some comparisons of the kinetic properties of femoral and splenic haemopoietic stem cells. *Cell and Tissue Kinetics*, **3**, 91—8.

Hagemann, R. F., 1976, Intestinal cell proliferation during fractionated abdominal irradiation. *British Journal of Radiology*, **49**, 56—61.

Hagemann, R. F. and Concannon, J. P., 1975, Time/dose relationships in abdominal irradiation: a definition of principles and experimental evaluation. *British Journal of Radiology*, **48**, 545—55.

Hagemann, R. F., Sigdestad, C. P. and Lesher, S., 1971, Intestinal crypt survival and total and per crypt levels of proliferative cellularity following irradiation: single X-ray exposures. *Radiation Research*, **46**, 533—46.

Hagemann, R. F., Sigdestad, C. P. and Lesher, S., 1972, Intestinal crypt survival and total and per crypt levels of proliferative cellularity following irradiation: role of crypt cellularity. *Radiation Research*, **50**, 583—91.

Hahn, G. M., 1982 (editor), *Hyperthermia and Cancer* (New York: Plenum Press).

Hall, E. J., 1978, *Radiology for the Radiologist* (Maryland, USA: Harper & Row), p. 460.

Ham, H. J., 1936, 13th Annual Report, British Empire Cancer Campaign, 134—55.

Hamilton, E., 1979, Diurnal variation in proliferative compartments and their relation to cryptogenic cells in the mouse colon. *Cell and Tissue Kinetics*, **12**, 91—100.

Hanks, G. E., Page, N. P., Ainsworth, E. J., Leong, G. F., Menkes, C. K. and Alpen, E. L., 1966, Acute mortality and recovery studies in sheep irradiated with cobalt-60 gamma rays or 1-MV X-rays. *Radiation Research*, **27**, 397—405.

Hayashi, S. and Suit, H. D., 1972, Effect of fractionation of radiation dose on skin contraction and skin reaction of Swiss mice. *Radiology*, **103**, 431 7.

Hegazy, M. A. H. and Fowler, J. F., 1973, Cell population kinetics and desquamation skin reactions in plucked and unplucked mouse skin. II. Irradiated skin. *Cell Tissue Kinetics*, **6**, 587—602.

Heinecke, H., 1903, 1904, Röntgenstrahlenwirkung auf Tiere. *Münchener Medizinische Wochenschrift*, **1903**, No. 48; **1904**, No. 31.

Hendry, J. H., 1972, A difference in haemopoietic stem cell repopulation after D-T neutrons or X-irradiation. *International Journal of Radiation Biology*, **22**, 279—83.

Hendry, J. H., 1973, Differential split-dose radiation response of resting and regenerating haemopoietic stem cells. *International Journal of Radiation Biology*, **24**, 469—73.
Hendry, J. H., 1978, The tolerance of mouse tails to necrosis after repeated irradiation with X-rays. *British Journal of Radiology*, **51**, 808—13.
Hendry, J. H., 1979a, The dose-dependence of the split-dose response of marrow colony-forming units (CFU-S): similarity to other tissues. *International Journal of Radiation Biology*, **36**, 631—7.
Hendry, J. H., 1979b, Regeneration of stem cells in intestinal epithelium after irradiation. *Proceedings of the 6th International Congress of Radiation Research*, edited by S. Okada, M. Imamura, T. Terashima and H. Yamaguchi (Tokyo: Japanese Association for Radiation Research), pp. 664—9.
Hendry, J. H., 1984a, The time course of split-dose sparing using radiation of different LET. *British Journal of Cancer*, **49**, (Suppl. VI), p. 313.
Hendry, J. H., 1984b, Correlation of the dose—response relationships for epidermal colony-forming units, skin reactions and healing, in the X-irradiated mouse tail. *British Journal of Radiology*, **57**, 909—18.
Hendry, J. H., 1985a, The cellular basis of long-term marrow injury after irradiation. *Radiotherapy and Oncology*, **3**, 331—8.
Hendry, J. H., 1985b, Mathematical aspects of colony growth, transplantation kinetics, and cell survival. In *Cell Clones: Manual of Mammalian Cell Techniques*, edited by C. S. Potten and J. H. Hendry (Edinburgh: Churchill-Livingstone), pp. 1—12.
Hendry, J. H., 1985c, Survival curves for normal-tissue clonogens: a comparison of assessments using *in vitro*, transplantation, or *in situ* techniques. *International Journal of Radiation Biology*, **47**, 3—16.
Hendry, J. H., 1987a, Lack of differential sparing of late ischaemic atrophy and early epidermal healing, by dose fractionation of mouse tails down to 2.6 Gy per fraction. *Radiotherapy and Oncology* (in press).
Hendry, J. H., 1987b, Considerations of long-term radiation injury in non-haemopoietic tissues. In *Bone Marrow Damage*, edited by N. G. Testa and R. P. Gale (New York, Marcel Dekker) (in press).
Hendry, J. H. and Fowler, J. F., 1986, Conclusions. Proceedings of the 12th L. H. Gray Conference. *British Journal of Cancer*, **53**, (Suppl. VII), pp. 390—1.
Hendry, J. H. and Lajtha, L. G., 1972, The response of haemopoietic colony-forming units to repeated doses of X-rays. *Radiation Research*, **52**, 309—15.
Hendry, J. H. and Lord, B. I., 1983, The analysis of the early and late response to cytotoxic insults in the haemopoietic cell hierarchy. In *Cytotoxic Insult to Tissue: Effect on Cell Lineages*, edited by C. S. Potten and J. H. Hendry (Edinburgh: Churchill-Livingstone), pp. 1—66.
Hendry, J. H. and Moore, J. V., 1985a, Deriving absolute values of $\alpha$ and $\beta$ for dose fractionation, using dose—incidence data. *British Journal of Radiology*, **58**, 885—90.
Hendry, J. H. and Moore, J. V., 1985b, Is the steepness of dose—incidence curves for tumour control or complications due to variation before, or as a result of, irradiation? *British Journal of Radiology*, **57**, 1045—6.
Hendry, J. H. and Scott, D., 1987, Loss of reproductive integrity of irradiated cells, and its importance in tissues. In *Perspectives on Cell Death*, edited by C. S. Potten (Oxford University Press) (in press).
Hendry, J. H. and Thames, H. D., 1986, The tissue-rescuing unit. (Letter to editor) *British Journal of Radiology*, **59**, 628—30.
Hendry, J. H., Moore, J. V. and Potten, C. S., 1984, The proliferative status of micro-colony forming cells in mouse small intestine. *Cell Tissue Kinetics*, **17**, 41—7.
Hendry, J. H., Testa, N. G. and Lajtha, L. G., 1974, Effect of repeated doses of X-rays or 14 MeV neutrons on mouse bone marrow. *Radiation Research*, **59**, 645—52.
Hendry, J. H., Major, D. and Greene, D., 1975, Daily D-T neutron irradiation of mouse intestine. *Radiation Research*, **63**, 149—56.
Hendry, J. H., Edmundson, J. M. and Potten, C. S., 1980, The radiosensitivity of hair follicles in mouse dorsum and tail. *Radiation Research*, **84**, 87—96.
Hendry, J. H., Potten, C. S. and Chadwick, C., 1982, Cell death (apoptosis) in the mouse

small intestine after low doses: effects of dose-rate, 14.7 MeV neutrons, and 600 MeV (maximum energy) neutrons. *International Journal of Radiation Biology*, 42, 611−20.
Hendry, J. H., Xu, C. X. and Testa, N. G., 1983a, A cellular analysis of residual haemopoietic deficiencies in mice after four graded doses of 4.5 Gy. *International Journal of Radiation Oncology Biology Physics*, 9, 1641−6.
Hendry, J. H., Potten, C. S. and Roberts, N. P., 1983b, The gastrointestinal syndrome and mucosal clonogenic cells: Relationships between target cell sensitivities, LD50 and cell survival, and their modification by antibiotics. *Radiation Research*, 96, 100−12.
Hendry, J. H., Schofield, R. and Bwire, N. E. B., 1986, Radiosensitivity of murine haemopoietic colony-forming units assayed *in situ* in the rib and in other marrow sites. *Radiation Research*, 105, 370−8.
Henk, J. M., 1986, Late results of trial of hyperbaric oxygen and radiotherapy in head and neck cancer: a rationale for hypoxic cell sensitizers? *International Journal of Radiation Oncology Biology Physics*, 12, 1339−41.
Henk, J. M. and Smith, C. W., 1977, Radiotherapy and hyberbaric oxygen in head and neck cancer. Interim report of second clinical trial. *Lancet*, 2, 104−5.
Henk, J. M., Kunkler, P. B. and Smith, C. W., 1977, Radiotherapy and hyperbaric oxygen in head and neck cancer. Final report of first controlled clinical trial. *Lancet*, 9, 101−3.
Henkelman, R. M., Lam, G. K. Y., Kornelsen, R. O. and Eaves, C. J., 1980, Explanation of dose-rate and split-dose effects on mouse foot reactions using the same time factor. *Radiation Research*, 84, 276−89.
Herbert, D. E., 1986, Clinical dose response models. I. Regression diagnostics and biased estimation. In *Multiple Regression Analysis − Applications in the Health Sciences*, edited by D. E. Herbert and R. H. Myers (New York: American Institute of Physics), pp. 208−306.
Hermens, A. F. and Barendsen, G. W., 1969, Changes in cell proliferation characteristics in a rat rhabdomyosarcoma before and after X-irradiation. *European Journal of Cancer*, 5, 173−89.
Hethcote, H. W., McLarty, J. W. and Thames, H. D., 1976, Comparison of mathematical models for radiation fractionation. *Radiation Research*, 67, 387−407.
Hill, R. P., 1983, Response of mouse lung to irradiation at different dose-rates. *International Journal of Radiation Oncology Biology Physics*, 9, 1043−7.
Hliniak, A., Maciejewski, B. and Trott, K-R., 1983, The influence of the number of fractions, overall treatment time and field size on the local control of cancer of the skin. *British Journal of Radiology*, 56, 596−8.
Hoffman, J. G. and Reinhard, M. C., 1934, Some mathematical aspects of radiation dosage. *Radiology*, 23, 737−42.
Holsti, L. R., 1969, Clinical experience with split-course radiotherapy: a randomized clinical trial. *Radiology*, 92, 591−6.
Holthusen, H., 1933, Vergleichende Untersuchungen uber die Wirkung von Röntgen- and Radiumstrahlen. *Strahlentherapie*, 46, 273−88.
Holthusen, H. and Braun, R., 1933, *Grundlagen und Praxis der Röntgenstrahlendosierung*. Leipzig 1933.
Holzknecht, G., 1902, Das Chromoradiometer. Presentation at Congresse International d'Electrologie.
Hopewell, J. W., 1980, The importance of vascular damage in the development of late radiation effects in normal tissues. In *Radiation Biology in Cancer Research*, edited by R. E. Meyn and H. R. Withers (New York: Raven Press), pp. 449−59.
Hopewell, J. W., 1986, Mechanisms of action of radiation on skin and underlying tissues. *British Journal of Radiology*, (Suppl. 19) 39−47.
Hopewell, J. W. and Wright, E. A., 1970, The nature of latent cerebral irradiation damage, and its modification by hypertension. *British Journal of Radiology*, 43, 161−7.
Horiot, J.-C., Fletcher, G. H., Ballantyne, A. J. and Lindberg, R. D., 1972, Analysis of failures in early vocal cord cancer. *Radiology*, 103, 663−5.
Horiot, J.-C., van den Bogaert, W., de Pauw, M., van Glabbeke, M., Gonzales, D. G. and van der Schueren, E., 1985, EORTC prospective trials of altered fractionation using multiple fractions per day (MFD). *Plenary Session Proceedings, XVI International Congress of Radiology*, Honolulu, Hawaii, pp. 95−8.

Hornsey, S., 1973a, The effectiveness of fast neutrons compared with low LET radiation on cell survival measured in the mouse jejunum. *Radiation Research*, 55, 58−68.

Hornsey, S., 1973b, The radiosensitivity of the intestine. *Strahlenschutz Forschung und Praxis*, 13, 79−87.

Hornsey, S. and Alper, T., 1966, Unexpected dose-rate effect in the killing of mice by radiation. *Nature*, 210, pp. 212−13.

Hornsey, S. and Vatistas, S., 1963, Some characteristics of the survival curve of crypt cells of the small intestine of the mouse deduced after whole-body irradiation. *British Journal of Radiology*, 36, 795−800.

Hornsey, S., Kutsutani, Y. and Field, S. B., 1975, Damage to mouse lung with fractionated neutrons and X-rays. *Radiology*, 116, 171−176.

Hornsey, S., Andreozzi, U. and Warren, P. R., 1977, Sublethal damage in cells of the mouse gut after mixed treatment with X-rays and fast neutrons. *British Journal of Radiology*, 50, 513−17.

Hornsey, S., Myers, R., Coultas, P. G., Rogers, M. A. and White, A., 1981a, Turnover of proliferative cells in the spinal cord after X-irradiation and its relation to time-dependent repair of radiation damage. *British Journal of Radiology*, 54, 1081−3.

Hornsey, S., Morris, C. C., Myers, R. and White, A., 1981b, Relative biological effectiveness for damage to the central nervous system by neutrons. *International Journal of Radiation Oncology, Biology, Physics*, 7, 185−9.

Hornsey, S., Myers, R. and Warren, P., 1982, Residual injury in the spinal cord after treatment with X-rays or neutrons. *British Journal of Radiology*, 55, 516−9.

Hornsey, S., Rogers, M. A. and Myers, R., 1983, Differences in time-dependent repair in brain and spinal cord. *British Journal of Radiology*, 56, 898 (abstract).

Howard, A. and Pelc, S. R., 1953, Synthesis of deoxyribonucleic acid in normal and irradiated cells and its relation to chromosome breakage. *Heredity* (Suppl.), 6, 261−73. Republished 1986 in *International Journal of Radiation Biology*, 49, 207−218.

Huczkowski, J. and Trott, K. R., 1984, Dose fractionation effects in low dose rate irradiation of jejunal crypt stem cells. *International Journal of Radiation Biology*, 46, 293−8.

Huczkowski, J. and Trott, K. R., 1987, Jejunal crypt stem-cell survival after fractionated $\gamma$-irradiation performed at different dose rates. *International Journal of Radiation Biology*, 51, 131−7.

Hunter, R. D. and Stewart, J. G., 1977, Tolerance to re-irradiation of heavily irradiated human skin. *British Journal of Radiology*, 50, 573−5.

ICRP 26, 1977, Recommendation of the International Commission on Radiological Protection. *Annals of the ICRP*, 1, No. 3 (Oxford: Pergamon Press).

ICRP 27, 1977, Problems involved in developing an index of harm. *Annals of the ICRP*, 1, No. 4 (Oxford: Pergamon Press).

ICRP 41, 1984, Nonstochastic effects of ionizing radiation. *Annals of the ICRP*, 14, No. 3, (Oxford: Pergamon Press).

Iliakis, G., 1980, Effects of $\beta$-arabinofuranosyladenine on the growth and repair of potentially lethal damage in Ehrlich ascites tumor cells. *Radiation Research*, 83, 537−52.

Iversen, O. H., Bjerknes, R., Iversen, U., Ziegler, J. L. and Bluming, A. Z., 1976, Cell kinetics in Burkitt's lymphoma. In *Growth Kinetics and Biochemical Regulation of Normal and Malignant Cells*, edited by B. Drewinko and R. M. Humphrey (Baltimore: Williams & Wilkins), pp. 675−86.

Jammet, H., Daburon, F., Gerber, G. B., Hopewell, J. W., Haybittle, J. L. and Whitfield, L., editors, 1986, Radiation damage to skin: fundamental and practical aspects. *British Journal of Radiology* (Supplement 19), 159.

Jampolis, S., Pipard, G., Horiot, J.-C., Bolla, M. and Lee Dorze, C., 1977, Preliminary results using twice-a-day fractionation in the radiotherapeutic management of advanced cancers of the head and neck. *American Journal of Roentgenology*, 129, 1091−3.

Jellinger, K. and Sturm, K. W., 1971, Delayed radiation myelopathy in man. *Journal of Neurological Sciences*, 14, 389−408.

Jirtle, R. L., McLain, J. R., Strom, S. C. and Michalopoulos, G., 1982, Repair of radiation damage in non-cycling parenchymal hepatocytes. *British Journal of Radiology*, 55, 847—51.

Joiner, M. C., Denekamp, J. and Maughan, R. L., 1986, The use of 'top-up' experiments to investigate the effect of very small doses per fraction in mouse skin. *International Journal of Radiation Biology*, 49, 565—80.

Jolles, B. and Mitchell, R. G., 1947, Optimal skin tolerance dose levels. *British Journal of Radiology*, 20, 405—9.

Joshi, G. P., Nelson, W. J., Revell, S. H. and Shaw, C. A., 1982, Discrimination of slow growth from non-survival among small colonies of diploid Syrian hamster cells after chromosome damage induced by a range of x-ray doses. *International Journal of Radiation Biology*, 42, 283—96.

Jüngling, O., 1924, *Röntgentherapie chirurgischen Krankheiten* (Leipzig), p. 237.

Kal, H. B., 1974, Responses of a rat rhabdomyosarcoma and rat skin to irradiation with gamma rays and 15 MeV neutrons at low dose rate. Ph. D. Thesis, University of Amsterdam, Radiobiological Institute TNO, Rijswijk.

Kal, H. B., Barendsen, G. W., Bakker-Van Hauwe, R. and Roelse, H., 1975, Increased radiosensitivity of rat rhabdomyosarcoma cells induced by protracted irradiation. *Radiation Research*, 63, 521—30.

Kappos, A. and Pohlit, W., 1972, A cybernetic model of radiation reactions in living cells. I. Sparsely ionizing radiations; stationary cells. *International Journal of Radiation Biology*, 22, 51—65.

Katz, H. R. and Alberts, R. W., 1983, A comparison of high-dose continuous and split-course irradiation in non-oat-cell carcinoma of the lung. *American Journal of Clinical Oncology*, 6, 445—57.

Kellerer, A. M. and Rossi, H. H., 1972, The theory of dual radiation action. *Current Topics Radiation Research Quarterly*, 8, 85—158.

Kerr, J. F. R., Wyllie, A. H. and Currie, A. R., 1972, Apoptosis: A basic biological phenomenon with wide-ranging implications in tissue kinetics. *British Journal of Cancer*, 26, 239—57.

Kienböck, R., 1900a, Absorptionsgesetz. *Wiener Klinische Wochenschrift*, No. 50.

Kienböck, R., 1900b, Über die Einwirkung der Röntgenlicht auf die Haut. *Wiener Klinische Wochenschrift*, 13, 1153—66.

Kienböck, R., 1901, Zur Pathologie der Hautveränderungen durch Röntgenbestrahlung bei Mensch und Thier. *Wiener Medizinische Presse*, 42, 873—1040.

Kim, J. H., Chu, F. C. H. and Hilaris, B., 1975. The influence of dose fractionation on acute and late reactions in patients with postoperative radiotherapy for carcinoma of the breast. *Cancer*, 35, 1583—6.

Kingery, L. B., 1920, Saturation in roentgen therapy: Its estimation and maintenance. *Archives of Dermatology*, 1, 423—33.

Kirk, J., Gray, W. M. and Watson, E. R., 1971, Cumulative radiation effect. Part I. Fractionated treatment regimes. *Clinical Radiology*, 22, 145—55.

Kirk, J., Gray, W. M. and Watson, E. R., 1972, Cumulative radiation effect. Part II. Continuous radiation therapy: long-lived sources. *Clinical Radiology*, 23, 93—105.

Kirk, J., Gray, W. M. and Watson, E. R., 1975, Cumulative radiation effect. Part V. Time gaps in treatment regimes. *Clinical Radiology*, 26, 159—76.

Knee, R., Fields, R. S. and Peters, L. J., 1985, Concomitant boost radiotherapy for advanced squamous cell carcinoma of the head and neck. *Radiotherapy and Oncology*, 4, 1—7.

Knospe, W. H., Blom, J. and Crosby, W. H., 1966, Local irradiation of bone marrow. I. Dose dependent, long-term changes in the rat with particular emphasis upon vascular and stromal effects. *Blood*, 28, 398—415.

Kogel, A. J. van der, 1977, Radiation tolerance of the rat spinal cord: time—dose relationship. *Radiology*, 122, 505—509.

Kogel, A. J. van der, 1979, *Late effects of radiation on the spinal cord*. Ph.D. Thesis, University of Amsterdam, Radiobiological Institute of the Organisation for Health Research TNO, Rijswijk, The Netherlands.

Kogel, A. J. van der, 1980, Mechanisms of late radiation injury in the spinal cord. In

Radiation Biology in Cancer Research, edited by R. G. Meyn and H. R. Withers (New York: Raven Press), pp. 461–70.

Kogel, A. J. van der, 1983, The cellular basis of radiation induced damage in the central nervous system. In *Cytotoxic Insult to Tissue: Effects on Cell Lineages*, edited by C. S. Potten and J. H. Hendry (Churchill-Livingstone: Edinburgh), pp. 329–52.

Kogel, A. J. van der, 1986, Radiation induced damage in the central nervous system: an interpretation of target cell responses. *British Journal of Cancer*, 53, (Suppl. VII), 207–17.

Kok, G., 1973, N. S. D. for treatment of carcinoma of the larynx. *International Journal of Radiation Biology*, 24, 317 (abstract).

Kolstad, L., 1964, *Vascularization, oxygen tensions and radiocurability in cancer of the cervix* (Stockholm: Scandinavian University Books).

Krause-Ziegler, H., 1906, Wirkung auf Tierisches Gewebe. Presented at Second Congress of the German Roentgen Society.

Krebs, J. S. and Jones, D. C. L., 1972, The LD50 and the survival of bone-marrow colony-forming cells in mice: Effect of rate of exposure to ionizing radiation. *Radiation Research*, 51, 374–80.

Krebs, J. S. and Leong, G. F., 1970, Effect of exposure rate on the LD50 of mice exposed to $^{60}$Co gamma rays or 250 kVp x-rays. *Radiation Research*, 42, 601–13.

Krönig, S. and Friedrich, W., 1918, Physikalische und biologische Grundlagen der Strahlentherapie. *Strahlentherapie*, Supplement 20.

Kummermehr, J., 1985, Measurement of tumour clonogens *in situ*. In *Cell Clones: Manual of Mammalian Cell Techniques*, edited by C. S. Potten and J. H. Hendry (Edinburgh: Churchill-Livingstone), pp. 215–22.

Kummermehr, J. and Trott, K. R., 1982, Rate of repopulation in a slow and a fast growing mouse tumour. In *Progress in Radio Oncology II*, edited by K. H. Karcher (New York: Raven Press), pp. 299–307.

Kummermehr, J., Schropp, K. and Neuner, M., 1986, Repopulation in squamous carcinoma AT 478 during daily irradiation. *Experimentelle Tumortherapie*, Annual Report 1985. Munich, GSF-Bericht 31/85, pp. 31–9.

Lahiri, S. K. and van Putten, L. M., 1972, Location of the G-phase in the cell-cycle of the mouse haematopoietic spleen colony forming cells. *Cell and Tissue Kinetics*, 5, 365–9.

Lajtha, L. G., 1963, On the concept of the cell cycle, *Journal of Cellular and Comparative Physiology*, 62, (Suppl. 1), 143–5.

Lajtha, L. G. and Oliver, R., 1961, Some radiobiological considerations in radiotherapy. *British Journal of Radiology*, 34, 252–7.

Lajtha, L. G., Gilbert, C. W. and Guzman, E., 1971, Kinetics of haemopoietic colony growth. *British Journal of Haematology*, 20, 343–54.

Lajtha, L. G., Oliver, R. and Gurney, C. W., 1962, Kinetic model of a bone-marrow stem-cell population. *British Journal of Haematology*, 8, 422–60.

Lange, C. S. and Gilbert, C. W., 1968, Studies on the cellular basis of radiation lethality. IV. The measurement of stem-cell repopulation probability. *International Journal of Radiation Biology*, 14, 373–88.

Langlois, D., Eschwege, F., Kramer, A. and Richard, J. M., 1985, Re-irradiation of head and neck cancers. *Radiotherapy and Oncology*, 3, 27–33.

Laurie, J. Orr, J. S. and Foster, C. J., 1972, Repair processes and cell survival. *British Journal of Radiology*, 45, 362–8.

Lea, D. E., 1938, A theory of the action of radiation on biological materials capable of recovery: Part I. The time–intensity factor. *British Journal of Radiology*, 11, 489–97.

Lea, D. E., 1947, *Actions of Radiations on Living Cells* (Cambridge: The University Press), p. 402.

Lesher, S. and Bauman, J., 1969, Cell kinetic studies of the intestinal epithelium: Maintenance of the intestinal epithelium in normal and irradiated animals. *National Cancer Institute Monographs*, 30, 185–95.

Lesher, S., Lamerton, L. F., Sacher, G. A., Fry, R. J. M., Steel, G. G. and Roylance, P. J., 1966, Effect of continuous gamma irradiation on the generation cycle of the duodenal crypt cells of the mouse and rat. *Radiation Research*, 29, 57–70.

Liechti, A., 1929, Über den Zeitfaktor der biologischen Strahlenwirkung. *Strahlentherapie*, **33**, 1–54.

Littbrand, B., Edsmyr, F. and Revesz, L., 1975, A low dose fractionation scheme for the radiotherapy of the carcinoma of the bladder. Experimental and preliminary results. *Bulletin of Cancer*, **62**, 241–50.

Little, J. B., 1971, Repair of potentially-lethal radiation damage in mammalian cells: enhancement by conditioned medium from stationary cultures. *International Journal of Radiation Biology*, **20**, 87–92.

Liversage, W. E., 1971, A critical look at the ret. *British Journal of Radiology*, **44**, 91–100.

Lord, B. I., 1964, The effect of continuous irradiation on cell proliferation in rat bone marrow. *British Journal of Haematology*, **10**, 496–507.

Lord, B. I., 1965, Cellular proliferation in normal and continuously irradiated rat bone marrow studied by repeated labelling with tritiated thymidine. *British Journal of Haematology*, **11**, 130–43.

Lord, B. I., 1968, *Effects of Radiation on Cellular Proliferation and Differentiation* (Vienna: IAEA), p. 247.

Lord, B. I., 1975, The control of cell proliferation in haemopoietic tissue. In *Radiation Research: Biomedical, Chemical and Physical Perspectives*, edited by O. F. Nygaard, H. R. Adler and W. K. Sinclair (New York: Academic Press) pp. 826–33.

Lord, B. I., 1986, Controls on the cell cycle. *International Journal of Radiation Biology*, **49**, 279–96.

Lord, B. I., Hendry, J. H., Keene, J. P., Hodgson, B. W., Xu, C. X., Rezvani, M. and Gordon, T. J., 1984, A comparison of low and high dose-rate radiation for recipient mice in spleen-colony studies. *Cell Tissue Kinetics*, **17**, 323–34.

Lu, C. C., Meistrich, M. L. and Thames, H. D., 1980, Survival of mouse testicular stem cells after gamma or neutron irradiation. *Radiation Research*, **81**, 402–15.

MacComb, W. S. and Quimby, E. H., 1936, The rate of recovery of human skin from the effects of hard or soft roentgen rays or gamma rays. *Radiology*, **27**, 196–204.

Maciejewski, B., Gunhild, P.-B. and Trott, K.-R., 1983, The influence of the number of fractions and of overall treatment time on local control and late complication rate in squamous cell carcinoma of the larynx. *International Journal of Radiation Oncology Biology Physics*, **9**, 321–8.

MacKillop, W. J., Ciampi, A., Till, J. E. and Buick, R. N., 1983, A stem cell model of human tumor growth: Implications for tumor cell clonogenic assays. *Journal of The National Cancer Institute*, **70**, 9–16.

McLarty, J. W., 1976, *Mathematical modeling methods in radiobiology*. Ph.D. Thesis, University of Texas at Houston Graduate School of Biomedical Sciences.

McNally, N. J. and de Ronde, J., 1976, Effect of repeated small doses of radiation on recovery from sub-lethal damage by Chinese hamster cells irradiated in the plateau phase of growth. *International Journal of Radiation Biology*, **29**, 221–34.

McNeese, M. and Fletcher, G. H., 1981, Retreatment of recurrent nasopharyngeal carcinoma. *Radiology*, **138**, 191–3.

McWhirter, R., 1935, 12th Annual Report, British Empire Cancer Campaign, p. 131–44.

Malaise, E. P., Charbit, A., Chavaudra, N., Combes, P. F., Douchez, J. and Tubiana, M., 1972, Change in volume of irradiated human metastases — investigation of repair of sublethal damage and tumour repopulation. *British Journal of Cancer*, **26**, 43–52.

Marcuse, W., 1896. Dermatitis und Alopecie nach Durchleuchtung mit Röntgenstrahlen. *Deutsche Medizinische Wochenschrift*, **22**, 481–3.

Marsden, J. J., Kember, N. F. and Shaw, J. E. H., 1980, Irregular radiation responses of a chondrosarcoma. *British Journal of Cancer*, **41** (Suppl. IV), 88–92.

Masuda, K., Reid, B. O. and Withers, H. R., 1977, Dose effect relationship for epilation and late effects on spinal cord in rats exposed to gamma rays. *Radiology*, **122**, 239–42.

Medini, E., Rao, Y., Kim, T., Jones, T. K. and Levitt, S. H., 1985. Radiation therapy for advanced head and neck squamous cell carcinoma using twice-a-day fractionation. *American Journal of Chemical Oncology*, **8**, 65–8.

Meistrich, M. L., Williams, M. V., Soranson, J., Fowler, J. F. and Denekamp, J., 1984, Increased collagen and fluid content of mouse kidneys at 9 months after single or fractionated X irradiation. *Radiation Research*, **99**, 185–201.

Meistrich, M. L., 1986, Relationships between spermatogonial stem cell survival and testis function after cytotoxic therapy. *British Journal of Cancer*, 53 (Suppl. VII), 89—101.

Meoz, R. T., Fletcher, G. H., Peters, L. J., Barkley, H. T. and Thames, H. D., 1984, Twice-daily fractionation schemes for advanced head and neck cancer. *International Journal of Radiation Oncology Biology Physics*, 10, 831—6.

Metting, N. F., Braby, L. A., Roesch, W. C. and Nelson, J. M., 1985, Dose-rate evidence for two kinds of radiation damage in stationary-phase mammalian cells. *Radiation Research*, 103, 204—18.

Michalowski, A., 1981, Effects of radiation on normal tissues: hypothetical mechanisms of limitations of *in situ* assays of clonogenicity. *Radiation Environmental Biophysics*, 19, 157—72.

Michalowski, A. and Hornsey, S., 1986, Assays of damage to the alimentary canal. *British Journal of Cancer*, 53, (Suppl. VII), 1—6.

Miescher, G., 1924, Das Röntgenerythem. *Strahlentherapie*, 16, 333—71.

Miescher, G., 1930, Gegenwartige methoden der Krebsstrahlung und ihre Erfolge. I. Einmalige Höchstdosis. *Strahlentherapie*, 37, 17—30.

Miescher, G., 1935, Tierexperimentelle Untersuchungen über den Einfluss der Fraktionierung auf den Späteffekt. *Acta Radiologica*, 16, 25—38.

Mijnheer, B. J., Battermann, J. J. and Wambersie, A., 1987, What degree of accuracy is required and can be achieved in photon and neutron therapy? *Radiotherapy and Oncology*, 8, 237—52.

Mitchell, J. B. and Bedford, J. S., 1977, Dose-rate effects in synchronous mammalian cells in culture. II. A comparison of the life cycle of HeLa cells during continuous irradiation or multiple-dose fractionation. *Radiation Research*, 71, 547—60.

Mitchell, J. B., Bedford, J. S. and Bailey, S. M., 1979, Dose-rate effects in mammalian cells in culture. III. A comparison of cell killing and cell proliferation during continuous irradiation for six different cell lines. *Radiation Research*, 79, 537—51.

Mohr, O. L., 1919, Röntgenstrahlenwirkung auf den Hoden von Dicticus *vernicivorus*. *Archiv fur Mikroskopische Anatomie*, 92,

Mole, R. H., 1984, The LD50 for uniform low LET irradiation of man. *British Journal of Radiology*, 57, 355—69.

Montague, E. D., 1968, Experience with altered fractionation in radiation therapy of breast cancer. *Radiology*, 90, 962—6.

Moore, J. L., 1972, Recent advances in radiotherapy. In *Modern Trends in Radiotherapy — 2*, edited by T. J. Deeley (London: Butterworths), p. 315.

Moore, J. V., 1983, Cytotoxic injury to cell populations of solid tumours. In *Cytotoxic injury to tissues: Effect on cell lineages*, edited by C. S. Potten and J. H. Hendry (Edinburgh: Churchill-Livingstone), pp. 368—408.

Moore, J. V. and Hendry, J. H., 1984, Relationship of clonogenic cells and tumour-rescuing cells modelled in irradiated spheroids *in vitro*. *British Journal of Radiology*, 57, 935—7.

Moore, J. V., Hendry, J. H. and Hunter, R. D., 1983, Dose—incidence curves for tumour control and normal tissue injury, in relation to response of clonogenic cells. *Radiotherapy and Oncology*, 1, 143—57.

Moore, J. V., Hasleton, P. S. and Buckley, C. H., 1985, Tumour cords in 52 human bronchial and cervical squamous cell carcinomas: Inferences for their cellular kinetics and radiobiology. *British Journal of Cancer*, 51, 407—13.

Moore, J. V., West, C. M. L. and Hendry, J. H., 1987, Radiation response of multicellular spheroids initiated from 5 human melanoma xenograft lines. *British Journal of Radiology*, 60, 302—3.

Moulder, J. E. and Fischer, J. J., 1976, Radiation reaction of rat skin: The role of the number of fractions and the overall treatment time. *Cancer*, 37, 2762—7.

Mulcahy, R. T., Gould, M. N. and Clifton, K. H., 1980, The survival of thyroid cells: In vivo irradiation and *in situ* repair. *Radiation Research*, 84, 523—28.

Munro, T. R. and Gilbert, C. W., 1961, The relation between tumour lethal doses and the radiosensitivity of tumour cells. *British Journal of Radiology*, 34, 246—51.

Nagasawa, H., Robertson, J. B., Arundel, C. S. and Little, J. B., 1984, The effect of X-irradiation on the progression of mouse 10T 1/2 cells released from density-inhibited cultures. *Radiation Research*, 97, 537—45.

Nather, K. and Schinz, H. R., 1923, Tierexperimentielle Studien zum Krebsproblem. I. Gibt es eine Reizdosis bei malignen tumoren? *Mitteilungen der Grenzgebiete Medizine und Chirurgie*, 36, 620–60.

Neal, F. E., 1960, Variation of acute mortality with dose-rate in mice exposed to single large doses of whole-body X-irradiation. *International Journal of Radiation Biology*, 2, 295–300.

Nelson, J. S. R., Carpenter, R. E. and Durboraw, D., 1976, Mechanisms underlying reduced growth rate in C3HBA mammary adenocarcinomas recurring after single doses of X-rays or fast neutrons. *Cancer Research*, 36, 524–32.

Nguyen, T. D., Demange, L., Froissart, D., Panis, X. and Loirette, M., 1985, Rapid hyperfractionated radiotherapy. *Cancer*, 56, 16–9.

Nias, A. H. W., 1963, Some comparisons of fractionation effects by erythema measurements on human skin. *British Journal of Radiology*, 36, 183–7.

Norin, T. and Onyango, J., 1977, Radiotherapy in Burkitt's lymphoma. Conventional or superfractionated regime – early results. *International Journal of Radiation Oncology Biology Physics*, 2, 399–406.

Nothdurft, W., Steinbach, K.-H. and Fliedner, T. M., 1983, *In vitro* studies on the sensitivity of canine granulopoietic progenitor cells (GM–CFC) to ionizing radiation: differences between steady state CM–CFC from blood and bone marrow. *International Journal of Radiation Biology*, 33, 133–40.

Okada, S., 1970, Radiation-induced death. In *Radiation Biochemistry, Vol. 1, Cells*, edited by K. I. Altman, G. B. Gerber and S. Okada (London: Academic Press Inc.), pp. 247–60.

Oliver, R., 1964, A comparison of the effects of acute and protracted gamma-radiation on the growth of seedlings of *Vicia faba*. II. Theoretical calculations. *International Journal of Radiation Biology*, 8, 475–88.

Orr, J. S., Wakerley, S. E. and Stark, J. M., 1966, A metabolic theory of cell survival curves. *Physics in Medicine and Biology*, 11, 103–8.

Orton, C. G., 1974, Time–dose factors (TDF) in brachytherapy. *British Journal of Radiology*, 47, 603–7.

Orton, C. G., 1985, A variable exponent TDF model, In *Optimization of Cancer Radiotherapy*. Proceedings of 2nd International Conference on Dose, Time, and Fractionation in Radiation Oncology, Madison, WI., Sept. 1984.

Orton, C. G. and Ellis, F., 1973, A simplification in the use of the NSD concept in practical radiotherapy. *British Journal of Radiology*, 46, 529–37.

Orton, C. G. and Webber, B. M., 1977, Time-dose factor (TDF) analysis of dose-rate effects in permanent implant therapy. *International Journal of Radiation Oncology, Biology and Physics*, 2, 55–60.

Overgaard, J., 1984a, (editor) *Hyperthermic Oncology 1984*, 2 volumes (London: Taylor & Francis).

Overgaard, M., 1984b, The clinical implication of non-standard fractionation. *International Journal of Radiation Oncology, Biology, Physics*, 11, 1225–9.

Overgaard, J., 1986, The role of radiotherapy in recurrent and metastatic malignant melanoma: a clinical radiobiological study. *International Journal of Radiation Oncology Biology Physics*, 12, 867–72.

Overgaard, J., Sand-Hansen, H., Jorgensen, K. and Hjelm-Hansen, M., 1986, Primary radiotherapy of larynx and pharynx carcinoma – an analysis of some factors influencing local control and survival. *International Journal of Radiation Oncology Biology Physics*, 12, 515–21.

Palcic, B. and Skarsgard, L. D., 1984, Reduced oxygen enhancement ratio at low doses of ionizing radiation. *Radiation Research*, 100, 328–39.

Pape, R. 1933, Zur Frage des Vergleichs der Hautreaktion unter verschiedenen Bestrahlungsbedingungen. *Strahlentherapie*, 48, 73–96.

Parkins, C. S. and Fowler, J. F., 1985, Repair in mouse lung of multifraction X-rays and neutrons: Extension to 40 fractions. *British Journal of Radiology*, 58, 1097–103.

Parkins, C. S., Fowler, J. F. and Yu, S., 1983, A murine model of lip epidermal/mucosal reactions to X-irradiation. *Radiotherapy and Oncology*, 1, 159–66.

Parkins, C. S., Fowler, J. F., Maughan, R. L. and Roper, M. J., 1985, Repair in mouse lung for up to 20 fractions of X-rays or neutrons. *British Journal of Radiology,* **58,** 225–41.

Parsons, J. T., Thar, T. L., Bova, F. J. and Million, R. R., 1980a, An evaluation of split course irradiation for pelvic malignancies. *International Journal of Radiation Oncology Biology Physics,* **6,** 175–81.

Parsons, J. T., Bova, F. J. and Million, R. R., 1980b, A re-evaluation of split-course technique for squamous cell carcinoma of the head and neck. *International Journal of Radiation Oncology Biology Physics,* **6,** 1645–52.

Parsons, J. T., Cassisi, N. J. and Million, R. R., 1984, Results of twice-a-day irradiation of squamous cell carcinomas of the head and neck. *International Journal of Radiation Oncology Biology Physics,* **10,** 2041–52.

Paterson, R., 1948, *Treatment of Malignant Disease by Radium and X-rays.* (Baltimore: Williams & Wilkins).

Paterson, R., 1952, Studies in optimum dosage. *British Journal of Radiology,* **25,** 505–16.

Paterson, R., 1963, *The Treatment of Malignant Disease by Radiotherapy,* 2nd edition (London: Edward Arnold).

Paterson, R., Tod, M. and Russell, M., 1945, The results of radium and X-ray therapy in malignant disease. Second Statistical Report from the Holt Radium Institute, Manchester, 1934–1938 (Edinburgh: E. S. Livingstone Ltd).

Paterson, R., Tod, M. and Russell, M., 1950, The results of radium and X-ray therapy in malignant disease, being the third statistical report from the Christie Hospital and Holt Radium Institute, Manchester (Edinburgh: E. S. Livingstone Ltd).

Patt, H., Tyree, E. B., Straube, R. L. and Smith, D. E., 1949, Cysteine protection against X-irradiation, *Science,* **110,** 213–14.

Payne, M. G. and Garrett, W. R., 1975a, Model of cell survival with low LET radiation. *Radiation Research,* **62,** 169–79.

Payne, M. G. and Garrett, W. R., 1975b, Some relations between cell survival models having different inactivation mechanisms. *Radiation Research,* **62,** 388–94.

Peacock, J. H., Steel, G. G. and Stephens, T. C., 1986, Radiation dose-rate dependent differences in cell kill and repopulation in murine bone-marrow CFU-S and CFU-C. *British Journal of Cancer,* **53** (Suppl. VII), 171–3.

Peperzeel, H. A. van, 1970, *Patterns of tumor growth after irradiation: a comparative study in men, dogs and mice.* Ph.D. Thesis, University of Amsterdam.

Peperzeel, H. A. van, 1972, Effects of single doses of radiation on lung metastases in man and experimental animals. *European Journal of Cancer,* **8,** 665–75.

Peracchia, G. and Salti, C., 1981, Radiotherapy with thrice-a-day fractionation in a short overall time: Clinical experiences. *International Journal of Radiation Oncology Biology Physics,* **7,** 99–104.

Perthes, G., 1904, Über die Behandlung des Karzinoms mit Röntgenstrahlen und über den Einfluss der Röntgenstrahlen auf die Zellteilung. *Münchener Medizinische Wochenschrift,* **51,** 282–3.

Peters, L. J. and Ang, K. K., 1987, Accelerated fractionation. In *Medical Radiology – Diagnostic Imaging and Radiation, Innovation in Radiation Oncology Research,* edited by L. J. Peters and H. R. Withers (Berlin, Heidelberg, New York, London, Paris, Tokyo: Springer-Verlag), (in press).

Peters, L. J. and Thames, Jr., H. D., 1984, Role of fraction size: correlation and discrepancies during calculations and available data. Presented at the 3rd Annual Meeting of ESTRO, September 9–15, 1984, Jerusalem, Israel.

Peters, L. J., Withers, H. R. and Thames, H. D., 1982, Radiobiological bases for multiple daily fractionation. In *Progress in Radio-Oncology II,* edited by K. H. Karcher, H. D. Kogelnik and G. Reinartz (New York: Raven Press), pp. 317–23.

Pfahler, G., 1927, Über die Sättigungsmethode in der Roentgentherapie tiefliegender maligner Geschwülste. *Strahlentherapie,* **25,** 597–610.

Phillips, R. A. and Tolmach, L. J., 1966, Repair of potentially lethal damage in X-irradiated HeLa cells. *Radiation Research,* **29,** 413–27.

Pierquin, B., Calitchi, E., Mazeron, J. J., Le Bourgeois, J. P. and Leung, S., 1985. A comparison between low dose rate radiotherapy and conventionally fractionated irradiation in moderately extensive cancers of the oropharynx. *International Journal of Radiation Oncology Biology Physics*, **11**, 431–9.

Pohlit, W. and Heyder, I. R., 1981, The shape of dose–survival curves for mammalian cells and repair of potentially lethal damage analyzed by hypertonic treatment. *Radiation Research*, **87**, 613–34.

Pointon, R. C. S., 1985, Treatment of the bladder. In *Radiotherapy of Malignant Disease*, edited by E. C. Easson and R. C. S. Pointon (Berlin: Springer-Verlag), p. 474.

Porteous, D. D.and Lajtha, L. G., 1966, On stem cell recovery after irradiation. *British Journal of Haematology*, **12**, 177–88.

Porter, E. H., Hewitt, H. B. and Blake, E. R., 1973, The transplantation kinetics of tumour cells. *British Journal of Cancer*, **27**, 55–62.

Potten, C. S., 1977, Extreme sensitivity of some intestinal crypt cells to X- and $\gamma$-irradiation. *Nature*, **269**, 518–21.

Potten, C. S., 1978, Small intestinal cryptogenic cells in W/W mutant mice. *Radiation Research*, **74**, 139–43.

Potten, C. S., 1981, The cell kinetic mechanism for radiation induced cellular depletion of epithelial tissue based on hierarchical differences in radiosensitivity. *International Journal of Radiation Biology*, **40**, 217–25.

Potten, C. S., 1985a, *Radiation and Skin* (London: Taylor & Francis).

Potten, C. S., 1985b, Cell death (apoptosis) in hair follicles and consequent changes in width of hair after irradiation of growing hairs. *International Journal of Radiation Biology*, **48**, 349–60.

Potten, C. S., 1986a, Cell cycles in cell hierarchies. *International Journal of Radiation Biology*, **49**, 257–278.

Potten, C. S., 1986b, The cellular basis of skin injury after cytotoxic insult. *British Journal of Cancer*, **53** (Supplement VII), 47–58.

Potten, C. S. and Hendry, J. H., 1975, Differential regeneration of intestinal proliferative cells and cryptogenic cells after irradiation. *International Journal of Radiation Biology*, **27**, 413–24.

Potten, C. S. and Hendry, J. H., 1983a, Stem cells in murine small intestine. In *Stem Cells: their Identification and Characterisation*, edited by C. S. Potten (Edinburgh: Churchill-Livingstone), pp. 155–99.

Potten, C. S. and Hendry, J. H. (editors), 1983b, *Cytotoxic Insult to Tissue: Effects on Cell Lineages* (Edinburgh: Churchill-Livingstone), p. 421.

Potten, C. S. and Hendry, J. H., (editors), 1985, *Cell Clones: Manual of Mammalian Cell Techniques*. (Edinburgh: Churchill-Livingstone).

Powers, E. L., 1962, Considerations of survival curves and target theory. *Physics in Medicine and Biology*, **7**, 3–28.

Powers, W. E. and Tolmach, L. J., 1963, Multicomponent X-ray survival curve for mouse lymphosarcoma cells irradiated *in vivo*. *Nature*, (London) **197**, 710–11.

Prempree, T., Amornmarn, R., Villasanta, V., Kwon, T. and Scott, R. M., 1984, Retreatment of very late recurrent invasive squamous cell carcinoma of the cervix with irradiation. II. Criteria for patients' selection to achieve the success. *Cancer*, **54**, 1950–5.

Proceedings of the 6th L. H. Gray Conference, 1975, *Cell survival after low doses of radiation: theoretical and clinical implications*, edited by T. Alper (The Institute of Physics/John Wiley and Sons).

Proceedings of the 12th L. H. Gray Conference, 1986, *British Journal of Cancer* **53** (Suppl. VII), p. 391.

Puck, T. T. and Marcus, P. I., 1956, Actions of X-rays on mammalian cells, *Journal of Experimental Medicine*, **103**, 653–66.

Puck, T. T., Marcus, P. I. and Cieciura, S. J., 1956, Clonal growth of mammalian cells *in vitro*: growth characteristics of colonies from single HeLa cells with and without 'feeder' layer. *Journal of Experimental Medicine*, **103**, 273–84.

Puro, E. A. and Clark, G. M., 1972, The effect of exposure rate on animal lethality and spleen colony cell survival. *Radiation Research*, **52**, 115–29.

Putten, L. M. van, Lelieveld, P. and Broerse, J. J., 1979. Effects of 300 kV X-rays and 15 MeV neutrons in single and fractionated doses on hemopoietic stem cells in mouse bone marrow. Proceedings of the NIH, AEC Meeting on: Time and dose relationships in radiation biology as applied to radiotherapy. Carmel, B. N. L. 50203 (C-57), p.162.

Putten, L. M. van, de Ruiter, J. and van der Vecht, B., 1985, Reoxygenation between radiotherapy fractions in an experimental osteosarcoma. *European Journal of Cancer and Clinical Oncology*, **21**, 1561−2.

Quastler, H., 1945, Studies on roentgen death in mice. I. Survival time and dosage. *American Journal of Roentgenology*, **54**, 449−56.

Quimby, E. H. and MacComb, W. S., 1937, Further studies on the rate of recovery of human skin from the effects of roentgen or gamma rays. *Radiology*, **29**, 305−12.

Rajewsky, B. and Danzer, H., 1934, Über einige Wirkungen von Strahlen. VI. Eine Erweiterung der statistischen Theorie der biologischen Strahlenwirkung. *Zeitschrift für Physik*, **89**, 412−20.

Rantanen, J., 1973, Radiation injury of connective tissue. A biochemical investigation with experimental granuloma. *Acta Radiologica Supplement*, **330**, 1−92.

Read, J., 1958, Aspects of radiation damage likely to be involved in tumour regression. *British Journal of Radiology*, **31**, 60−9.

Redpath, J. L., Peel, D. M. and Hopewell, J. W., 1984, Implications of tissue target-cell survival-curve shape for values of split-dose recovery doses; late versus early effects. *International Journal of Radiation Biology*, **45**, 133−7.

del Regato, J. A., 1986, Antoine Lacassagne. *International Journal of Radiation Oncology Biology Physics*, **12**, 2165–73.

Regaud, C., 1921, Sur la radio-immunisation des tissus cancéreux et sur le mécanisme de l'action des rayons X et des rayons gamma de radium sur les cellules et les tissus vivants en géneral. *Bulletin de l'Académie de Paris*, **91**, 604.

Regaud, C. 1927, Principes du traitement des epithéliomas épidermoides par les radiations. Application aux épidermoides de la peau et de la bouche. *Journal de Radiologie et de l'Electrologie*, **7**, 297.

Regaud, C. and Ferroux, R., 1927, Disordance des effets de rayons X, d'une part dans le testicule, par le fractionnement de la dose. *Comptes Rendus Societé Biologique*, **97**, 431.

Regaud, C. and Ferroux, R., 1929, Über den Einfluss des Zeitfaktors auf neoplastischen Zellnachwuchs durch die Radiotherapie. *Strahlentherapie*, **31**, 495−508.

Reinhoid, H. S. and Buisman, G. H., 1975, Repair of radiation damage to capillary endothelium. *British Journal of Radiology*, **48**, 727−31.

Reinhold, H. S. and Visser, A. G., 1986, Multiple fractions per day in retrospect; the L−Q model and the tolerance profile. *Radiotherapy and Oncology*, **5**, 259−64.

Reisner, A., 1933, Hauterythem und Roentgenstrahlung. *Ergebrisse der Medizinischen Strahlenforschung*, **6**, 1−60.

Reitan, J. B. and Kaalhus, O., 1980, Radiotherapy of liposarcomas. *British Journal of Radiology*, **53**, 969−75.

Resouly, A. and Svoboda, V. H. J., 1982, Management of advanced head and neck squamous carcinoma by multiple daily sessions of radiotherapy and surgery. In *Progress in Radio-Oncology, II*, edited by K. H. Karcher, H. D. Kogelnik and G. Reinartz (New York: Raven Press), pp. 339−47.

Revell, S. H., 1983, Relationships between chromosome damage and cell death. In *Radiation-induced Chromosome Damage in Man*, edited by T. Ishilara and M. S. Sasaki, pp. 215−34.

Reynaud, A. and Travis, E. L., 1984, Late effects of irradiation of mouse jejunum. *International Journal of Radiation Biology*, **49**, 125−34.

Robinson, C. V., 1968, Relationship between animal and stem cell dose−survival curves. *Radiation Research*, **35**, 318−44.

Roesch, W. C., 1978, Models of the radiation sensitivity of mammalian cells. In *Third Symposium on Neutron Dosimetry in Biology and Medicine*, edited by G. Burger and H. G. Ebert (Luxembourg: Commission of the European Communities), pp. 1−27.

Rojas, A-M., Joiner, M. C., Ninis, J. and Johns, H., 1987, Rate of repair of radiation injury. *Gray Laboratory Annual Report (1986)*, Cancer Research Campaign, U.K.

Röntgen, W. C., 1895, Über eine neue Art von Strahlen. Erste Mitteilung. *Sitzungsberichte der Physikalische-Medizinschen Gesellschaft in Würzburg*, 132−41.

Rous, P. and Jones, F. S., 1916, A method of obtaining suspensions of living cells from the fixed tissues, and for the plating out of individual cells. *Journal of Experimental Medicine*, **23**, 549–55.

Sasaki, T., Sato, Y. and Sakka, M., 1980, Cell population kinetics of human solid tumors. a statistical analysis in various histological types. *Gann*, **71**, 520–9.

Sause, W. T., Stewart, J. R., Plenk, H. P. and Leavitt, D. D., 1981, Late skin changes following twice-weekly electron beam radiation to post-mastectomy chest walls. *International Journal of Radiation Oncology, Biology, Physics*, **7**, 1541–4.

Scanlon, P. W., 1963, Split-course radiotherapy: follow-up in 50 cases. *American Journal of Roentgenology*, **90**, 280–93.

Schenken, L. L., and Hagemann, R. F., 1975, Time/dose relationships in experimental radiation cataractogenesis. *Radiology*, **117**, 193–8.

Schinz, H. R., 1930, Gegenwärtige Methoden des Krebsbestrahlung and ihre Erfolge. II. Verteilte Dosis. *Strahlentherapie*, **37**, 31–49.

Schinz, H. R., 1937, Die fraktionierte und protrahiert-fraktionierte Bestrahlung. Zürcher Erfahrungen. *Strahlentherapie*, **58**, 373–405.

Schueren, E. van der, Ang, K. K., Horiot, J. C., Gonzalez, D. G., Glabbeke, M. van and de Pauw, M., 1985, Concentrated radiotherapy schedules: role of repair and repopulation. *Proceedings of the XVI International Congress of Radiology, Hawaii*, pp. 99–103.

Schwarz, G., 1909, Desensibilisierung gegen Röntgen-und Radiumstrahlen. *Münchener Medizinische Wochenschrift*, No. 24.

Schwarz, G., 1914a, Dauerbestrahlung mit täglichen kleinen Dosen. *Wiener Medizinische Wochenschrift*, No. 52; 1914b, *Münchener Medizinische Wochenschrift*, **61**, 317; 1914c, Heilung tiefliegender Karzinome durch Röntgenbestrahlung von der Körperoberflache aus. *Münchener Medizinische Wochenschrift*, **61**, 1733.

Schwarz, G., 1924, Zur Kenntnis der Roentgenreaktion der Haut. Der Begriff der Schädigungsquotienten. *Strahlentherapie*, **18**, 845–8.

Schwarz, G., 1930, Über die theoretischen und praktischen Grundlagen einer Langschwachbestrahlungsmethode. *Strahlentherapie*, **37**, 709–18.

Schwarz, G., 1937, Entwicklung, Prinzipien, und biologischen Grundlagen der röntgentherapeutischen Bestrahlungsmethodik. *Strahlentherapie*, **58**, 523–44.

Scott, D., Gellard, P. A. and Hendry, J. H., 1984, Differential rates of loss of chromosome aberrations in rat thyroid after X-rays or neutrons. *Radiation Research*, **97**, 64–70.

Seitz, A. and Wintz, H., 1920, Unsere Methode der Röntgentherapie und ihre Erfolge. *Strahlentherapie*, Supplement 22.

Seydel, H. G., Diener-West, M., Urtasun, R., Pdolsky, W. J., Cox, J. D., Zinninger, M., Francis, M. E. and Radiation Therapy Oncology Group (RTOG), 1985, Hyperfractionation in the radiation therapy of unresectable non-oat cell carcinoma of the lung: preliminary report of a RTOG pilot study. *International Journal of Radiation Oncology Biology Physics*, **11**, 1841–7.

Seymour, C. B., Mothersill, C. and Alper, T., 1986, High yields of lethal mutations in somatic mammalian cells that survive ionizing radiation. *International Journal of Radiation Biology*, **50**, 167–79.

Shipley, D. U., Stanley, J. A., Courtenay, V. D. and Field, S. B., 1975, Repair of radiation damage in Lewis lung carcinoma cells following *in situ* treatment with fast neutrons and γ-rays. *Cancer Research*, **35**, 932–8.

Sigdestad, C. P., 1975, Correlation of animal, crypt and stem cell survival in fission neutron irradiated mice. A chemical protection study, US Army Med. Rc. and Development Command, Contract No. DADA-17-72-C-2038.

Simpson, W. J. and Platts, M. E., 1976, Fractionation study in the treatment of glioblastoma multiforme. *International Journal of Radiation Oncology Biology Physics*, **1**, 639–44.

Sinclair, W. K., 1969, Protection by cysteamine against lethal x-ray damage during the cell cycle of the Chinese hamster cell. *Radiation Research*, **39**, 135–53.

Sinclair, W. K. and Morton, R. A., 1966, X-ray sensitivity during the cell generation cycle of cultured mammalian cells. *Radiation Research*, **29**, 450–74.

Singh, K., 1978, Two regimes with the same TDF but differing morbidity used in the treatment of stage III carcinoma on the cervix. *British Journal of Radiology*, 51, 357—62.

Sjögren, T., 1901, Die Röntgenbehandlung des Ulcus rodens. *Fortschritte Röntgenstrahlen*, 5, 37—9.

Skolyszewski, J., Korzentowski, S. and Reinfuss, M., 1980, The irradiation of recurrences of head and neck cancer. *British Journal of Radiology*, 53, 462—5.

Sodicoff, M., Pratt, N. E. and Sholley, M. M., 1974, Ultrastructural radiation injury of rat parotid gland: a histopathologic dose—response study. *Radiation Research*, 58, 196—208.

Sonntag, C. von, 1987, *The Chemical Basis of Radiation Biology* (London: Taylor and Francis, Ltd).

Spanos, W. J., Shukovsky, L. J. and Fletcher, G. H., 1976, Time, dose and tumor volume relationships in irradiation of squamous cell carcinomas of the base of tongue. *Cancer*, 37, 2591—9.

Spencer, H. and Shorter, R. G., 1962, Cell turnover in pulmonary tissues. *Nature*, 194, 880.

Stearner, S. P. and Christian, E. J. B., 1978, Long-term vascular effects of ionizing radiations in the mouse: capillary blood flow. *Radiation Research*, 73, 553—67.

Steel, G. G., 1968, Cell loss from experimental tumours. *Cell and Tissue Kinetics*, 1, 193—207.

Steel, G. G., 1977, *Growth Kinetics of Tumours: Cell Population Kinetics in Relation to the Growth and Treatment of Cancer* (Oxford: Clarendon Press).

Steel, G. G., 1986, Autoradiographic analysis of the cell cycle. Howard and Pelc to the present day. *International Journal of Radiation Biology*, 49, 227—35.

Steel, G. G. and Stephens, T. C., 1983, Stem cells in tumours. In *Stem Cells, Their Identification and Characterization*, edited by C. S. Potten (Edinburgh: Churchill-Livingstone), pp. 271—93.

Steel, G. G., Down, J. D., Peacock, J. H. and Stephens, T. C., 1986, Dose-rate effects and the repair of radiation damage. *Radiotherapy and Oncology*, 5, 321—31.

Steel, G. G., Deacon, J. M., Duchesne, G. M., Horwich, A., Kelland, L. R. and Peacock, J. H., 1987, The dose-rate effect in human tumor cells. *Radiotherapy and Oncology* (in press).

Stefani, S., Chandra, S. and Tonaki, H., 1977, Ultrastructural events in the cytoplasmic death of lethally-irradiated human lymphocytes. *International Journal of Radiation Biology*, 31, 215—25.

Stell, P. M. and Morrison, M. D., 1973, Radiation necrosis of the larynx. *Archives of Otolaryngology*, 98, 111—13.

Stenbeck, T., 1900, Ein Fall von Hautkrebs geheilt durch Röntgenbestrahlung. *Mitteilungen der Grenzgebiete Medizine und Chirurgie*, 6, 347.

Stenstrom, W. and Mattick, W. L., 1926, Study of skin reactions after divided roentgenray-dosage. *American Journal of Roentgenology*, 15, 513—19.

Stephens, L. C., Ang, K. K., Schultheiss, T. E., King, G. K., Brock, W. A. and Peters, L. J., 1986, Target cell and mode of radiation injury in rhesus salivary glands. *Radiotherapy and Oncology*, 7, 165—74.

Stephens, T. C. and Steel, G. G., 1980, Regeneration of tumors after cytotoxic treatment. In *Radiation Biology in Cancer Research*, edited by R. E. Meyn and H. R. Withers (New York: Raven Press), pp. 385—95.

Stephens, T. C., Currie, G. A. and Peacock, J. H., 1978, Repopulation of $\gamma$-irradiated Lewis lung carcinoma by malignant cells and host macrophage progenitors. *British Journal of Cancer*, 38, 573—82.

Stewart, F. A., 1986, Mechanism of bladder damage and repair after treatment with radiation and cytostatic drugs. *British Journal of Cancer*, 53, Supplement VII, 280—291.

Stewart, F. A., Denekamp, J. and Hirst, D. G., 1980, Proliferation kinetics of the mouse bladder after irradiation. *Cell and Tissue Kinetics*, 13, 75—89.

Stewart, F. A., Rojas, A. and Denekamp, J., 1983, Radioprotection of two mouse tumours by WR-2721 in single and fractionated treatments. *International Journal of Radiation Oncology Biology Physics*, 9, 507—13.

Stewart, F. A., Randhawa, V. S. and Michael, B. D., 1984a, Multifraction irradiation of mouse bladders. *Radiotherapy and Oncology*, 2, 131–40.
Stewart, F. A., Sorenson, J. A., Alpen, E. L., Williams, M. V. and Denekamp, J., 1984b, Radiation induced renal damage: The effects of hyperfractionation. *Radiation Research*, 98, 407–20.
Stewart, F. A., Oussoren, Y., Luts, A., Begg, A. C., DeWit, L., Lebesque, J. and Bartelink, H., 1987, Repair of sublethal radiation injury after multiple small doses in mouse kidney: an estimate of flexure dose. *International Journal of Radiation Oncology Biology Physics*, 13, (in press).
Stewart, J. G. and Jackson, A. W., 1975, The steepness of the dose response curve both for tumour cure and normal tissue injury. *Laryngoscope*, 85, 1107–11.
Strandqvist, M., 1944, Studien über die kumulative Wirkung der Röntgenstrahlen bei Fraktionierung. *Acta Radiologica*, 55, (Suppl.), 1–300.
Suit, H. D., 1977, Superfractionation (editorial). *International Journal of Radiation Oncology Biology Physics*, 2, 591–2.
Suit, H. D., 1984, Modification of radiation response. *International Journal of Radiation Oncology Biology Physics*, 10, 101–8.
Suit, H. D., Shalek, R. J. and Wette, R., 1965, Radiation response of C3H mouse mammary carcinoma evaluated in terms of cellular radiosensitivity. *Cellular Radiation Biology* (Baltimore: Williams & Wilkins), pp. 514–30.
Suit, H. D., Howes, A. E. and Hunter, N., 1977, Dependence of response of C3H mammary carcinoma to fractionated irradiation on fraction number and intertreatment interval. *Radiation Research*, 72, 440–54.
Svoboda, V. H. J. 1975, Radiotherapy by several sessions a day. *British Journal of Radiology*, 48, 131–3.
Svoboda, V. H. J., 1978, Further experience with radiotherapy by multiple daily sessions. *British Journal of Radiology*, 51, 363–9.
Svoboda, V. H. J. 1984, Accelerated fractionation: the Portsmouth experience 1972–1984. *Proceedings of Varian's Fourth European Clinac Users Meeting, Varian, Zug, Switzerland*, pp. 70–75.
Swann, W. F. G. and del Rosario, C., 1931, The effect of radioactive emanations upon Euglena. *Journal of Franklin Institute*, 211, 303–17.
Szczepanski, L. V. and Trott, K. R., 1975, Post-irradiation proliferation kinetics of a serially transplanted murine adenocarcinoma. *British Journal of Radiology*, 48, 200–8.
Szechter, A. and Schwarz, G., 1977, Dose-rate effects, fractionation, and cell survival at lowered temperatures. *Radiation Research*, 71, 593–613.
Szechter, A., Schwarz, G. and Barsa, J. M., 1978, Continuous and fractionated irradiation of mammalian cells in culture – I. The effect of growth rate. *International Journal of Radiation Oncology Biology Physics*, 4, 991–1000.
Tannock, I. F., 1986, Experimental chemotherapy and concepts related to the cell cycle. *International Journal of Radiation Biology*, 49, 335–55.
Tates, A. D., Broerse, J. J., Neuteboom, I. and de Vogel, N., 1982, Differential resistance of chromosomal damage induced in resting rat-liver cells by x-ray and 4.2 MeV neutrons. *Mutation Research*, 92, 275–90.
Taylor, J. M. G. and Withers, H. R., 1985, Estimating the parameters in the two-component model for cell survival from experimental quantal response data. *Radiation Research*, 104, 358–64.
Terry, N. H. A. and Denekamp, J., 1984, RBE values and repair characteristics for colo-rectal injury after caesium-137 gamma-ray and neutron irradiation. II. Fractionation up to ten doses. *British Journal of Radiology*, 57, 617–29.
Terry, N. H. A., Denekamp, J. and Maughan, R. L., 1983, RBE values for colo-rectal injury after caesium-137 gamma-ray and neutron irradiation. I. Single doses. *British Journal of Radiology*, 56, 257–65.
Testa, N. G., Hendry, J. H. and Lajtha, L. G., 1973, The response of mouse haemopoietic colony-forms to acute or continuous gamma irradiation *Biomedicine*, 19, 183–6.
Testa, N. G., Hendry, J. H. and Lajtha, L. G., 1974, The response of mouse haemopoietic colony forming units to repeated whole body X-irradiation. *Biomedicine (Express)*, 21, 431–4.

Testa, N. G., Hendry, J. H. and Molineux, G., 1985, Long-term bone marrow damage in experimental systems and in patients after radiation or chemotherapy. *Anticancer Research*, 5, 101–10.

Thames, H. D., 1984, Effect-independent measures of tissue responses to fractionated radiation. *International Journal of Radiation Biology*, 45, 1–10.

Thames, H. D., 1985, An 'incomplete-repair' model for survival after fractionated and continuous irradiations. *International Journal of Radiation Biology*, 47, 319–39.

Thames, H. D., 1987a, Repair of radiation injury and the time factor in radiotherapy. In *Cancer Modeling*, edited by J. M. Thompson and B. W. Brown (New York: Marcel Dekker) (in press).

Thames, H. D., 1987b, Does the LQ model fail at very low doses per fraction? *International Journal of Radiation Biology* (submitted).

Thames, H. D. and Suit, H. D., 1986, Tumor radioresponsiveness versus fractionation sensitivity. *International Journal of Radiation Oncology Biology Physics*, 12, 687–91.

Thames, Jr., H. D. and Withers, H. R. 1980, Test of equal effect per fraction and estimation of initial clonogen number in microcolony assays of survival after fractionated irradiation. *British Journal of Radiology*, 53, 1071–7.

Thames, H. D., Peters, L. J., Spanos, W. and Fletcher, G. H., 1980, Dose response of squamous cell carcinomas of the upper respiratory and digestive tracts. *British Journal of Cancer*, 41, (Suppl. IV), 35–8.

Thames, H. D., Withers, H. R., Mason, K. A. and Reid, B. O., 1981, Dose-survival characteristics of mouse jejunal crypt cells. *International Journal of Radiation Oncology Biology Physics*, 7, 1591–7.

Thames, H. D., Withers, H. R., Peters, L. J. and Fletcher, G. H., 1982, Changes in early and late radiation responses with altered dose fractionation: implications for dose-survival relationships. *International Journal of Radiation Oncology Biology Physics*, 8, 219–26.

Thames, H. D., Peters, L. J., Withers, H. R., and Fletcher, G. H., 1983, Accelerated fractionation vs. hyperfractionation: rationales for several treatments per day. *International Journal of Radiation Oncology Biology Physics*, 9, 127–38.

Thames, H. D., Withers, H. R. and Peters, L. J., 1984, Tissue repair capacity and repair kinetics deduced from multifractionated or continuous irradiation regimens with incomplete repair. *British Journal of Cancer*, 49, (Suppl. VI), 263–9.

Thames, H. D., Grdina, D. J. and Milas, L., 1985, On the $\alpha/\beta$ ratio and OER for clonogenic tumor cells. *International Journal of Radiation Oncology Biology Physics*, 11, 1572–3.

Thames, H. D., Brock, W. A., Bock, S. P. and Dixon, D. O., 1986a, Effect of dose per fraction on the division potential of lethally irradiated plateau-phase CHO cells exposed to isoeffective fractionation regimens. *British Journal of Cancer*, 53 (Suppl. VII), 376–81.

Thames, H. D., Rozell, M. E., Tucker, S. L., Ang, K. K., Fisher, D. R. and Travis, E. L., 1986b, Direct analysis of quantal radiation response data. *International Journal of Radiation Biology*, 49, 999–1009.

Thames, H. D., Hendry, J. H., Moore, J. V., Ang, K. K. and Travis, E. L., 1987a, The greater steepness of dose-response curves for late- than for early-responding normal tissues. *International Journal of Radiation Oncology Biology Physics*, 13, (in press).

Thames, H. D., Turesson, I., Withers, H. R. and Peters, L. J., 1987b, Changes in fractionation sensitivity of acutely responding tissues following radiation-induced compensatory regeneration. *Radiotherapy and Oncology* (submitted).

Thomlinson, R. H., 1967, Oxygen therapy — biological considerations. In *Modern Trends in Radiotherapy*, edited by T. J. Deeley and C. A. P. Wood (London: Butterworths), pp. 52–72.

Thomlinson, R. H. and Gray, L. H., 1955, The histological structure of some human lung cancers and the possible implications for radiotherapy. *British Journal of Cancer*, 9, 539–49.

Thompson, L. H. and Suit, H. D., 1969, Proliferation kinetics of x-irradiated mouse-L cells studied with time-lapse photography. II. *International Journal of Radiation Biology*, 15, 347–62.

Thrasher, J. D., 1967, Age and the cell cycle of the mouse colonic epithelium, *Anatomical Record*, 157, 621–5.
Till, J. E. and McCulloch, E. A., 1961, A direct measurement of the radiation sensitivity of normal mouse bone marrow cells. *Radiation Research*, 14, 213–22.
Tobias, C. A., Blakely, E. A. Ngo, F. Q. H. and Yang, T. C. H., 1980, The repair—misrepair model and cell survival. In *Radiation Biology in Cancer Research*, edited by R. Meyn and H. R. Withers (New York: Raven Press), pp. 195–230.
Travis, E. L. and Tucker, S. L., 1986, The relationship between functional assays of radiation response in the lung and target cell depletion. *British Journal of Cancer*, 53 (Suppl. VII), 304–19.
Travis, E. L., Peters, L. J., McNeill, J., Thames, H. D. and Karolis, C., 1985, Effect of dose-rate on total body irradiation: lethality and pathologic findings. *Radiotherapy and Oncology*, 4, 341–51.
Travis, E. L., Thames, H. D., Helbing, S. J., Kiss, I. and Watkins, T. L., 1987, Kinetics of repair in mouse lung after fractionated radiation. *International Journal of Radiation Biology* (submitted).
Trott, K. R., 1984, Chronic damage after radiation therapy: challenge to radiation biology. *International Journal of Radiation Oncology Biology Physics*, 10, 907–13.
Trott, K. R. and Hug, O., 1970, Intraclonal recovery of division probability in pedigrees of single X-irradiated mammalian cells. *International Journal of Radiation Biology*, 17, 483–6.
Trott, K. R. and Kummermehr, J., 1985, What is known about tumour proliferation rates to choose between accelerated fractionation or hyperfractionation? *Radiotherapy and Oncology*, 3, 1–9.
Trott, K. R., von Lieven, H., Kummermehr, J., Skopal, D., Lukacs, S., Braun-Falco, O. and Kellerer, A. M., 1981, The radiosensitivity of malignant melanomas, Part II: Clinical Studies. *International Journal of Radiation Oncology, Biology, Physics*, 7, 15–20.
Trott, K. R., Maciejewski, B., Preuss-Bayer, G. and Skolyszwski, J., 1984, Dose—response curve and split dose recovery in human skin cancer. *Radiotherapy and Oncology*, 2, 123–30.
Tsubouchi, S. and Matsuzawa, T., 1973, Correlation of cell transit time with survival time in acute intestinal radiation death of germ-free and conventional rodents. *International Journal of Radiation Biology*, 24, 389–96.
Tubiana, M., Frindel, E. and Malaise, E., 1968, The application of radiobiologic knowledge and cellular kinetics to radiation therapy. *American Journal of Roentgenology*, 102, 822–30.
Tucker, S. L., 1984, Tests for the fit of the linear—quadratic model to radiation isoeffect data. *International Journal of Radiation Oncology Biology Physics*, 10, 1933–9.
Tucker, S. L. and Thames, H. D., 1983, Flexure dose: the low-dose limit of effective fractionation. *International Journal of Radiation Oncology Biology Physics*, 9, 1373–83.
Tucker, S. L., Withers, H. R., Mason, K. A. and Thames, Jr., H. D., 1983, A dose-surviving fraction curve for mouse colonic mucosa. *European Journal of Cancer Clinical Oncology*, 19, 433.
Tucker, S. L., Thames, H. D., Mason, K. A., Hunter, N. and Withers, H. R., 1987, Direct analysis of *in vivo* colony survival after single and fractionated doses of radiation. *International Journal of Radiation Biology* (submitted).
Turesson, I. and Notter, G. 1984a, The influence of fraction size in radiotherapy on the late normal tissue reaction – I. Comparison of effects of daily and once-a-week fractionation on human skin. *International Journal of Radiation Oncology Biology Physics*, 10, 593–8.
Turesson, I. and Notter, G., 1984b, The influence of the overall treatment time in radiotherapy on the acute reaction: comparison of the effects of daily and twice-a-week fractionation on human skin. *International Journal of Radiation Oncology Biology Physics*, 10, 607–19.
Turesson, I. and Notter, G., 1986, Dose—response and dose—latency relationships for human skin after various fractionation schedules. *British Journal of Cancer*, 53 (Suppl. VII), 67–72.

Ullrich, R. L. and Casarett, G. W., 1977, Interrelationship between the early inflammatory response and subsequent fibrosis after radiation exposure. *Radiation Research*, 72, 107–21.
UNSCEAR, 1977. *United Nations Scientific Committee on the Effects of Atomic Radiation. Report to the General Assembly*, Vienna, p. 773.
UNSCEAR, 1982, *Annex J — Non-stochastic effects of irradiation. United Nations, Committee on the Effect of Atomic Radiation. Report to the General Assembly, New York*, pp. 571–654.
UNSCEAR, 1986, *United Nations Scientific Committee on the Effects of Atomic Radiation. Genetic and Somatic Effects of Ionizing Radiation, Report to the General Assembly, New York*.
Utsumi, H., Hill, C. K., Berkur, E. and Elkind, M. M., 1981, 'Single hit' potentially lethal damage: evidence of its repair in mammalian cells. *Radiation Research*, 87, 576–92.
Valeriote, F. A., Collins, D. C. and Bruce, W. R., 1968, Hematological recovery in the mouse following single doses of gamma radiation and cyclophosphamide. *Radiation Research*, 33, 501–511.
Vassort, F., Winterholer, M., Frindel, E. and Tubiana, M., 1973, Kinetic parameters of bone marrow stem cells using *in vivo* suicide by tritiated thymidine or by hydroxyurea. *Blood*, 41, 789–96.
Vegesna, V., Withers, H. R., Thames, H. D. and Mason, K. A., 1985, Multifraction radiation response of mouse lung. *International Journal of Radiation Biology*, 47, 413–22.
Villard, P., 1908, Instrument de mésure a lecture directe pour les rayons X. *Archives d'Electrologie Medicale*.
Vriesendorp, H. M. and van Bekkum, D. W., 1984, Susceptibility to total body irradiation. In *Response of Different Species to Total Body Irradiation* edited by J. J. Broerse and T. J. MacVittie (The Netherlands: Martinus Nijhoff Publishers), pp. 43–57.
Wachsmann, F., 1943a, Grundsätzliches zur Frage der Fraktionierung bei der Roentgenbehandlung bösartiger Geschwülste. *Strahlentherapie*, 73, 636–48.
Wachsmann, F., 1943b, Experimentelle Untersuchungen an einem Fall von multiplem Hautkarzinom unter besonderer Berücksichtigung der Frage der Zweckmässigkeit der Fraktionierung. *Strahlentherapie*, 73, 649–62.
Wald, N., 1971, Hematological parameters after acute radiation injury. In *Manual on Radiation Haematology* (Vienna: IAEA).
Wambersie, A., Dutreix, J. G. and Lellouch, J., 1974, Early recovery for intestinal stem cells, as a function of dose per fraction, evaluated by survival rate after fractionated irradiation of the abdomen of mice. *Radiation Research*, 58, 498–515.
Wambersie, A., Dutreix, J., Stienon-Smoes, M. R. and Octave-Prignot, M., 1978, Effect of dose rate on intestinal tolerance in mice. Implications in radiotherapy. *Journal de Radiologie et de l'Électrologie*, 59, 315–22.
Wambersie, A., Stienon-Smoes, M.-R., Octave-Prignot, M. and Dutreix, J., 1979, Effect of dose rate on intestinal tolerance in mice. Implications in radiotherapy. *British Journal of Radiology*, 52, 153–5.
Wang, C. C., 1985, Improved local control for advanced oropharyngeal carcinoma following twice daily radiation therapy. *American Journal of Clinical Oncology*, 8, 512–16.
Wang, C. C. and Schultz, M. D., 1966, Management of locally recurrent carcinoma of the nasopharynx. *Radiology*, 86, 900–3.
Wang, C. C., Blitzer, P. H. and Suit, H. D., 1985, Twice-a-day radiation therapy for cancer of the head and neck. *Cancer*, 55, 2100–4.
Wang, C. C., Suit, H. D. and Blitzer, P. H., 1986, Twice-a-day radiation therapy for supraglottic carcinoma. *International Journal of Radiation Oncology Biology Physics*, 12, 3–7.
Wangenheim, K.-H. von, 1976, A mechanism for endocellular control of cell differentiation and cell proliferation. *Journal of Theoretical Biology*, 59, 205–22.
Wara, W. M., Phillips, T. L., Margolis, L. W. and Smith, V., 1973, Radiation pneumonitis — a new approach to the derivation of time–dose factors. *Cancer*, 32, 547–52.
Watson, E., Halnan, K. E., Dische, S., Saunders, M. I., Cade, I., McEwen, J. B., Wiernik, G., Perrins, D. J. D. and Sutherland, I., 1978, Hyperbaric oxygen and radiotherapy: a

Medical Research Council trial in carcinoma of cervix. *British Journal of Radiology*, 51, 879—87.
Weiss, K., 1966, Dem Gedenken an österreichs grosse Röntgenpioniere. *Radiologia Austriaca*, 16 (Supplement), 37—44.
Wheeler, K. T. and Nelson, G. B., 1987, Saturation of a DNA repair process in dividing and nondividing mammalian cells. *Radiation Research*, 109, 109—17.
Wheldon, T. E., 1980, Can dose-survival parameters be deduced from *in situ* assay? *British Journal of Cancer*, 41 (Suppl. IV), 79—87.
Wheldon, T. E., Michalowski, A. and Kirk, J., 1982, The effect of irradiation on function in self-renewing normal tissues with differing proliferative organisation. *British Journal of Radiology*, 55, 759—66.
Wheldon, T. E., Abdelaal, A. S. and Nias, A. H. W., 1977, Tumour curability cellular radiosensitivity and clonogenic cell number (Letter to Editor), *British Journal of Radiology*, 50, 843—4.
White, D. C., 1976, The histopathologic basis for functional decrements in late radiation injury in diverse organs. *Cancer*, 37, 1126—43.
White, A. and Hornsey, S., 1978, Radiation damage to the rat spinal cord: the effect of single and fractionated doses of x-rays. *British Journal of Radiology*, 51, 515—523.
Wichtl, O., 1986, 90 Jahre Röntgenstrahlen: ein Beitrag zu den Anfangen der Röntgenologie in Wien. *Österreichische Röntgengesellschaft-Mitteilungen*, 1986, (1), 5—41.
Wiernik, G., Bleehen, N., Brindle, J., Bullimore, J., Churchill-Davidson, I. F. J., Davidson, J., Fawler, J. R., Francis, P., Hadden, R. C. M., Haybittle, J. F., Howard, N., Lansley, I. F., Lindup, R., Phillips, D. L. and Skeggs, D., 1978, Sixth interim progress report of the British Institute of Radiology fractionation study of 3F/week versus 5F/week in radiotherapy of the laryngo-pharynx. *British Journal of Radiology*, 51, 241—50.
Wilkinson, J. M., Hendry, J. H. and Hunter, R. D., 1980, Dose-rate considerations in the introduction of low-dose-rate afterloading intracavity techniques for radiotherapy. *British Journal of Radiology*, 53, 890—3.
Williams, M. V., 1986, The cellular basis of renal injury. *British Journal of Cancer*, 53 (Suppl. VII), 257—64.
Williams, M. V. and Denekamp, J., 1984, Radiation induced renal damage in mice: influence of fraction size. *International Journal of Radiation Oncology, Biology, Physics*, 10, 885—94.
Williams, M. V., Denekamp, J. and Fowler, J. F., 1985, A review of $\alpha/\beta$ values for experimental tumors: implications for clinical studies of altered fractionation. *International Journal of Radiation Oncology Biology Physics*, 11, 87—96.
Winston, B. M., Ellis, F. and Hall, E. J., 1969, The Oxford NSD calculator for clinical use. *Clinical Radiology*, 20, 8—11.
Wintz, H., 1937, Die Einzeitbestrahlung. *Strahlentherapie*, 58, 545—51.
Withers, H. R., 1967a, Recovery and repopulation *in vivo* by mouse skin epithelial cells during fractionated irradiation. *Radiation Research*, 32, 227—39.
Withers, H. R., 1967b, The effect of oxygen and anaesthesia on radiosensitivity *in vivo* of epithelial cells of mouse skin. *British Journal of Radiology*, 40, 335—43.
Withers, H. R., 1971, Regeneration of intestinal mucosa after irradiation. *Cancer*, 28, 75—81.
Withers, H. R., 1972, Cell renewal system concepts and the radiation response. In *Frontiers of Radiation Therapy Oncology*, Vol. 6, edited by J. M. Vaeth and B. Kager (Baltimore: University Park Press), pp. 93—107.
Withers, H. R., 1975a, Cell cycle redistribution as a factor in multifraction irradiation. *Radiology*, 114, 199—202.
Withers, H. R., 1975b, Responses of some normal tissues to low doses of radiation. In *Cell Survival after Low Doses of Radiation: Theoretical and Clinical Implications*, edited by T. Alper (London and New York: John Wiley & Sons, Ltd.), pp. 369—75.
Withers, H. R., 1975c, Isoeffect curves for various proliferative tissues in experimental animals. In *Proceedings of Conference on Time-Dose Relationships in Clinical Radiotherapy*. Madison, Wisconsin, Madison Printing and Publishing, pp. 30—8.
Withers, H. R., 1977, Response of tissues to multiple small dose fractions. *Radiation Research*, 71, 24—33.

Withers, H. R. and Elkind, M. M., 1968, Dose–survival characteristics of epithelial cells of mouse intestinal mucosa. *Radiology*, 91, 998–1000.
Withers, H. R. and Elkind, M. M., 1969, Radiosensitivity and fractionation response of crypt cells of mouse jejunum. *Radiation Research*, 38, 598–613.
Withers, H. R. and Elkind, M. M., 1970, Microcolony survival assay for cells of mouse intestinal mucosa exposed to radiation. *International Journal of Radiation Biology*, 17, 261–7.
Withers, H. R. and Mason, K. A., 1974, The kinetics of recovery in irradiated colonic mucosa of the mouse. *Cancer*, 34, 896–903.
Withers, H. R. and Peters, L. J., 1980, Biologic aspects of radiotherapy. In *Textbook of Radiotherapy*, edited by G. H. Fletcher (Philadelphia: Lea & Febiger).
Withers, H. R., Hunter, N., Barkley, H. T. and Reid, B. O., 1974, Radiation survival and regeneration characteristics of spermatogenic stem cells of mouse testis. *Radiation Research*, 57, 88–103.
Withers, H. R., Chu, A. M., Reid, B. O. and Hussey, D. H., 1975, Response of mouse jejunum to multifraction radiation. *International Journal of Radiation Oncology Biology Physics*, 1, 41–52.
Withers, H. R., Thames, H. D., Flow, B. L., Mason, K. A. and Hussey, D. H., 1978, The relationship of acute and late skin injury in 2 and 5 fraction/week γ-ray therapy. *International Journal of Radiation Oncology Biology Physics*, 4, 595–601.
Withers, H. R., Peters, L. J. and Kogelnik, H. D., 1980, The pathobiology of late effects of irradiation. In *Radiation Biology in Cancer Research*, edited by R. E. Meyn and H. R. Withers (New York: Raven Press), pp. 439–48.
Withers, H. R., Peters, L. J., Thames, H. D. and Fletcher, G. H., 1982a, Hyperfractionation. *International Journal of Radiation Oncology Biology Physics*, 8, 1807–9.
Withers, H. R., Thames, H. D. and Peters, L. J., 1982b, Biological bases for high RBE values for late effects of neutron irradiation. *International Journal of Radiation Oncology Biology Physics*, 8, 2071–6.
Withers, H. R., Thames, H. D. and Peters, L. J., 1982c, Differences in the fractionation response of acutely and late-responding tissues. In *Progress in Radio-Oncology*, Vol. II., edited by Karcher et al. (New York: Raven Press), p. 287.
Withers, H. R., Thames, H. D. and Peters, L. J., 1983, A new isoeffect curve for change in dose per fraction. *Radiotherapy and Oncology*, 1, 187–91.
Withers, H. R., Mason, K. A. and Thames, H. D., 1986, Late radiation response of kidney assayed by tubule-cell survival. *British Journal of Radiology*, 59, 587–95.
Withers, H. R., Hunter, N., Tucker, S. L. and Thames, H. D., 1987, Response of resting and proliferating hair follicle cells in the mouse to multi-fraction X-rays. *International Journal of Radiation Biology* (submitted).
Witte, E., 1939, Über die Umrechnung der r-Dosis auf Einheiten biologischer Wirkung bei der protrahiert-fraktionierten Bestrahlung unter besonderer Berücksichtigung der Bestrahlung mit kleinen Raumdosen. *Strahlentherapie*, 65, 630–8.
Witte, E., 1942, Dosierung im biologischen Mass. *Strahlentherapie*, 72, 177–94.
Wright, N. and Allison, M., 1984, *The Biology of Epithelial Cell Populations* Volumes I and II (Oxford: Clarendon Press).
Wu, C. and Lajtha, L. G., 1975, Haemopoietic stem-cell kinetics during continuous irradiation. *International Journal of Radiation Biology*, 27, 41–50.
Wyklicky, H., 1980, Zur Geschichte der Strahlentherapie in Österreich. *Wiener Klinische Wochenschrift*, 92 (5), 165–71.
Wyllie, A. H., 1985, The biology of cell death in tumours. *Anti-Cancer Research*, 5, 131–136.
Xu, C. X., Hendry, J. H. and Testa, N. G., 1986, Residual deficiencies in haemopoietic precursor cell populations after repeated irradiation of mice with X-rays or neutrons: dose–response relationships. *Experimental Hematology*, 4, 230–3.
Xu, F. X., van der Schueren, E. and Ang, K. K., 1984, Acute reactions of the lip mucosa of mice to fractionated irradiations. *Radiotherapy and Oncology*, 1, 369–74.
Yan, J.-H., Hu, Y.-H. and Gu, X.-Z., 1983, Radiation therapy of recurrent nasopharyngeal carcinoma. *Acta Radiologica Oncology Radiation Therapy Physics and Biology*, 22, 23–8.

Zeman, W., 1971, Effect of irradiation on the nervous system. In *Pathology of Irradiation*, edited by C. C. Berdjis (Baltimore: Williams & Wilkins), pp. 213–67.
Zeman, E. M. and Bedford, J. S., 1984, Changes in early and late effects with dose per fraction: alpha, beta, redistribution and repair. *International Journal of Radiation Oncology Biology Physics*, **10**, 1039–47.
Zeman, E. M. and Bedford, J. S., 1985a, Dose fractionation effects in plateau-phase cultures of C3H 10T1/2 cells and their transformed counterparts. *Radiation Research*, **101**, 373–93.
Zeman, E. M. and Bedford, J. S., 1985b, Loss of repair capacity in density-inhibited cultures of C3H 10T1/2 cells during multifraction irradiation. *Radiation Research*, **104**, 71–7.
Zuppinger, A., 1941, Spätveranderungen nach protrahiert-fraktionierte Rontgenbestrahlung im Bereich der oberen Luft-und Speisewege. *Strahlentherapie*, **70**, 361–442.
Zuppinger, A., 1960, Die Hypopharynxtumoren. In *11th International Congress of Radiology Transactions (Georg Thieme Verlag – Stuttgart)*, pp. 626–35.

# Index

α/β
  late effects 93
  normal tissues 72
  tumours 76
Accelerated
  fractionation 127, 128, 129, 225, 237
  growth 112, 115
  growth, tumours 118
  proliferation 102
Acceleration of regeneration in the skin 116
Accumulation
  models 85
  of sublethal injury 185
Alpha particles 174
Altered fractionation 224
Alveolar cells 17, 239
Amplifying divisions 3
Angiogenesis 208
Apoptosis 5, 216
Arterial occlusions 16
Assays of tissue injury 180
Autonomic nervous system 238
Autoradiography 200
Avalanche 216

BFU-E 103
Baclesse technique 148
Biological hazards 237
Biologically effective dose 148
Bone marrow 14, 29, 42
  proliferation 103
  syndrome 14, 205
  residual injury 131

Brachytherapy 233
Breast 78
  disease 99
British Institute of Radiology Study 120
Bromodeoxyuridine 197, 203

CFU-E 103
CNS 19
CRE 161, 221
Carcinogenesis 240
Carcinoma 107
  bladder 96
  cervix 147
Cataracts 240
Cell
  and tissue kinetics 200
  cycle time 101, 200, 209, 223
  death 4
  loss 5, 105
  loss factor 6, 105, 125, 209, 223
  population kinetic (CPK) model 164
  production 2
  survival 177
Charged particles 176
*Chlamydomonas reinhardi* 86
Chromoradiometer 139
Chromosomal injury 58
Chronic hypoxia 211
Clinical hyperfractionation 96, 98
Clone 178
Clonogenic cells 178
Clonogens 178
  hair follicle 123

292

# Index

regeneration 124
tumour 124
Cohen's analysis 157
Colonic mucosa 113
Colony 178
  assay 180
Colony-forming
  cells 178
  efficiency 178
  units 43
  units (CFU-S) 103
Colony-size distributions 81
Compensatory proliferation 8, 102
Compton
  effect 171
  scattering 173
Concentrated treatment 141
Conditional renewal (flexible) tissues 216
Connective tissue tolerance 163
Continuous
  exposure 84, 162
  irradiation 50
  labelling 9
  repair factors 234, 235
Coutard's technique 144
Cumulative radiation effect 221
Curability of tumours 210
Curie Institute 142

$D_0$ 27, 185
$D_2$-$D_1$ 46
DNA 176
Damage fixation 60, 188
Direct
  action 175, 192
  effects 174
Division delay 109
Dog GM-CFC 32
Dosage factor 226, 232
Dose rate to stop growth 109
Dose-equivalent
  incomplete repair 83
  limits 242
Dose-incidence curve 217
Dose-modifying factor 45, 193
Double-log
  plots 156
  representation 152
Doubling
  rate 125
  time 103

$D_q$ 64, 185

ED50 69
ERC 103
Elastic scattering 173
Electron-affinic sensitizers 197
Electronic excitation 173
Elkind recovery 160
Ellis NSD formula 160
Embryo 240
Endogenous colonies 179
Endothelial cells 17
Energy-average LET 177
Epidermis 46
  residual injury 133
Epithelial nests, tumours 211
Erlangen School 141, 219
Erythema 16, 120, 150
  dose 152
Erythema-ometer 149
Excitation 171
Expedited method 142
Exponential decay factor 162
Exponential-repair
  kinetics 83
  model 85
Exposure-time
  coefficient 255
  exponent 49, 51
Extrapolated total dose (ETD) 168
Extrapolation number 185

F-type tissues 13
Fast-repair 159
Fat pad assays 182
Fertility 41
Fetus 240
Fibrosis of the lung 17
Field-size effect 16
First-order repair 82, 85, 143
Fixation points 254
Flagyl 198
Flexible tissues 2, 216
Flexure dose 47, 90, 91

Flow cytometry 203
Four R's of radiotherapy 222
Fraction labelled mitoses (FLM) 201
Fraction-size exponent 254
Fractionation
  dosage factor (FDF) 226
  dose rate 38

factor 226, 232
parameters 74
sensitivity 64, 223
sensitivity, accelerated growth 119
sensitivity, human tumours 80
sensitivity, normal tissues 70
tumours 74
Free radicals 174
Freundlich formula 154

G2 block 223
GI
  syndrome 32, 44, 205
  tract, proliferation 102
GM-CFC 30, 103
Gastrointestinal syndrome 15, 239
Genotype 178
Germ-free mice 15
Glutathione 198, 199
Goitrogen 182
Granulocytopenia 14, 239
Growth
  delay 105, 106, 213
  fraction 4, 105, 209, 222
Gut 43

Haematopoietic
  stem cells 43
  system 103
Hair follicle 122
  clonogens, fractionation sensitivity 123
Hairy nevus 138
Halogenated pyrimidines 197
Harm 241
Head and neck cancer 98
Hereditary effects 242
Hierarchical tissues 2, 204
High-LET radiation 62
Hoechst 33258 203
Holding recovery 61
Holzknecht units 139
Human tumours 36
Hyperbaric oxygen 121, 214
Hyperfractionation 94, 95, 225, 232
Hypofractionation 121, 225
Hypopharynx tumours 146
Hypoxia 211, 224

IR model 248
Incomplete repair 87, 232
  factors 232, 233

models 83
Incremental dose per fraction 90
isoeffect 90
Indirect action 175, 192
Induced resistance 133
Infertility 240
Initial slope 61, 187, 188
Interaction of radiation with matter 170
Intercept-to-slope ratio 70
Interphase death 5
Interstitial therapy 233
Intestine 32
  crypts 179
  residual injury 132
  syndrome 13
Ionization and excitation 171
Ionization chamber 139
Isoeffect relationships 225

K
  value 198
  values, tissues 37
Kidney colonies 182

LD50/30 30, 43
LD50/7 15, 32, 44
LPL model 86, 251
LQ isoeffect models 166
Labelling index 209
Langmuir absorption formula 154
Late
  complications 78
  effects, $\alpha/\beta$ 94
Latency period 217
Lewis lung tumours 106
Life shortening 241
Limiting fraction size, effective fractionation 90
Linear energy transfer (LET) 176
Linear-quadratic model 47, 68, 166, 187, 246
Lip mucosa
  fractionation 116
  proliferation 104
Liposarcomas 80
Low dose-rate fractionation 145
Low-dose limit of effective fractionation 164
Lumbar cord 69
Lung 17
Lymphopenia 14

Macromolecules 176
Macroscopic
  colonies 182
  necrosis 208
Massive-dose treatment 140
Maturing cells 103
Maximum-likelihood analysis 86
Mean lethal dose 185
Metronidazole 198
Microcolony assay 182
Microdosimetry 177
Microencephaly 240
Microscopic necrosis 208, 211
Misonidazole 198, 214, 231
Misrepair 60, 85, 188, 252
Mitotic
  death 5, 6
  delay 6, 101
  harvest 200
Mucosal reaction 104
Multi-target single-hit model 167
Multiple daily fractions 138
Musculo-skeletal tissues 216
Myeloid leukemia 240
Myelopathy 19, 231

$N$-exponent 68
NSD 221, 225
  concept 219
  formula 89, 161
Negative feedback 2, 8
Nerve-root necrosis 20
Neural control mechanism 238
Neurological syndrome 238
Neutron absorption reactions 174
Neutrons 63, 172, 177
Nominal standard dose 64, 161, 221
Non-standard fractionation 224
Nonstochastic effect 206, 242
Normal tissue
  endpoints 183
  tolerance 218, 229
Number-of-fractions 221
  exponent 47, 49, 64, 163, 254
  versus overall time 159

Optimum dose 147
Overall treatment time 127
Oxygen
  electrode measurements 214
  enhancement ratio (OER) 199

PLDR 57, 61, 189, 217, 223
Pair production 171
Palliation 235
Paralysis 69, 86
Partial
  effect (PE) 227
  hepatectomy 182
  tolerance 162
Pathogenesis 10
Percent labelled mitoses (PLM) 201
Peyers (lymphoid) patches 182
Phenotype 178
Photoelectric effect 171
Pigskin 159
Plateau-phase cultures 112
Plating efficiency 178
Pleural effusions 17
Pneumonitis 17, 18, 93, 239
Poisson distribution 179, 183
Pool model 85
Population doubling time 109
Potential doubling time 118, 125, 209
Potentially lethal damage 57, 223
Power-law models 137, 148, 151, 152, 163
Pre-GM-CFC 103
Precursor cells 103
Probability curve 24
Prodromal phase 15, 238
Progression 83
Proliferative
  organization 4, 204
  organization, tumours 208
  responses 100, 101
Protective agents 199
Protraction factors 150
Protraction-fractionation method 144
Pulse labelling 200

Q
  cells 105
  factor 60
Quasi-threshold dose 185

Rabbit ear 149
Radiation protection 241
Radical
  production 175
  reactions 175
  scavengers 199
Radiobiology of tumours 208

Radiosensitivity and the cell cycle 196
Radium treatments 219
Rat skin, fractionated irradiation 122
Reaction scores 86
Reciprocal-dose
  graphs 251
  technique 70
Recoil protons 171, 173
Recovery
  factors 148, 149, 150
  of tolerance 136
Recurrences, squamous cell carcinomas 125
Redistribution 82, 95, 222, 223
Reflectance spectrophotometry 120
Regaud technique 219
Regeneration during fractionated radiotherapy 124
Relative
  biological effectiveness (RBE) 193
  effect (RE) 226
Renewing normal tissues 204
Reoxygenation 75, 211, 213, 222
Repair 222, 246
  halftime 233, 234
  kinetics 82, 86, 169
  models 60, 188, 223
  of potentially lethal damage 189
  of sublethal damage 190
  rate constant 255
  saturation 60
Repair-type models 192
Repopulation 160, 222, 223
Reproductive integrity 5, 22, 178
Residual injury
  different tissues 135
  retreatment 130
Response of renewing tissues 205
Responsiveness of tumours 210
Reverse dose-rate effect 110
Rhabdomyosarcoma 105
Ro-03-8799 198
Ro-07-0582 198
Röntgen 139

SLDR 54, 190
Sarcomas 107
Saturation method 143
Schwann cells 20
Schwarzschild law 150, 220

Self-renewal
  of survivors 7
  probability 8
Seminiferous epithelium 143
Sensitizing agents 197
Shoulder 222
Sieverts 242
Sigmoid curve 25
Simple fractionation 144, 146
Single-hit multitarget equation 186
Skin 16, 33
  erythema 219
  proliferation 101
Slope
  of chord 65, 256
  of tangent 68, 256
Slopes of isoeffect curves 46, 64, 73
Slow repair 106, 159, 223
Spermatogenetic colonies 182
Spermatozoa 205
Spheroids 213
Spinal cord 19, 93
Spleen colonies 103, 178
Split-course treatment 119
Split-dose recovery 38, 54, 82, 190
Squamous cell carcinomas 98
Stem cells 2, 103, 204
Sterility 41
Stochastic effect 206, 242
Stockholm technique 141
Strandqvist monograph 153
Sublesion-interaction processes 85
Sublethal damage and repair 54
Sulphydryl compounds 199
Superfractionation 148
Surfactant 17
Survival curves 183
Survival-curve models 163
Synchronous cultures 200

TDF (time-dose factors) 162, 221, 225
TRU 74
Target theory 176, 186
Target-cell 11, 22
  depletion 22
  hypothesis 22, 29, 40
  population 180, 183
Telangiectasia 16, 152
Testis 41, 143
Therapeutic
  gain 96, 224
  ratio 142

## Index

Thiols 199
Threshold erythema 150
Thrombocytopenia 14
Time
  coefficient 161
  dose factor 221, 225
  exponent 220
  factor 137, 140, 147, 219, 245, 255
  factor: slopes of isoeffect graphs 254
Time-dose formula 220
Tissue
  isoeffect and cell survival 164
  repair 160
  repair half-times 88
Tissue-rescuing unit (TRU) 27
Tissues
  at long-term risk 216
  flexible 108
Total
  body irradiation 236, 239
  effect (TE) 226
Tourniquet hypoxia 214
Track-average LET 177
Transient hypoxia 212
Transit
  cells 3, 204
  times 202
Transplantation assays 57

Tritiated thymidine 200
Tumour-related complications 218
Tumours 35
  angiogenic factor 208
  bed effect 212
  clonogen proliferation 124
  control probability 124
  cord 208
  growth delay 212
  proliferative response 105
  regeneration during treatment 117
Turnover kinetics 101
Two-component
  model 68, 166
  multitarget equation 187

UV irradiation 102
Unpaired electron 174

Vasculature 105
  recovery 136
Viable cells 178
Vibrational excitation 173
Volume doubling time 106, 117, 209

WR-2721 41, 199
Weber–Fechner law 154
White-matter necrosis 20
Whole-body syndromes 237